BLACK WOMEN IN WHITE

Blacks in the Diaspora

Darlene Clark Hine, John McCluskey, Jr., and David Barry Gaspar
General Editors

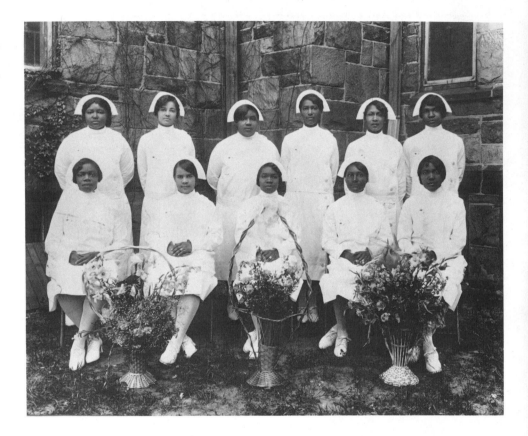

The 1930 graduating class of Mercy Hospital School of Nursing in Philadelphia. Collection of the Mercy-Douglass Alumnae Association. Courtesy of the Center for the Study of the History of Nursing, University of Pennsylvania.

BLACK WOMEN IN WHITE

Racial Conflict and Cooperation in the Nursing Profession 1890–1950

Darlene Clark Hine

INDIANA UNIVERSITY PRESS
Bloomington & Indianapolis

Manufactured in the United States of America

Library of Congress Cataloging-in-Publication Data

Hine, Darlene Clark.
  Black women in white : racial conflict and cooperation in the nursing
profession. 1890–1950 / Darlene Clark Hine.
     p. cm. — (Blacks in the diaspora)
  Bibliography: p.
  Includes index.
  ISBN 0–253–32773–3. — ISBN 0–253–20529–8 (pbk.)
  1. Afro-American nurses—History.   2. Nursing—United States—
History.   3. United States—Race relations—History.   I. Title.
II. Series.
  RT83.5.H56   1989
  362.1'73'08996073—dc19   88–46023
                                                                      CIP

  2   3   4   5   93   92   91   90

In loving memory of my father,
Levester Clark,
and brother,
Orlando Stanley Clark

Contents

Preface

Since the abolition of slavery, each generation of Afro-Americans has waged a valiant struggle to eradicate the multifaceted manifestations of racism. There have been many casualties and few black victories. For the most part, racism still exists. This study of the successes, and to a limited extent the failures, of black nurses from the 1890s to 1950 is yet another chapter in this seemingly endless confrontation.

Though it is much too simple a definition, in the interest of brevity, I define racism as the system of beliefs and practices promulgated by certain whites to maintain an unequal distribution of power and resources between themselves and black Americans. The central unifying focus of this book is the efforts of Afro-American health-care professionals to assemble an institutional and organizational arsenal with which to combat the racism inside the health-care establishment.

Being the product of a society which views men's work as more important and interesting than women's, and that of subordinate black women as least significant of all, when I first began to study the history of black health-care professionals I focused on physicians, intending to pay only cursory attention to nurses. Gradually, as my research unfolded and I sought to understand the connection between health-care delivery and black morbidity and mortality, my attention shifted almost completely to the nurses.

To understand fully the link between health-care delivery and the albeit minuscule improvement in black health over the past century requires a close examination of the role played by the black nurse. Whereas physicians were trained to treat the specific ailments of the patient as individual, from the very outset nurses were expected to deal with the patient as part of a broader social system. During the course of the training experience in the early black hospital and nursing schools, the student was taught to accord equal significance to preventive care and instruction. Her special sphere, first as a private-duty and then in the 1930s as a public-health nurse, embraced the entire black community. The dependence was mutual. Without the institution-building initiative of black leaders and the material and moral support of the black community, the trained black nurse would not have existed. As a consequence, the black nurse belonged to the community; she labored within and on behalf of the community. This is not to suggest that black medical men were inconsequential in the still-raging war for improved black health-care delivery. To make such an assertion would be unfair and inaccurate.

Nevertheless, as I grew more familiar with the compelling careers and struggles of several exemplary nurses, most notably Mabel K. Staupers, M. Elizabeth Carnegie, Frances Davis, Eunice Rivers Laurie, and Estelle Massey Riddle, I was persuaded that the first volume in an envisioned multivolume exploration of black health-care professionals had to concentrate on black nurses. And by the end of my research I resolved that this study must have as its central construct the examination of the powerful impact of racism on the nursing experience for black women.

It is not the aim of this book to create new stereotypes or to paint sentimental portraits of the long-suffering, much-exploited, self-sacrificing but heroic black women nurses at the expense of black physicians. Nor is it the intent to make of white nurses racist villains. But it is important to reveal the causes and consequences of the racial conflict that characterized the first half-century of black women's entry into the nursing profession. To its credit, organized nursing, unlike medicine and law, actually proved more willing to remove color bars and to embrace integration in the post–World War II years. But then, black nurses seemed more determined to raise hell to get what they wanted—that is, to end segregation—than did members of other professions.

In 1950 black nurses voted to dissolve the National Association of Colored Graduate Nurses, a separate professional organization founded in 1908 both to promote their advance and to win integration into the mainstream of American nursing. Once the black nurse leaders achieved the goal of integration, a victory aided by many white nurses and philanthropists and the larger black community, they did what no other black professional or protest organization had ever done: they voluntarily went out of business. Whatever has been the history of race relations in nursing since 1950, the post–World War II era began with a promise of cooperation in the nursing profession.

This book is part of the ongoing enterprise of nursing-history scholars to develop new interpretations and fresh insights to explain the evolution and transformations of American health care. I have taken many cues from the excellent nursing histories that have appeared in the past decade. I would be remiss, however, not to mention that far too many of the revisionist and pathbreaking works that have opened new vistas for research into the social, political, and economic underpinnings of nursing have failed to incorporate an analysis of race. Bluntly put, all professions look different when viewed from the black woman's angle, and even more so when she belongs to the working poor.

In 1910 and 1920 black women constituted less than 3 percent of trained nurses. They were, however, 17.6 and 24.0 percent, respectively, of the total female population. This gross underrepresentation alone suggests much about the structure of the nursing profession and the nature of race relations in the larger society. To ignore black women, however small their numbers, while endeavoring to study the experiences of women in the professions, as well as in other aspects of American life and culture, will continue to yield, at best, partial truths.

Acknowledgments

I have worked on this project longer than I wish to remember. But in so doing, I have incurred enormous debts which it now gives me pleasure to recall. It is with considerable relish, therefore, that I savor conclusion and embrace this opportunity to express sincere appreciation for the many kindnesses and invaluable assistance I received from my family, friends, and colleagues in nursing, women's studies, and Afro-American history. It is with gratitude that I acknowledge the Racial Ethnic Minority Fellowship Program and the Cabinet on Human Rights of the American Nurses' Association for giving me the Women's Honor in Public Service Award in June 1988.

There exists a small but growing community of revisionist nursing and medical-history scholars characterized by a willingness to share documents and copies of works in progress, and to offer words of encouragement when most needed. I have benefited most particularly from the pioneering work of the late Janet Wilson James, Barbara Melosh, Patricia Sloan, Vanessa Gamble, Stephanie Shaw, Karen Buhler-Wilkerson, Nancy Tomes, and particularly Susan Reverby. Susan read the entire manuscript, and it is a much better work because of her insightful, indeed brilliant, criticisms. I am grateful also to D'Ann Campbell, Anne Hudson Jones, Judith Walzer Leavitt, Rima Apple, Carol Gino, Todd Savitt, James Jones, and Vern Bullough for the example of their excellent work.

Without the assistance of archivists and librarians, this book would not exist. I am especially grateful to Esme Bhan of the Moorland-Spingarn Library at Howard University in Washington, D.C.; Howard Dodson and the staff of the Schomburg Center for Research in Black Culture in New York City; Daniel T. Williams at the Hollis Burke Frissell Library at Tuskegee University in Tuskegee, Alabama; Clifton Johnson of the Amistad Research Center at Tulane University in New Orleans, Louisiana; William Hess of the Rockefeller Archive and Research Center in Tarrytown, New York; Archie Motley of the Chicago Historical Society; Fritz Mal Val at Hampton University, and Patricia Sloan at the M. Elizabeth Carnegie Nursing History Archives, also at Hampton University, Hampton, Virginia; Ruth Rothenberg in the interlibrary loan department at Purdue University; Joan Lynaugh of the Center for the Study of the History of

Nursing; and Rebecca Vargas of the National Humanities Center. Likewise, I am grateful to the staffs of the Western Reserve Historical Society in Cleveland; the Library of Congress in Washington, D.C.; the National Archives in Suitland, Maryland; the South Carolina Medical Library in Charleston; and Fisk University in Nashville, Tennessee.

Several black women historians whose works and conversations helped to crystalize my thoughts on the intersection of race, class, and gender deserve special accolades. They included Gwendolyn Keita Robinson, Elsa Barkley Brown, Deborah Gray White, Jacqueline Rouse, Tiffany Patterson, Wilma King, Sharon Harley, Lillian S. Williams, Rosalyn Terborg-Penn, Adrienne Lash Jones, and Cynthia Nerverdon-Morton. I appreciated the gifts of books on black nursing history received from Beverly Guy-Sheftall, Meredith Woods, Valinda Rogers, and Janet Sims-Woods.

Several agencies provided the two things most scholars find in short supply, money and time. I was fortunate to receive two fellowships, one from the Rockefeller Foundation for Minority Scholars Fellowship Program and the other from the American Council of Learned Societies. Equally appreciated were the Eleanor Roosevelt Institute Research Grant and the Rockefeller Archive and Research Center Award. A yearlong resident fellowship at the National Humanities Center in Research Triangle Park, North Carolina, provided the ideal intellectual environment in which to complete the writing of this study.

Among my dearest friends are some of the most supportive scholars in the academy. A special bouquet of heartfelt thanks is due James D. Anderson, Aldon D. Morris, D. Barry Gaspar, William C. Hine, Betty Brandon, Robert Hall, Jacqueline Goggins, and, especially, John Hope Franklin for their comments on various drafts of the manuscript.

I appreciate the extensive comments of August Meier and Harold Woodman on the original version of this study. My former Purdue University colleagues deserve special thanks for their provocative comments during the early stages of my research and writing: Donald J. Berthrong, Linda Levy Peck, Regina Wolkoff, Lois Magner, Jon Teaford, Lester Cohen, Charles Ingrao, and Philip VanderMeer.

No acknowledgment would be complete without words of gratitude to a group of very special secretaries, Joyce Good and Cynthia FitzSimmons of Purdue University and Peggy Jeffrey of Michigan State University. MSU graduate student Pamela Smoot assisted me with the preparation of the bibliography.

I also thank the editors of the *Journal of Negro Education* and the *Journal of Negro History* for permission to use material here that first appeared in their publications.

Several individual black nurses with whom I talked over the years deserve my deepest appreciation. I would especially like to thank for their scholarship and encouragement M. Elizabeth Carnegie, Patricia Sloan, Gloria Smith, Rhetaugh Dumas, Helen Miller, Mabel K. Staupers, Verdelle B. Bellamy, and Hattie Bessent.

My family is a constant source of inspiration and caring. All that I do acquires added significance because of their faith, trust, and unquestioning devotion. It is impossible to name every member of my extended family; some will have to await the next book. For always being there, I thank especially my grandmother Fannie Venerable Thompson, mother Lottie Mae Thompson Clark, daughter Robbie Davine, sisters Barbara Clark and Alma Mitchell, and cousins Bridgie Alexis Ford, Diane Adams, LaMar Ford, and Herbert King, Jr.

I share all that is good and empowering in this book with the friends, colleagues, nurses, and family members mentioned above. I would be willing to share any errors in the book with them as well, but perhaps that is asking too much.

Introduction

Nurses are special. They are essential to the smooth operation of the entire health-care establishment. But like so many of the other human, material, and environmental resources abundant in our society, we take nurses for granted. It is perhaps only a small exaggeration to suggest that without them hospitals would collapse; physicians would find it difficult, if not impossible, to heal; and patients would be doomed to endure the pain, despair, and fear of their illnesses in not-so-splendid isolation.

There are many reasons for our society's disregard of nurses. First, and perhaps foremost, nursing is the most female of all professions. As Barbara Melosh has pointed out, every nurse, in our collective imagination, and in keeping with the sexual division of labor in American health care, is a woman.[1] Thus, it is daunting to see beyond nurses' femaleness, to move beyond the ingrained tendency to devalue the labor performed by women, and to develop an appreciation for the special skill they bring to their work. Second, we seldom encounter nurses as professionals until we are devastated by disease and incapacity. However, once health is regained nurses are quickly, perhaps gratefully, forgotten.

In the black community, nurses historically have enjoyed a level of respect and responsibility unusual in the larger society. Indeed, in some black communities nurses have been regarded much more favorably than physicians. The majority of black people perceive nurses to be the one group of health-care professionals most responsive and sympathetic to their needs. This is especially the case among those blacks who, for reasons of racism, poverty, and powerlessness, continue to experience limited access to quality health care, and who register a higher incidence of morbidity and mortality than any other segment of the population. For many Afro-Americans in the closing decade of the nineteenth and first half of the twentieth centuries, nursing was the most accessible of all the professions. It provided the one comparatively open gateway through which young black women of working-poor backgrounds could cross toward dignified employment, and a middle-class lifestyle, while rendering much-needed service to their people.

Black women had their own reasons for becoming trained nurses. While the sheer diversity of motivations defies easy generalization, there were clusters of aspirations, including a determination to escape poverty and a yearning for occupational mobility. For some black women, an early identification with a nurse role model was the only inspiration necessary. Others sought self-fulfillment while attempting to make real the frustrated aspirations of their parents and kin. And, of course, there was the altruistic desire simply to care for others, to serve a suffering humanity, to make a difference, to help people to live better lives.

Often sex-role stereotyping eased black women into nursing. When Estelle Massey Riddle, destined to become one of the most important black nurse leaders in the first half of the twentieth century, confided to her brother, a dentist practicing in St. Louis, a desire to follow in his footsteps and become a dentist, she met resistance. Her brother advised that inasmuch as she did not have enough money to pay for a medical education, it would be better if she entered nurse training. He considered it a more appropriate and less demanding occupation for a woman.[2]

Where sex-role proscriptions and racial exclusion failed to dissuade determined black women bent on professional careers, often dire poverty or limited family support propelled them toward nursing. In January 1918, Mary L. Steele Reives entered Lincoln Hospital School for Nurses in New York City simply because her mother was "unable to pay college tuition."[3] The decision of yet another nurse, Elizabeth Sharpe, similarly reflected the role poverty played in shaping her career choices. She lamented, "I always had aspiration of being a doctor." But like Riddle, Sharpe was unable to pursue her real interest. She recalled, "The fact is, I came from a family which could not afford to send me anywhere else." She added, "When I went into training, that was the cheapest."[4] For Lillian Kemp, a 1912 graduate of the Dixie Hospital nursing school, neither poverty nor sexism influenced her initial decision to enter nurse training. She declared, "My mother wanted me to be a nurse—she was a good nurse although she never took nurses' training but she knew exactly what to do and she didn't lose her head with sick people and I didn't either. She stayed calm and could follow a doctor's directions."[5] This discussion of the reasons black women chose to enter nurse training is continued in chapter seven.

This history of black women nurses necessarily probes questions of the relationship between class and race, and seeks to explain precisely how they acquired agency, that is, the power and resources to bring down the wall of racial exclusion, segregation, and discrimination erected at the dawn of professional nursing. The entrenched racism of late-nineteenth-century America operated to deny to the vast majority of black women access to the new schools and hospitals responsible for training nurses. Moreover, the racism of elite white leaders within the profession dictated that black graduate nurses be prohibited from membership in the organizations created to promote the status of nursing and wrest autonomy from the tyranny of male physicians and hospital administrators. The professionalization impulse and class divisions separating black practitioners and elite white nurse leaders overshadowed the potentially powerful bonds of sisterhood and work in modern nursing. In other words, the structure of the nursing profession combined with the leaders' obsessive preoccupation with status to preclude the development of a sorority of consciousness across racial and class barriers.

Given the starkly drawn battle lines of race and class, the equation was a simple one. If black women were to become trained nurses, the black community had to create the requisite institutions to provide training. Undaunted, beginning in the 1890s and continuing through the 1920s, Afro-Americans established a national network of approximately two hundred black hospitals and nurse training schools. Significantly, black women's clubs and auxiliaries and resources from poor black communities contributed substantially to the start-up of and initial operating funds to create and sustain this emerging institutional system. Accordingly, the first generations of graduate nurses were expected to repay the community's investment—in exchange for the opportunity to become "trained" nurses, they accepted the burden of racial obligation. Black nurses, more so than any other black health-care professional, were to bear the bulk of the responsibility to provide health-care services for, and to lift up from the bottom of the American social scale, the entire black race.[6] By their example of altruistic caring, self-discipline, and personal sacrifice, they would teach lessons of moral rectitude, cleanliness, order, proper diet, and deference to and respect for authority.

In addition to both the community's and their own personal expectations and desires to provide quality health-care service and education, the first generation of trained black nurses were expected to be models of feminine decorum. Thus, to a certain extent, black nurses were not immune to the hardening of social conventions and normative attitudes concerning gender roles in an increasingly industrialized society. The ideology of "virtuous womanhood" sharply and oppressively defined women's proper actions and behaviors in very restricted terms. Women were considered to be repositories of moral sensibility, purity, refinement, and maternal affection in a male-dominated society. Thus, woman's highest calling consonant with her biological destiny was to be a mother and nurturer. Accordingly, women were consigned to the private sphere of the home while men functioned in the public sphere of paid employment and politics. To be sure, the black woman, owing to a constellation of reasons, always inhabited the outer realms of woman's proper sphere.[7]

Throughout the post-Reconstruction years and well into the twentieth century, a devastating combination of poverty and the marginal and seasonal jobs available to most black men dictated that black women work both inside and outside the home. Whether she was wife, daughter, or sister, the black woman's income was critical to family survival, so much so that she never enjoyed the option of retreating into the so-called private sphere. In reality, an increasing number of turn-of-the-century white women sought exit from the private sphere. Thus the tension between the theory of the public/private sphere dichotomy and reality created a paradox. As certain occupations closed their doors to women, other female-stereotyped professions opened. White women, but not black women, found employment in an expanding number of sex role–stereotyped jobs in department stores, factories, and offices. In short, within this ideological and economic context, nursing seemed the best possible avenue for aspiring black women possessed of few other means to achieve the moral status, self-fulfillment, and economic autonomy so fervently desired.

The social construction of gender roles within the black community could not afford to confine black women to as narrow a band of occupations and jobs as was the case in the larger white society. Actually, the larger reality of race and class oppression confined and restricted them more. Still, many black male professionals, especially the founders of hospitals and nursing training schools and those concerned with black education, emphasized women's suitability for nursing because of their "special" nurturing talents. However, because they were to be black women nurses—a triple index of inferiority in the minds of some black men and most whites—they were denied opportunities to occupy administrative and leadership positions within their chosen profession. Such positions were considered the preserve of either black male physicians or white female administrators. For example, Adah Belle Samuels Thoms served as acting director of the Lincoln Hospital School for Nurses in New York from 1906 through 1923. Although this institution trained black women, the white managers were unwilling to defy custom and promote a black woman to a major administrative post.[8]

By the turn of the century, self-conscious elite white nurse leaders heralded nursing as ideal work for middle-class women. They argued that formal nurse training and practice provided an attractive outlet to white, native-born, middle-class, private sphere–restricted women, especially those respectable ladies who needed something to do before marriage or who were widowed. This had not always been the case. Prior to the Civil War, nursing, as historian Janet Wilson James has pointed out, was a "low-paid, low-status job for laboring-class women, who, over a twelve-hour day, attended to the physical needs of the patients while doing the heavy domestic work on the wards."[9] The opening of the first nursing schools, in 1873, launched the movement to upgrade nursing, to obliterate any identification with domestic service, and to attract a "higher-class woman" into the profession. Of course, few truly middle-class women with other options for meaningful employment were willing to enter the restricted and exploitative world of hospital nurse training. Obvious discrepancies existed between the expressed ideal and the actual social status of the student nurse probationers.

The vast majority of the first generations of black student nurses, like their white counterparts, were from working-poor backgrounds. It was precisely this class origin, and a desire to escape it, that enabled student nurses unquestioningly to endure the arduous tasks and the paternalism and military regimentation characteristic of all hospital training schools. However, the class origins and social status of most black women, while making them easy recruits for nursing, undoubtedly exacerbated tensions with elite white nurse leaders, who were laboring to distance the profession from any taint of domestic servitude.

When elite white nurses embraced the ideology of professionalization, black nurses encountered increased hostility and restricted access both to training schools and to the professional organizations. Their tenuous presence in the profession was seriously threatened. To be sure, the process of professionalization in America, regardless of the profession, inclined to exclude blacks, women, and lower-class white males. Such purging of those deemed unfit by middle-class white males was generally achieved either through outright denial of admission to training institutions on racial and gender grounds, or through the implementation of more subtle barriers such as increasing the educational requirements and lobbying for the adoption of state licensing legislation.[10]

Elite white nurse leaders mirrored their male counterparts in law and medicine in their insensitivity to and lack of concern for the special barriers and problems confronting their black colleagues. Indeed, some of the policies they adopted effectively denied black nurses opportunities for professional advance. Most white nursing schools in the North adopted racial quotas, while all such schools in the South denied admission to black women. The American Nurses' Association, as it was reorganized in 1916, instituted the policy of accepting members through state associations. Unfortunately, sixteen southern states and the District of Columbia denied black nurses membership in their local associations. Thus only those black nurses who had been members of the national organization prior to 1916 belonged; the vast majority were professional outcasts. Few hospitals and settlement houses employed more than a token black woman nurse. In every instance where black and white nurses performed the same jobs, the black nurse was paid substantially less.[11]

Given the racist burdens placed on black nurses, it is imperative to examine the processes whereby they became agents for social change and professional integration. The founding in 1908 of the National Association of Colored Graduate Nurses was the first step in the acquisition of agency. Although the NACGN did not employ an executive director until 1934, it did launch black nurses on the path of professionalization and fortified their resolve to destroy racial segregation in nursing. In 1932 black nurses formed a second national organization, the Chi Eta Phi sorority of registered nurses. One of its major purposes was "to provide continuous identification of nursing leaders within the membership who will function as agents of change on all levels."[12] After the NACGN dissolved in 1950, Chi Eta Phi was for two decades the only independent black nursing organization. During its first decade of existence the sorority concentrated heavily on health projects for the black community of Washington, D.C. The Sorors formed girls' and mothers' clubs, immunized children against diphtheria, equipped the first-aid room of the Metropolitan Boys' Club #2, and raised money for the Eye Glass Fund of Public Schools.[13]

As black and white nurse leaders engaged in their separate but parallel quests for professional status, greater autonomy, and power, they sought increased control over the selection of students, extension and standardization of curriculum, stricter admission requirements, and state licensing legislation. To be sure, black nurse leaders had the more difficult or ambiguous dilemma. Indeed, the sheer complexity of their situation threatened severe internal group ruptures.

In order to win full recognition and acceptance into the mainstream of American nursing, black nurse leaders had to embark upon their own distinct process of professionalization, which at some level could not avoid exclusionary practices. Thus professionalization risked provoking a hardening of class divisions within the group. On the other hand, black nurse leaders who were determined to eradicate racial barriers occupied an adversarial relationship vis à vis organized nursing. To be sure, intractable white hostility undoubtedly helped to cement black solidarity. It was important for black nurse leaders to maintain the support of their own group while they adopted confrontational poses publicly, focusing attention on the racism informing the very profession in which they sought acceptance and integration. These complex themes are explored in chapters five and eight.

Regional variations, including the differences in racial relations and demographics manifested in the North and South, affected the development of black nursing. Northern black nurses seemed relentless in their determination to fight against institutional separatism and all vestiges of discrimination. Southern black nurses, while never fully conceding the futility of struggling to integrate nursing schools and professional organizations in that region, devoted tremendous energy to addressing the urgent health-care needs of the region's black poor. An exception to this regional distinction, however, was revealed in the career of Ludie Clay Andrews of Atlanta.

Andrews was born in 1875 in Milledgeville, Georgia. On her 1901 application for admission to the MacVicar Hospital School of Nursing,

Spelman College, she wrote that she could not count on any financial assistance from her family "because my mother is poor with a large family to support and also an old flicted husband." Her biological father was dead, and although she was married she explained that she did not live with her husband. Her reference letters from reputable businessmen in her home town attested to her "good moral character" and described her as "an industrious, straightforward and intelligent woman." Andrews received her diploma in 1906. She later recalled, "I had decided while in training that I wanted to work for my people, how or where this was to be done I did not know; however, it was not long before my fondest hopes were realized." She elaborated,

> After having nursed two white patients through a siege of severe typhoid fever I accepted a position as superintendent of the Lula Grove Hospital and Training School for colored nurses and patients. This hospital was operated by a group of white physicians that composed the faculty of the Atlanta School of Medicine, Atlanta, Ga., and closed after seven years of operation to merge with a larger medical school and i(s) n(o)w Emory University for whites only.[14]

Andrews's major contribution to black nursing history, however, was neither her superintendency of the Lula Grove Hospital nor her founding of the Municipal Training School for Colored Nurses at Grady Hospital in Atlanta in 1917. (The original nursing school at Grady, founded in 1892, was for white women only.) Rather, it was the result of her ten years of struggle with the Georgia Board of Nurse Examiners. She wrote in 1926, "I worked unceasingly for almost ten years against tremendous odds to secure state registration for colored nurses in Georgia, and finally succeeded in nineteen twenty with the result that all colored nurses graduating from certified training schools are permitted to take the examinations and register."[15] Until this victory, black nurses were denied the opportunity to take the same registration examination administered to white nurses. The point, as Andrews's career illustrates, is that black nurses had to fight for every bit of recognition and fair treatment they received. Throughout the period from 1900 through 1950, professionalization for them was synonymous with struggle.

Unlike Andrews, most southern black graduate nurses tended to work for long stretches of time in isolated communities, and in private practice in black and white families. Such isolation undoubtedly engendered a greater sense of autonomy and control. Northern black nurses congregated in the more densely populated cities and towns. Beginning with the Great Depression and the distribution of government funds to state governments and agencies, southern black nurses had perhaps a slightly better chance than their northern counterparts of securing employment in public and voluntary health operations. Moreover, when the nursing profession pushed for the development of bachelor's-degree programs, black nurses in the South were better situated, because of the regional difference in the black institutional infrastructure, to establish at black colleges several new baccalaureate programs. The development of one such program is discussed in chapter four.

Again as Ludie Andrews's life and career exemplify, any recounting of the history of black women in the nursing profession must of necessity include their political struggles against segregation and discrimination. In this regard, black nursing history mirrors the unending quest of all Afro-Americans for societal recognition of their contributions, open access to equal educational opportunities, and acceptance as competent professionals. The history of black nursing is therefore a microcosm of the history of Afro-Americans. It is a complex, and often contradictory, history of conflict and cooperation.

Not all white nurses were hostile to the strivings of their black counterparts; in fact, influential whites have occasionally aided the black struggle against oppression. White philanthropies, most notably the Julius Rosenwald Fund, the General Education Board, and the Rockefeller Foundation, played a significant role in the development of black nursing. At critical junctures in this history, the foundations provided the requisite funds to sustain black hospitals and nurse training schools, to pay the salaries of black nurse leaders engaged in the long struggle to integrate the profession, and to provide scholarships for students seeking advanced degrees. To be sure, philanthropic largesse was not always sought or welcomed by black recipients, especially when the foundation managers interfered with the internal affairs of the institutions under black control. Moreover, it is quite likely that the foundations were playing a subtle game of social control. These themes are explored in chapters one, two, and three.

The study of the history of nursing, including black nursing, must take into account the evolution of hospitals. The second and third chapters focus specifically on the development of black hospitals in the North and South and examine the nature of the training made available to black women, as well as the larger ideological debates concerning the efficacy of establishing and preserving separate black institutions. Throughout the first century of trained nursing, the hospitals played a critical role in the development of this profession. Yet the advantages were not all one-sided. As the urban middle classes demanded quality health care away from the home and indicated a willingness to pay for such services, the hospital system grew.[16]

The political economy of the hospital depended upon a constant supply of obedient, disciplined, and inexpensive workers willing to provide up to seventy hours a week of unremitting labor. Student nurses were therefore essential to the institution's existence and function. For the network of black hospitals created during the 1890s and the opening decades of the twentieth century, the establishment of nurse training schools was mandatory.[17] Within these institutions the nurse apprentices developed a distinctive work culture that affected their subsequent careers and lives. These themes are developed more fully in chapters three and seven.

This work is divided into two parts. The first four chapters concern the development of the institutional infrastructure of black nursing, examining the founding of black hospitals and nurse training schools in the North and South and tracing the emergence of black collegiate nursing education, as well as exploring the internal world of the training schools. In part two the focus is on the rise of black professional nursing. The primary emphasis is on an institution of a different sort: the National Association of Colored Graduate Nurses and the leaders who orchestrated the relentless struggle to elevate the status of black nurses and to achieve for their group greater social acceptance and complete integration into the mainstream of professional nursing. This work is grounded on an analysis of white racism and black efforts to overcome its manifestations as a key to understanding the evolution of the black nursing profession in particular and nursing history in general.

PART ONE

The Institutional Infrastructure of Black Nursing

Origins of the Black Hospital and Nurse Training School Movement: An Overview

1 The movement to create a national network of black hospitals and nurse training schools began in the 1890s and peaked during the 1920s. Entrenched racial antipathy characterized the late nineteenth century. Its closing decades witnessed the complete subordination of black Americans. Political and educational institutions in both the North and South adopted and perpetuated the dogmas of racial segregation and white supremacy. The racial fortress that imprisoned blacks in a separate world of poverty, powerlessness, disease, and despair seemed increasingly invulnerable to attack.

The discrepancies in the status and treatment of the two races were most apparent in the area of health-care delivery and in the virtual absence of educational and career opportunities for black women and men in the nursing and medical professions. Left with little recourse, the first generation of post-slavery black physicians, educators, and community leaders developed within their enclosed world a number of health-care institutions. Through them they launched a nationwide movement to provide educational opportunities for black women who desired to become nurses. Moreover, these new hospitals aimed to improve the health care available to black citizens while facilitating the professional development of physicians and nurses.

Since their arrival in the Americas, black women had always provided health care. They were nurturers of the sick, both black and white, on slave plantations. As granny midwives they helped to deliver most of the babies born during slavery and in the early years of freedom, especially in the rural South. Indeed, some black women even in the antebellum era achieved widespread recognition for their nursing and curative skills. As early as the 1820s, Jensey Snow, for example, became a living legend in her native Petersburg, Virginia. After earning her freedom, Snow opened a hospital and continued for over thirty years to provide health-care services for the community. Black abolitionist and women's-rights activist Sojourner Truth (1797–1881) served as an unpaid nurse to wounded civilians and soldiers during the Civil War in Washington, D.C., while Harriet Tubman (1820–1913) performed in a similar capacity in the Sea Islands off the coast of South Carolina. During the Civil War, Susie King Taylor (1848–1912), an ex-slave who possessed an extensive knowledge of the curative properties of various flora, provided treatment for dysentery and other ailments for black soldiers in Camp Saxton, South Carolina. Taylor, in commenting on her nursing activities, wrote: "I gave my services willingly for four years and three months without receiving a dollar. I was glad, however, to be allowed to go with the regiment, to care for the sick and afflicted."[1]

The Civil War left many impressions upon Americans, one of which was the importance of effective medical care. In response to the lack of trained nurses, women in the North and South formed voluntary associations, erected makeshift hospitals, and scrounged for supplies and medicines to alleviate some of the misery and pain of the wounded soldiers. The shockingly high morbidity and mortality rates during the war demonstrated the critical shortage of medical personnel and treatment.[2]

Shortly after the Civil War, in 1869, an American Medical Association committee evaluated and made recommendations concerning the training of nurses. Following a lengthy enumeration of the preferred qualifications of a good nurse and discussion of the duties she should be required to perform in hospitals and in private duty, the committee suggested that the nurse should be a woman who possessed so many positive traits that she was virtually perfect. She should be "of sound constitution, of good muscular strength, and of great power of endurance, capable of bearing up manfully under fatigue and loss of sleep." In addition, she should be "literate, courageous, patient, temperate, punctual, cheerful, discreet, honest, sympathetic, refined, selfless, and devoted." She should not be younger than twenty-two or older than thirty-five. The nurse should be able to notice the "character of the secretions and excretions, and the changes in the patient's physical countenance." She should be adept in the application of "leeches, blisters, bandages and other dressings." Finally, the committee asserted that the nurse should be "proficient in making up beds, changing sheets, and handling patients exhausted by disease and injury." The report included the suggestion that each state medical association work to establish schools for the training of such nurses for work in hospitals and with private families.[3]

The connection between the Crimean War and Florence Nightingale's movement in the 1850s in Great Britain to establish an organized system of rigorous training of female nurses and exacting standards of recruitment is a familiar tale in need of little elaboration here. It is worthwhile to note, however, that one black West Indian nurse, Mary Grant Seacole of Jamaica, did provide, at her own expense, some nursing service during the Crimean War, though she was never accepted or given an official position by Florence Nightingale. The first three American nursing schools were founded in 1873: Massachusetts General Hospital in Boston, Bellevue Hospital in New York, and the New Haven Hospital in Connecticut. Each adhered to the "Nightingale Tradition," emphasizing uniforms and military discipline. Each evidenced an overriding concern for attracting middle-class students into the program. There were 15 nursing training schools in 1880; by 1900 there were 432. (See Appendix, table 1.) Some of these early schools were quasi-independent, with separate sources of funding enabling faculty to enjoy some measure of autonomy. Actually, even these very early institutions were surrounded by hospitals, and the power of the women administrators was not as absolute as they preferred.[4]

Within a remarkably short time, hospitals acquired dominance in nursing education and soon eclipsed the seemingly autonomous nurse training schools. Two factors among many others aided hospital administrators in gaining complete hegemony in nursing training: insufficient capital and lack of endowment of the fledgling schools, and the increased demand for more scientifically based instruction. Additional factors included unchecked urbanization, revolutionary scientific discoveries, and steady improvements in medicine and surgery. Moreover, the increasing demand of patients for treatment away from the home dramatically fueled the expansion of hospitals.[5] The history of the growth and development of the nursing profession is inextricably tied to the emergence and maturation of the modern American hospital. Nursing history is therefore as much a study of the evolution of hospitals as health-care institutions as it is an examination of the experiences, deeds, and struggles of the trained nurse.

Beginning in the last decade of the nineteenth century, hospitals gradually acquired more respectability, prestige, and acceptance as the previously skeptical, indeed hostile, public came to perceive them as places of effective care as opposed to dens of death. This transformation in public attitudes did not occur overnight. Throughout much of American medical history, the general hospital, using untrained nurses, provided treatment almost exclusively to the rootless poor. White middle-class Americans did not consider hospitalization a viable alternative to home care. Most often they were treated in their homes by an attending physician and female family members.

The growing urbanization of the American population and advances in late-nineteenth-century medicine, including the discovery of germicides and the development of more appropriate therapeutics, spurred the modernization of hospitals. This modernization dictated that administrators not only rationalize services but also cease to rely on poverty-stricken patients and the unrefined, uneducated nurses who provided the necessary hospital services and performed all of the domestic and maintenance chores. Instead of requiring the ambulatory patients to care for one another, hospital administrators recognized the need for a constant, obedient, and efficient supply of cheap labor. The best solution was to use student nurses. The rise of nursing as a profession stimulated the growth of the late-nineteenth-century hospital movement.

In 1873 there had been 178 hospitals in the United States; in 1909 there were 4,359. By the close of the first decade of the twentieth century, therefore, "not only had the hospital become more evenly distributed throughout the United States, it had become a potential recourse for a much larger proportion of Americans; the respectable and prosperous as well as the indigent might be treated in hospitals, frequently by their regular physicians."[6] By 1923 there were 6,830 hospitals, and fully one-quarter of them included a nursing school. By the mid-1920s these schools had graduated 17,000 trained nurses. (See Appendix, table 1.) As white physician Alfred Worcester observed in 1909, "Hospitals are everywhere springing up, not merely because their advantages were made so apparent in war times, nor only because the germs that formerly killed have themselves met their destroyer. An even greater cause is to be found in the development of the art of nursing."[7] In some schools the students received a modest stipend, but most simply received rudimentary nursing instruction, room and board, and a bolt of cloth with which to make their uniforms. In return they pledged to serve the hospital for a period of from eighteen months to three years.

Although black women for generations had borne primary responsibility for providing nursing care in their communities, few were admitted to the new training schools. Most of the hospital nursing schools in the North imposed racial quotas, while institutions in the South excluded black women. Mary E. Mahoney was the first black woman to graduate from a nursing school. In August 1879 she received her diploma from the New England Hospital for Women and Children in Boston. The charter of this pioneering nursing school stipulated that only *one* Negro and *one* Jewish student be accepted each year. By 1899 only five other black women had been graduated: Lavinia Holloway, Josephine Braxton, Kittie Toliver, Ann Dillit, and Roxie Dentz Smith.[8]

Southern black women possessed scant opportunity to become "trained" nurses. The patterns and practices of racial segregation received the highest sanction when in 1896 the United States Supreme Court delivered a decision destined to have profound implications for all black Americans. In *Plessy* v. *Ferguson* the Court promulgated the doctrine of "separate but equal," which provided the legal basis for the whole system of segregation. This decision and the one delivered in the 1899 case *Joseph W. Cumming, James Harper, and John C. Ladevez* v. *School Board of Richmond County, Georgia* became the cornerstone for segregated education, housing, and health care.[9] Although the Court insisted

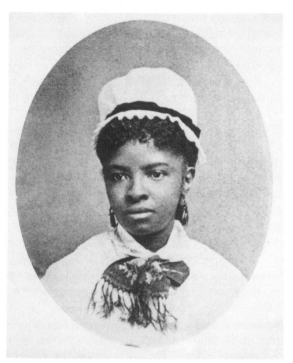

Mary Eliza Mahoney (1845–1926), the first black professional nurse in America. She earned her diploma from the New England Hospital for Women and Children on August 1, 1879. Courtesy of the Schomburg Center for Research in Black Culture, New York Public Library.

that equal facilities be provided for blacks, none of the southern states deigned to do so. Black patients were either excluded from or segregated within publicly supported municipal hospitals, while racial discrimination denied black physicians access to internships, residencies, and hospital staff appointments.

By the turn of the century, many contemporary observers linked the general deterioration in the health of black Americans to the absence of adequate health care–delivery systems, the lack of trained black medical practitioners, and the increased migration of black people from rural South to urban North. A brief examination of the black morbidity and mortality rates of one southern city, New Orleans, is illustrative of prevailing conditions in cities across the nation. Severe food shortages and unsanitary and overcrowded living arrangements repeatedly contributed to the spread of contagious diseases in urban America. During the Civil

War the United States government had established the Freedmen's Bureau, which in turn had constructed approximately fifty makeshift hospitals to treat illnesses born of poverty and racial oppression. Three of these hospitals were located in Louisiana. By the collapse of Reconstruction in 1877, however, all of the Louisiana facilities were closed.[10] Only the Freedmen's Hospital in Washington, D.C., would survive into the twentieth century.

The morbidity and mortality rates of New Orleans blacks and whites diverged sharply as thousands more blacks contracted tuberculosis, pneumonia, influenza, typhoid fever, whooping cough, malaria, syphilis, and pellagra. Among black women, puerperal (or childbirth) fever and complications associated with premature births took a deadly toll. Between 1890 and 1900 the death rate in New Orleans dropped modestly from 25.4 to 23.8 per thousand among whites. For blacks, however, the rate increased significantly from 36.6 to 42.4 per thousand. Infant mortality throughout the South remained high for both races, but blacks registered greater losses. In 1920 in South Carolina, 159 babies out of every 1,000 died before they reached one year of age, as compared to 86 white infants per 1,000.

Unsanitary water supplies and inadequate sewage systems contributed to the excessively high black mortality not only in New Orleans but throughout the urban South. Black urbanites in Chicago, Cleveland, Philadelphia, Detroit, and New York, like their counterparts in southern cities, lived in overcrowded, poorly ventilated, vermin-infested housing. Their children suffered from malnutrition, and whole families relied far too heavily on diets of fat pork, grits, and molasses. Yet even had blacks known (and many did not have sufficient knowledge of nutrition) what to eat, procuring adequate fare on meager, often nonexistent, earnings proved difficult, if not impossible.[11]

A convergence of critical forces including the high incidence of black morbidity and mortality gave impetus to the creation of a separate network of black hospitals and nursing schools. A major factor shaping their development was the simultaneous emergence of private philanthropic foundations organized by John D. Rockefeller, Andrew Carnegie, and particularly Julius Rosenwald, the president of Sears, Roebuck and Company. Through the Julius Rosenwald Fund, Rosenwald distributed a small fortune to "his chief philanthropic interest," the Negro.[12] Before blacks could enjoy adequate health care and before black women could have access to formal nursing training, black leaders and these white philanthropists had to replicate the health-care system then developing within the white communities. John D. Rockefeller and his wife, Laura Spelman Rockefeller, financed the establishment of the nation's first black nursing training school. They contributed the funds necessary to establish in 1881 the Atlanta Baptist Female Seminary, subsequently renamed Spelman College, a private black women's school, and to create a department of nursing in 1886. It was the first two-year program leading to a diploma in nursing established within an academic institution. By 1901, Dr. Malcolm MacVicar had amassed sufficient funds to construct a thirty-one-bed hospital on the Atlanta campus to serve as a school infirmary and practice facility for the student nurses.

By the turn of the century, although the student nurses followed a four-year course of study, only one year was devoted to the study of nursing theory. The remaining three were spent on duty at the MacVicar Hospital and in private cases. One Rockefeller Foundation official described the school as being "devoted to the most conventional training of negro girls, practically all of whom go into private duty in white families."[13] In 1905 John D. Rockefeller gave $25,000 to the program to build a new nurses' home. Money failed to solve all of the schools' problems. In spite of the early Rockefeller financial support, the college's trustees voted on December 15, 1927, to close the nursing training program. According to Florence M. Read, a former president of Spelman College, the decision was made because "it had become apparent that first-class training could not be offered with the facilities provided by MacVicar Hospital. The hospital contained too small a number of beds; the variety of cases was too limited; and the equipment was insufficient for modern techniques."[14]

During the 1890s and the opening years of the twentieth century, white racism, black self-help initiatives, and white philanthropic largesse led to the founding of about a dozen major black hospitals and nursing training schools: the Provident Hospital School of Nursing, Chicago (1891); the Dixie Hospital Training School, Hampton, Virginia (1891); the Tuskegee Institute nursing training course, which began in 1892 in connection with the school's hospital and later evolved into the John A. Andrew Hospital (built in 1913) and School of Nursing, Tuskegee, Alabama; the Freedmen's Hospital Nursing School, later affiliated with Howard University in Washington, D.C. (1894); the Lincoln School for Nurses, New York City (1896); St. Agnes Hospital and Nurse Training School, Raleigh, North Carolina (1896); the Phillis Wheatley Sanitarium and Training School for Nurses, renamed in the late teens the Flint-Goodridge Hospital School of Nursing, New Orleans (1896); the Hospital and Training School for Nurses, Charleston, South Carolina (1897); Hubbard Hospital and School of Nursing, Meharry Medical College, Nashville, Tennessee (1900); Lincoln Hospital in Durham, North Carolina (1901); and the Mercy Hospital School of Nursing, Philadelphia (1907). By 1928 these schools had produced 2,238 graduates, accounting for 80.3 percent of the total of 2,784 black graduate nurses. (See Appendix, tables 2, 3, 4.)

By the mid-1920s, at the height of the black hospital movement, over 25 new nursing schools and almost 200 black hospitals in the South, Mid-

west, and Northeast existed. Some were supported by municipal governments.[15] By 1940 only 110 black hospitals remained, with a total bed
capacity of approximately 10,000. More than 70 percent of these institutions were privately owned. Only 22 black hospitals had received full
approval by the American College of Surgeons, while 5 others were provi-
sionally approved. The number of black schools of nursing had decreased
to 20, although a few of the predominantly white institutions occasionally admitted black women.[16]

No single philosophical rationale impelled those who founded the early
black hospitals and nurse training schools. To be sure, even the most dis-
passionate observers acknowledged that something had to be done to improve the system of health-care delivery for blacks. The type of institution created reflected to a great extent, however, the nature of the
connections between the motives of founders, the financial resources provided by white philanthropists, and the level of black community support
and interest. Many of the individual creators of black hospitals and nurse
training schools acted out of a complex array of motives ranging from al-
truism, to professional self-aggrandizement, to a commitment to the preservation of racial segregation. Perhaps the white philanthropist Julius
Rosenwald best typifies this combination of motives.

At the height of the movement to develop black hospitals and nursing
training facilities, Julius Rosenwald (1862–1936) donated large sums of
money to select institutions: Provident Hospital in Chicago, Hubbard
Hospital in Nashville, and the nursing school at Hampton Institute. Between 1929 and 1942 the Julius Rosenwald Fund under the direction of
president Edwin R. Embree expended $1,701,928 on a variety of efforts
designed to promote black professional development and to improve black
health. At least seventeen black hospital and nursing school–development projects received Rosenwald funds. Rosenwald combined his altruistic interest in improving black educational programs with a desire
to protect and preserve the health of the white population, to shield
whites as much as possible from contamination by black germ carriers.
The most effective way to preserve white health, he reasoned, was to improve black health. He declared on one occasion, "If colored doctors and
nurses are to have the teaching and stimulus which will enable them to
reach high standards, white physicians must encourage them by counsel
and service; white citizens must help if adequate funds are to be provided
for Negro hospitals and health." And he added, "It is well to remember
that germs recognize no color lines and the disease in one group threat-
ens the health of all."[17]

A 1922 interoffice memorandum circulated among the officers of
Rockefeller's General Education Board captures well the prevailing sentiments concerning the relationship between black and white health and
the reasons for philanthropic largesse:

The GEB's interest is neither sentimental nor merely humanitarian, it is practical. The Negro race is numerous and widely scattered; it is with us to stay. Aside from any concern which on humanitarian grounds might be felt for the Negro for his sake, it is clear that the welfare of the South, not to say the whole country—its prosperity, its sanitation, and its morale—is affected by the condition of the Negro race.[18]

When white philanthropists Benjamin N. and James B. Duke joined with their father, Washington Duke, to finance the establishment in 1901 of Lincoln Hospital in Durham, North Carolina, they were largely motivated out of a desire to erect a monument "to the memory of the southern slaves and their loyalty to the southern people during the Civil War." The entrance to Lincoln Hospital bore a marble tablet inscribed, in part, "With grateful appreciation and loving remembrance of the fidelity and faithfulness of the Negro slaves to the Mothers and Daughters of the Confederacy, during the Civil War. . . . Not one act of disloyalty was recorded against them."[19] The sustaining benefaction of the Duke Endowment and subsequent annual contributions from the city of Durham helped Lincoln to become one of the best black institutions in the South.

Black physicians, male and female, who founded nursing schools often married professional interests and concern for their own advancement within the medical hierarchy with a desire to make available health-care facilities for the black community and to provide new career opportunities for black women, especially those who belonged to or aspired to membership in the small but growing black middle class. In a 1910 report, a committee of black physicians succinctly summarized the diverse reasons why individual black medical doctors had founded fifteen private hospitals: "to care for the sick under his charge; . . . to develop his talent as a surgeon, a clinician, an obstetrician, or a pathologist . . . to enable his patients to enjoy the advantages of modern methods of treatment." Responding after the committee's presentation, black physician J. H. Burney of Athens, Georgia, provided another motive. He explained, "In Savannah we have a hospital which is supported by contributions from churches and from the city." Burney emphasized one point in particular: "We have a Nurse Training School and find it quite a lucrative business; and every hospital in Savannah has a Nurse Training Department." To underscore the urgency of the committee's recommendation that a black hospital be erected in every community, another physician declared,

The reason why we should recommend more hospitals is based on the ground that in every community where there are white physicians they are trained in thorough investigation along all lines of new endeavor by having the advantage of hospital training; and in a community where there is a large number of Negroes, unless the Negro physician has had this training, we must admit that the white man has had better training than we have.[20]

In the minds of these early black physicians, the creation of a hospital enhanced their professional development, provided much-needed health care for the community, and through the establishment of a companion training school helped to earn money.

Daniel Hale Williams was a prominent black physician in Chicago who founded two black nursing schools: Provident in 1891, and Freedmen's in Washington, D.C., in 1894. He became a key figure in the turn-of-the-century crusade to establish a black hospital and nursing training school in every black community. He railed against the exclusion of black women from white nursing schools, attacked the inadequacies of segregated hospitals, and blasted those white physicians who treated black patients with contempt. Williams challenged fellow black physicians and community leaders to "not waste time trying to effect changes or modifications in the institutions unfriendly to us, but rather let us seek to promote the doctrine of helping and stimulating our race."[21] Although he issued this strong call for black self-help, Williams readily accepted contributions from leading white citizens in Chicago when he launched Provident.

Actually, Williams's views and sentiments echoed those of many blacks and some whites who rallied to the call to establish hospitals and nursing schools. To be sure, while some black professionals were skeptical about the motives of whites who participated in and supported black hospital development, Williams believed that the black community in conjunction with white philanthropic groups should share the work of raising the start-up costs for buildings and other facilities. At one level his use of black-self-help rhetoric was employed to elicit the maximum support from an already overtaxed and largely impoverished but increasingly urban and unhealthy black population.

A careful reading of Williams's speeches and writings illuminates both his own and the larger society's image of black nurses. Williams informed potential supporters of black hospital training schools that "the servant class no longer furnishes the nurses." Ironically, and especially before white audiences, he was prone to invoke the ubiquitous slave mammy image of black women to substantiate his claims that the black woman was a "natural nurse possessed of a long heritage, in slavery and freedom, of caring for the sick of both races." He declared that "more than two hundred years before Florence Nightingale began the work of training as scientific nurses, the black 'mammy' was the accepted nurse in the country."[22] After extolling black women as natural nurturers, Williams contended that the "trained" nurse was even more special. He viewed the "trained" black nurse as an object lesson who "teaches the people cleanliness, thrift, habits of industry, sanitary housekeeping, the proper care of themselves and of their children." He continued, "She teaches them how to prepare food, the selection of proper clothing for the sick and well and how to meet emergencies."[23]

This concern with the perception of and imagined role of black women nurses begs further attention, for it informs much of the ambiguous rhetoric used by late-nineteenth-century black physicians and educators to justify the creation of black hospitals and nurse training schools. The rhetoric also served another, perhaps even more important, function. Williams and others had to persuade young black women to pursue nursing training. Skeptical black women understandably had to be convinced that nursing was neither domestic service nor a "warmed-over slavery." Furthermore, the leaders of this movement felt the need to impress upon black women the notion that they were somehow ideally suited for nursing, indeed that they were imbued with inherent or "natural" proclivities for the kind of work nursing entailed.

When Booker T. Washington launched nursing training at Tuskegee Institute in Alabama in 1892, he viewed it on the one hand simply as an extension of the school's industrial and vocational thrust. Yet he took pains to claim that "colored women have always made good nurses. They have, I believe, a natural aptitude for that sort of work."[24] Two wooden structures on the campus were used as quarters for treating the sick, one for men and the other for women. In addition there was another one-room structure which served as a dispensary for drugs for those ailing members of the faculty and student body who did not require hospitalization. In 1900 the institute erected a new two-story frame building large enough to accommodate twenty-five beds and extended its services to include members of the entire community. The building was made possible by a gift from a white benefactor, Mrs. Thomas J. Bennett of New Haven, Connecticut. In 1902 Washington hired black physician John A. Kenney, a graduate of Hampton Institute who had completed his medical education the previous year at the Leonard Medical School of Shaw University in Raleigh, North Carolina, to become resident physician and superintendent of the hospital and nursing training school.[25]

Washington justified the opening of the new program on the grounds that nursing training would enable the black woman to enjoy a career prior to marriage, but one which would also make her a better wife, mother, and homemaker. In fact, the 1896 Tuskegee Institute catalogue offers somewhat contradictory but revealing testimony regarding the reasons the nursing training program was launched in the first place and the expectations it held of its graduates: "Many of our young women who take the course will never become professional nurses, but take it with a view to being better prepared for the responsibilities of family life." Washington, like most black Americans, expected the women of the race to work before and after marriage and to contribute economically to the well-being of the family. Unlike their white middle-class sisters, then, black women occupied places in both the sphere of men working in the public arena and that of women looking after the domestic domain.

Yet, images seldom conform completely to reality. Thus, the fact that black women had historically performed double duty and would continue to labor both within and outside the home did not prevent some black male leaders from espousing idealized views of what constituted the "proper" woman's place in American society. Like the majority of whites in Victorian America, black male physicians and educators viewed woman's proper role as a vital but subordinate helpmate to the men in the family and a crucial resource for the total community. Washington insisted that "the course in child nurture and nursing has been established to complete the training in home building which is carried on as part of the industrial training of young women at Tuskegee." Ever the pragmatist, he added that should hard times befall a family, the trained nurse would always be able to earn some money.[26] Washington and Williams stressed the vocational dimensions and economic value of nurse training even when such training was made available in an academic institution. Williams had declared: "We must not lose sight of the fact that college education is not so much the need of the hour for our women as practical education, breadwinning education, education that will maintain them in independent and honorable positions."[27]

John A. Kenney, the new superintendent of the renamed John A. Andrew Hospital at Tuskegee Institute, also unabashedly lauded the black nurses' many womanly virtues of "devotion, endurance, sympathy, tactile delicacy, unselfishness, tact, resourcefulness, [and] willingness to undergo hardship." This sentimentalized portrait conjured up notions and reinforced visions of the black nurse as primarily a mother-nurturer figure. Of course, these images were identical to those of white nurses. It was as if Kenney wanted to reassure himself and others that the "trained" black nurse would remain essentially unchanged by the instruction she received in these new structures. He recalled: "Regardless of the demand made upon her [his mother] by the exacting duties of her own household, if there was a case of serious illness among her friends, white or colored, even miles away she thought it her duty to go and care for them night after night if necessary."[28]

The implications of these reminiscences were unmistakable. Tuskegee nurses would replicate the same selfless, devoted soul of Kenney's mother. Consistent with prevailing Victorian ideas and images of separate spheres, Kenney believed that training black women to become nurses merely honed and enlarged their female virtues. Whether she was at work outside the home or within it, the black nurse, at heart, represented a fulfillment of those traditional roles and obligations expected of her by the black community and her family, and posed little threat to distinct gender spheres. Examples abound of black male founders of hospital training schools who molded the idealized Florence Nightingale archetype nurse to fit their own and the communities' image of the black nurse as a self-sacrificing, dutiful, warm, caring mother figure. Some of these men deliberately downplayed any depiction of the black nurse as an efficient, autonomous, and assertive professional.

On the other hand, several black male physicians established hospital training schools precisely because they wanted to produce a cadre of level-headed, skilled, and resourceful black nurses, and proudly proclaimed their intent. Alonzo C. McClennan, born May 1, 1855, in Columbia, South Carolina, completed one year of study at South Carolina College (1876–1877) before going on to earn his medical degree in 1880 from the Howard University Medical School in Washington, D.C. He began the practice of medicine in Augusta, Georgia, but moved to Charleston in 1884. In 1892 he opened the first black pharmacy in the city, the People's Pharmacy.

In 1896, McClennan called a meeting of the five other black physicians and dentists in Charleston to protest their being denied staff privileges at the city's public hospitals. During the meeting they lamented the lack of nurse training opportunities for black women. After long discussions, the black doctors, with the support of prominent black businessmen and religious leaders organized into the Hospital Association, resolved to found a separate black hospital and nursing school with McClennan elected chief of staff. In subsequent appeals for money to the black community through the monthly publication the *Hospital Herald*, McClennan declared, "Physicians get better results from the treatment of the sick in the hospitals or in private practice when they have to aid them competent nurses who are able to carry out intelligently whatever directions may be given them, and who can detect the changes in the progress of disease under treatment."[29] He then added: "It would be a great monument to the people of this State if it could be said to their honor and credit that the institution at least was paid for through money collected from them."[30]

Another black physician, J. Edward Perry, an 1895 graduate of Meharry Medical College and founder of the small proprietary Wheatley Provident Hospital and Nurse Training School in Kansas City, Missouri, shared McClennan's sentiments. Perry declared: "The nurse is a co-partner of the doctor. Without her, in many instances, his efforts in the battle of disease would be futile." Perry acknowledged that "since the inception of the work of Wheatley Provident Hospital the nurses have played a conspicuous part." He concluded, "But for their loyalty and devotion, the institution would early have been grounded upon a sandbar of disaster and chaos."[31]

Women, whether white or black, who founded hospital training schools seldom spoke in terms of the trained nurse as being a physician's helper. Moving beyond this limited perspective, they envisioned nursing training as one significant means to an end, to wit, the delivery of better health care for black people and the simultaneous production of autonomous professionals. In June 1891 Alice Mabel Bacon, white, from Massachusetts, founded the Dixie Hospital and Hampton Training School for Nurses "in a little yellow-washed building" with ten beds in Hampton, Virginia. It opened with a resident physician, a superintendent of nursing, and its first students, one of whom was Anna De Costa Banks, a Hampton Institute graduate.

Bacon justified her action as a means "to retain in the hands of trained colored women a profession for which even without training, the Negro women have always shown themselves especially adapted." She argued that black women could not "long retain a hold upon the profession of

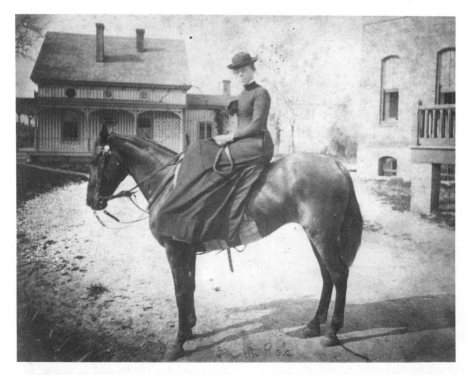

Alice Mabel Bacon on her horse, Dixie, in the 1890s. Hampton Training School for Nurses was commonly called "Dixie Hospital" because Bacon would go out, with Dixie hitched to a surrey, to bring patients into the hospital. Courtesy of the Hampton University Archives, Alice Mabel Bacon Collection.

nursing without training at least equal to that enjoyed by white women."
She insisted, "It is to keep open for them [black women] a means of livelihood which they are in danger of losing that the school was founded."[32]
Perhaps Bacon was inspired to undertake this work by the example set
by her brother, Francis Bacon, head surgeon at the New Haven Hospital,
and his wife, who was the director of its training school for nursing.

Four months after opening Dixie, Bacon described the training-school
operation and the role of the pupil nurses:

> Two girls enlisted in the service last June, immediately after the close of
> school, and have shown, during the three months of training, promising
> material from which good nurses can be made. Their training in the hospi-
> tal has been varied by visits to outside cases of interest, and one of them
> has just returned from a pay case in a white family three miles from Hamp-
> ton. There seems no doubt that we could find profitable employment for
> all the nurses we could train even before they have fully finished their
> training, and our graduates will be started in an honorable and lucrative
> profession as soon as they leave school. Class work with the nurses has not
> yet begun, but we hope soon to start the daily lectures or lessons, in which
> we have the promise of aid from neighboring physicians.[33]

Bacon then detailed the layout of Dixie Hospital and its training school,
emphasizing both its strengths and weaknesses:

> The hospital contains two wards, airy and bright and sunny, each pleas-
> antly furnished, and with five beds. A nurse's room between the two wards
> at the front of the building and a square hall at the back, opening into the
> wards, the nurse's room, and the covered way that leads to the detached
> kitchen—these are all the rooms that the Dixie can boast. The dining table
> must be set in the back hall, one of the wards, the nurse's room, or on the
> front piazza, for there is no dining room. The nurses off duty must sleep
> in one of the empty rooms in the Whittier School building [across the
> street] for there is only room for the one in charge of the wards to sleep
> in the little front room; and there is no dispensary, no room for the doctor,
> no privacy or rest for tired nurses until in some way we obtain a six room
> cottage connecting by covered way with the kitchen, and in which we can
> have a home for nurses and doctor, as well as a dispensary for out-
> patients.[34]

In the neighboring state of North Carolina, white churchwomen assumed the responsibility of establishing two black hospitals and training
schools. Mrs. John Wilkes and the white ladies of the Episcopal Church
of Charlotte had served as untrained nurses in the local Confederate hospital during the Civil War. After the war these women established the
St. Peter's Hospital for the city's white citizens. Then, as an act of charity,
beginning in 1882 they initiated a fundraising campaign to purchase an
unused school building, formerly a Presbyterian mission, and a neighbor-

ing lot which was to be the site of a hospital for black people. In June 1891 the new building, spacious enough to accommodate twenty patients, was completed, and on September 23, 1891, it was opened to the public. A matron was employed, and one white and two black doctors served as the staff. Not until 1903 did the all-white female board of managers open a school of nursing "in order that carefully selected young Negro women might be prepared to render efficient service to their race and to earn a living in an honored profession."[35]

Similarly, in Raleigh, North Carolina, five white women on October 18, 1896, established St. Agnes Hospital in a private residence on the grounds of St. Augustine College (for Negroes). They were led in this endeavor by Sara Hunter, wife of the principal of the college. Serving on the staff during the early years were Dr. Catherine P. Hayden (M.D., Colorado, 1894), first resident physician and superintendent; Dr. Jennie A. Duncan (M.D., Illinois, 1910); Dr. Mary V. Glenton (M.D., Northwestern

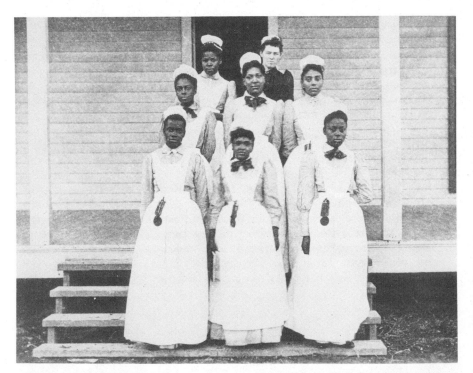

This is the second (1894) class of nurses to receive their diplomas from the Hampton Training School. *Left to right, back to front*: Alberta Boyd, Dr. Conacher; Gnni(?) Walker, Annie Taylor Smith, Sallie Anderson; Ella Gaines, Ella Thomas, unknown. Courtesy of the Hampton University Archives, Dixie Hospital Collection.

Woman's Medical College, 1893); and Miss Edna H. Wheeler, who served as matron and general supervisor of lay matters from 1900 until her death in 1922. The National Women's Auxiliary of the Episcopal Church provided the necessary operating expenses. The institution, housed in a four-story stone building, had a seventy-five-bed capacity. During the first two months of operation, however, it had only four patients and four student nurses. The first commencement, held on April 21, 1898, graduated two nurses. In 1915 the training period was increased from two and a half to three years. By 1922 116 black nurses had been graduated, with 33 then in training.[36]

Staff physician Mary V. Glenton provided a candid and illuminating description of the harsh working conditions endured by student nurses at St. Agnes:

> No water in the house, except one faucet in the kitchen.
> No hot water, but what could be heated on the ward stoves.
> Whole house heated by wood.
> Two small steamers for sterilizers (the results untrustworthy) formed the operating room equipment—a probationer stationed outside of the operating room door, to hand in hot water when called for, and to empty buckets of used water.
> No screens in windows or doors, and flying things innumerable, with wings small and great.
> Laundry equipment—three ordinary wash tubs, flat iron heater, and a big iron kettle in the yard for boiling clothes.
> Ice only in extreme emergency, and it had to come from town. Automobiles were not invented, and trolleys were still an oddity, and Mr. Hunter's horse Mellie with a two-wheeled cart had to carry the ice and other things from Raleigh—four miles.
> Cool water was brought by hand from the spring to bathe Typhoid patients, and the nurses carried it. And that was for old-fashioned Typhoid treatment before the days of vaccine. There was no sewerage.
> The Office was Reception Room, Doctor's Living Room, Dining Room, Surgeon's Dressing Room on operating days, and sometimes the Morgue.
> No plumbing anywhere—only earth closets.
> No Diet Kitchen—the trays kept on a shelf in the kitchen.
> No gas for cooking nor for lighting; simply oil lamps.
> Not always enough food for patients; nor the proper kind for nurses and staff.[37]

Black clubwomen in many southern communities played a major role in launching and sustaining black hospitals and nursing schools. On October 31, 1896, the members of the Phillis Wheatley Club founded the only such institution in New Orleans. The Phillis Wheatley Sanitarium and Training School for Nurses began rather inauspiciously in a private residence with seven beds and five student nurses. The clubwomen founded the institution in part out of a desire to do something socially useful, and to alleviate excessive suffering, morbidity, and mortality among New Orleans blacks. From its inception, therefore, the sanitarium had a dual mission: to serve the health-care needs of black New Orleans and to provide facilities for the training of black nurses and other health-care personnel.[38] The role of black women in providing health care to the masses of blacks and making available nurse training opportunities for their sisters encompassed more than the establishment of the Phillis Wheatley Sanitarium. In every community, regardless of geographic locale, black women organized groups and clubs and occupied leadership positions in raising funds to furnish and sustain the hospitals and training schools, whether established by black physicians, educators, or municipalities, white philanthropists, or white women.

It was propitious that the national mobilization of black women in 1896 resulting in the formation of the National Association of Colored Women's Clubs coincided with the launching of the Negro hospital and nursing training movement. Throughout the ensuing decades organized groups of black women such as the Lucy Brown Club of Charleston, South Carolina, named after the black woman physician who had assisted McClennan in launching the Hospital and Training School for Nurses, supplied black hospitals "with linen for surgical work, and the different wards of the hospital with pillow slips, sheets and gowns." Furthermore, the club members helped to recruit nursing students and even raised money to pay the salary of a graduate nurse.[39] This record of involvement and support was repeated in hundreds of black communities around the country. Indeed, raising funds and providing supplies for a local hospital and nursing school became one of the most popular club activities of black community women.[40]

Municipal governments did not enter into the movement to establish hospitals and nursing training schools for blacks until well into the twentieth century. They did so reluctantly and often more to appease black protesters than out of a generous spirit of humanitarian concern for black citizens. As the number of black migrants swelled urban populations, the demands placed on municipal health-care facilities drastically increased. Many cities, from New Orleans with its Charity Hospital to Kansas City, Missouri, initially solved the problem of providing hospital services and facilities for blacks by reserving a separate floor, a basement, or part of a ward in an existing institution. When urban governments yielded to political pressure exerted by black politicians and leaders, they created separate black hospitals, usually with white administrators and staff. Even this limited response occurred only after the city had constructed a new hospital for whites. Blacks then inherited the abandoned, dilapidated, and obsolete structures. Still, the third stage, requiring more pressure and protest, often took years to reach, winning for black professionals the right and privilege of administering and staffing the hospitals set up for black patients.

Kansas City General Hospital No. 2 in Missouri was one of the larger municipal hospitals and training schools founded between 1905 and 1925. One black writer, in 1919, bitterly described the process: "When a magnificent new building was erected in Kansas City, Mo., in 1906, the general Hospital, and the white patients transferred there, the old building was thrown open to Negro patients, where they had formerly only been allowed in the basement. But the institution remained under white management with white doctors, nurses and employees."[41] One of the primary reasons for the establishment of separate facilities at No. 2 was the desire of white authorities to keep the races apart and thereby, they hoped, reduce potential conflict.

The price of maintaining racial segregation and the illusion of white supremacy was the erection of a dual health care–delivery system complete with separate and unequal facilities for the training of black nurses. To be sure, not all urban communities supplied even separate health-care and training facilities for blacks. Excluded entirely from institutions which their taxes supported, blacks in most northern communities had to marshal additional resources with which to meet group needs. In the case of Kansas City General Hospital No. 2, however, segregation worked to blacks' advantage. Black physician William J. Tompkins successfully convinced both the mayor of the city and the white president of the hospital a⁻.d health board that it was in the interests of all concerned to place the institution entirely in the hands of black health-care personnel.[42]

Whether academically affiliated, voluntary, or municipal, controlled by whites or blacks, operated out of a spirit of humanitarianism or professional self-interest, black hospitals and nursing training schools had to prove their value to the masses of black people. Thus it is not surprising that the first generation of hospital administrators, black physicians, and educators confronted a major challenge in attracting black patients into the hospitals, especially those who could afford to pay for medical services. It is hard to exaggerate the difficulties encountered in the attempt to dispel the fear and superstitions deeply entrenched within the black population. As late as 1930 black physician Peter Marshall Murray of New York lamented that "the unfair practice well nigh general in this country of excluding negro physicians from the staff of hospitals where negroes are patients imposes a distinct psychologic handicap on the negro patient and makes the result of treatment given him less effective." Marshall elaborated, "He [the Negro] is less inclined to apply for hospital service for preventive and early treatment and too often submits only after he has become a grave risk."[43]

Murray's remarks are an accurate reflection of blacks' historical distrust of hospitals. Further substantiation of this almost universal black

fear is gleaned from accounts recalling the circumstances under which
the first black patients received care at the Good Samaritan Hospital of
Charlotte, North Carolina. Frank Wilkes, son of Mrs. John Wilkes,
founder of the institution, described the first two patients attended in the
hospital:

> The first patient was found lying just inside the gate, unconscious, almost
> naked in the final stages of pneumonia. Those who had brought him were
> evidently too frightened to knock on the door. His case was hopeless but
> he had care and comfort in his last hours and a decent burial.
>   The next patient, protesting and struggling violently, was brought in by
> two policemen. His physician had advised his coming, his family approved,
> but he had heard rumors that people were carved up with butcher knives
> in hospitals, so he rebelled.[44]

While much of the progress toward allaying such anxiety was due to
the growing presence of black student nurses on hospital wards, even
they could do little to increase the ability of black people to pay for such
services. During the first eighteen months of operation, 1896–98, the
Hospital and Training School for Nurses in Charleston treated approximately two hundred cases. According to nurse Anna De Costa Banks, as
the patient load increased, only one-half of those treated were able to pay
the three-dollars-a-week charge. She elaborated: "Our hospital work is
entirely among the poor, ignorant, and superstitious class of colored people of Charleston and its counties—people who are without homes, money
and friends, and who believe in all kinds of signs and conjuration."[45]

Banks admitted that even poor patients reluctantly entered the hospital, and when they did so, their anxiety was often mixed with fear that
they had been voodooed. Complaints ran the gamut from "snakes under
their skins" to "frogs in their throats," wrote Banks. Many were convinced that there was really nothing of substance that the doctors or
nurses could do to treat their ailments. Nevertheless, out of desperation
they came. In repayment for services, those short of cash gave rice, corn,
eggs and chickens in the place of money."[46]

Not only were hospitals and nursing training schools new kinds of
black community institutions, but the nursing schools, in particular,
were unique and significant institutions through which thousands of
black women passed on their journey toward professional careers. Each
institution possessed a rigid internal hierarchical structure. Hospital administrators were almost exclusively male, and the superintendent of
nurses was, with rare exception in the early decades, if not male then
certainly white. Only the student body comprised young black women.
These women ranged in age from eighteen to thirty-five. Administrators
generally preferred the younger women because of the severe and often
excessive work loads, which required tremendous stamina, and the train-

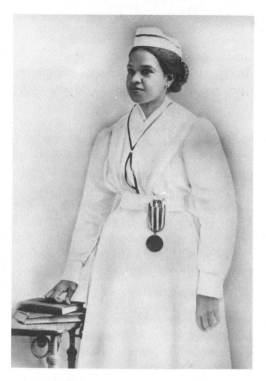

Anna De Costa Banks (1869–1930) received her diploma in 1893 from the Hampton Training School for Nurses. She served as the superintendent of nurses at the Charleston Hospital and Training School, worked as a public-health nurse for the Ladies' Beneficial Society of Charleston, and acted as a Collector for black policyholders for the Metropolitan Life Insurance Company. Courtesy of the Waring Historical Library, Medical University of South Carolina.

ing-school culture, which mandated blind, unquestioning obedience. Older women were deemed too unyielding and thus difficult to discipline. Regardless of the quality of instruction or the status of the institution, students enrolled in these enclosed worlds shared the common experience of nurses' distinctive training. Their experiences within the schools undoubtedly shaped their professional aspirations, racial and political ideologies, and personal identities, and their relationship to the work they would perform in the black and white communities upon receipt of the diploma and white cap.

After graduation, many of the nursing students lived in close proximity to the schools for varying lengths of time. Friendships forged during their apprenticeships, initiations, and training often lasted a lifetime. The training experience was a period during which they had looked out for each other, had shared frustrations and exhaustion, and had frequently conspired to escape the ever-vigilant eye of the supervisors to win moments of respite from endless toil. In order to survive the two or three years' training, they banded together and on occasion protested overly severe exploitation as they made do with insufficient supplies, inadequate food, and overcrowded shelters. In spite of it all, identification with the school and relationships with fellow alumni remained strong throughout their subsequent careers.

What these hospital training schools seemed to have imparted most effectively to their graduates was a sense of commitment to and responsibility for the black community and its health-care institutions. The nurses trained in these black community–supported schools were expected to owe primary allegiance to black people. Their work and position in the community as nurses were an extension of their place in the family. Bessie B. Hawes, a 1918 graduate of Tuskegee Institute's nursing program, wrote Kenney of her pride and elation in providing good patient care under impossible circumstances, which thus reflected well on her alma mater. As the following passage from the letter reveals, black nurses had to be resourceful, alert, fearless, and able to act autonomously if they were to render high-quality service:

> I shall tell you of an experience of which I am very proud. Eight miles from Talladega [Alabama] in the back woods, a colored family of ten were in bed and dying for the want of attention. No one would come near. I was glad of the opportunity. As I entered the little country cabin, I found the mother in bed. Three children were buried the week before. The father and the remainder of the family were running a temperature of 102–104. Some had influenza, others had pneumonia. No relatives or friends would come near. I saw at a glance I had work to do. I rolled up my sleeves and killed chickens and began to cook. I forgot I was not a cook, but I only thought of saving lives. I milked the cow, gave medicine, and did everything I could to help conditions. I worked day and night trying to save them for seven days. I had no place to sleep. In the meantime, the oldest daughter had a miscarriage and I delivered her without the aid of any physicians. I didn't realize how tired I was till I got home. I sat up at night alone, and one night with a corpse in the house. The doctor lived about twenty miles away. He came every other day. He thought I was very brave. I didn't realize till it was over just how brave I was. I did feel happy when they were out of danger. I only wished that I could have reached them earlier and been able to have done something for the poor mother.[47]

Hawes's experiences mirrored those of countless other southern black nurses who endured hours of isolated labor in backwater communities. Further, her career following the 1918 influenza epidemic demonstrates the contributions of black nurses to the general health care of their race. Born in Macon, Georgia, in the late 1890s, Bessie Hawes was graduated from Ballard Normal School before entering the John A. Andrew Hospital training school. In 1920 she entered Lincoln Hospital in New York City to take a postgraduate course in general nursing. While there she met Belle Davis, a graduate of Fisk University who then was the executive secretary of the National Health Circle for Colored People, Incorporated (a black counterpart of the American Red Cross which promoted public-health work in southern rural black communities). Davis assisted Hawes by granting her a Circle scholarship to Columbia University, where she completed a course in public-health nursing. The Circle then dispatched Hawes to Palatka, Florida, a small, isolated lumber town. On her own, Hawes had to overcome considerable opposition and fear, but she prevailed and soon proved her usefulness. She conducted a mothers' club, lectured on health issues in the local schools, visited homes of the sick, and mobilized the community to build a health center, from which she directed her work. After a few years Hawes moved on to Jacksonville, Florida, where she continued her work as a public-health nurse.[48]

Launched in response to racial segregation and the lack of professional opportunities, the black hospital and nursing-school movement of the late nineteenth and twentieth centuries was a graphic illustration of black initiative and the social-control efforts of white philanthropists. Once these new institutions were established, however, their leaders confronted the larger and more difficult challenges of maintaining an adequate financial base, providing sound training for black nursing students, and winning the confidence of the people served. Questions about the internal pressures and external forces, differences created by regional locale, and the role white philanthropists played in the growth and development of, and indeed some failures among, institutions founded in the early decades of the hospital and nursing school movement must be answered. An examination of representative hospital training schools in the South and the North during the period from 1891 to 1930 enlarges this discussion of the effect regional variation and racism had on the growth and development of black nursing.

Northern Black Hospitals
and Nurse Training Schools

2 Problems of inadequate finances, dilapidated physical plants, insufficient supplies, and exploitation of student nurses plagued both northern and southern black hospitals and nurse training schools. In this regard, regional location mattered little. All of the northern-based institutions, like their southern counterparts, suffered from a lack of a uniform or standardized instructional program. The acquisition of modern facilities and equipment and a trained staff of teaching personnel constituted the most critical challenge.

Not until the major philanthropic foundations—the General Education Board, the Rockefeller Foundation, and the Julius Rosenwald Fund— engaged in the upgrading of black hospitals and training schools would improvements occur. Their contributions, however, proved a mixed blessing. The involvement of white philanthropies in the black hospital movement of the 1920s and 1930s provoked controversy and exacerbated ideological rifts between the founders of the southern and northern institutions. Even among northern hospital founders and nursing-school administrators, the debates were heated. Some blacks argued that philanthropic largesse merely preserved and strengthened segregation. Others insisted that inasmuch as segregation existed, it was incumbent upon black leaders and professionals to create separate institutions to serve their race's needs and to accept assistance from white philanthropies whenever the opportunity arose. For the most part, southern black leaders reasoned that their fight was not against segregation, but rather it was to prevent total exclusion from nursing and medicine. Although there were exceptions, most health-care professionals in the South believed that by providing and controlling their own clinical facilities essential for development and advancement, blacks would eventually achieve integration.

At the turn of the century, three important northern black nurse-training centers existed: Daniel Hale Williams's Provident Hospital School of Nursing in Chicago (1891–1966); and in Philadelphia, the Frederick Douglass Memorial Hospital Nurse Training School (1895–1923), founded by black physician Nathan F. Mossell, and the Mercy Hospital School of Nursing (1907–1949), founded by a group of black physicians. At midcentury these two merged to become Mercy-Douglass Hospital School of Nursing (1949–1960). The third northern center consisted of the nursing schools at Lincoln Hospital (1896–1961) and Harlem Hospital (1923–1977) in New York City. An examination of the special histories of these institutions illuminates the context in which the black nursing profession emerged. Moreover, such histories demonstrate the effects of racism on the development of sites for black health care and professional training in both nursing and medicine.

Of these five northern institutions, three were basically proprietary (Provident, Douglass, and Mercy), one was sponsored by a private charity (Lincoln), and the remaining one (Harlem) was municipally controlled. The three proprietary nurse training schools were founded by black physicians and remained under black control throughout their existence. Both Lincoln and Harlem operated under white management. Only Provident experienced a tension-filled period of unsuccessful affiliation with a larger, more resourceful white institution. During the 1930s, at the behest of leaders of the Julius Rosenwald Fund, Provident Hospital and the University of Chicago experimented with the idea of turning the black institution into a teaching and training facility for black nurses and interns then enrolled at the University of Chicago.[1]

The founders of the proprietary schools came from similar backgrounds. Daniel Hale Williams, born on January 18, 1858, in Hollidaysburg, Pennsylvania, the son of Daniel and Sarah Price Williams, began his study of medicine under the tutelage of Henry Palmer in 1878 and subsequently entered the Northwestern University Medical School. After he completed his studies in 1883, he practiced medicine in Chicago. In 1884, Williams took up active surgical work in connection with the Southside Dispensary, located near the area where most of the city's black population was concentrated. A year later, he accepted an appointment as assistant physician at the Protestant Orphan Asylum and worked his way up to the position of attending physician. For four years he served as a demonstrator of anatomy at the Northwestern Medical School. In 1887 he was appointed a member of the Illinois State Board of Health. Unlike most black physicians, Williams developed an integrated practice. He is credited with, and is perhaps best known for, performing, in 1893, the first successful open-heart suture. In spite of Williams's privileged professional career, he was dismayed by the denial of nursing-training opportunities to black women. Furthermore, he disdained the common policy adhered to by white hospitals of denying staff or consulting privileges to practically all of Chicago's black physicians. His being an exception to this policy did not appease him. Most of these institutions refused even to accept black patients, unless, that is, the attending physician was white.[2]

When Emma Reynolds, the sister of a prominent black minister in Chicago, arrived in 1890 from Kansas City with hopes of attending nurse training school, she quickly discovered the doors of the existing institutions closed. Denied admission into every nursing school in the city, Reynolds spoke to her brother, who in turn sought advice and assistance from Williams. A group of black ministers, physicians, and businessmen failed in their attempts to pry open the doors of the white nursing schools. Williams appealed to the Reverend Jenkins Lloyd Jones, pastor of All Soul's Church, for aid. Jones placed the issue squarely before the members of his congregation. Fortuitously, the indefatigable black clubwoman and organizer Fannie Barrier Williams numbered among the congregation. With her usual verve, Williams, along with other black clubwomen, eventually played a major role in mobilizing community support and raising money for the establishment of a nurse training school for black women.

Actually, the black nurse Nanahyoke Sockum Curtis, who later would help to organize a small contingent of black nurses to serve during the Spanish-American War, became involved in the movement to create a new hospital and nurse training school. The wife of a young physician in the city, Curtis proved quite instrumental in piquing the interest of white businessman Philip D. Armour. Contributions from wealthy white elites and the not-inconsequential donations from blacks enabled Daniel Hale Williams, on January 22, 1891, to open the twelve-bed Provident Hospital in a two-story frame building on the corner of Twenty-ninth and Dearborn streets. To be sure, the equipment was not only meager and crude, but the building was ill suited for this new venture.[3]

Undaunted, Williams declared the primary purpose of the new institution to be the opening of "a new field for noble and useful employment for colored women who are otherwise barred from lucrative and respectable occupations." He personally selected, from 175 applicants, the first class of seven student nurses. Under Williams's direction, the hospital admitted patients of both races, and maintained an interracial staff of white consulting doctors and black attending and resident physicians.[4]

In time, Williams's insistence on an integrated institution with whites occupying key positions angered members of the black community, particularly those who believed Provident Hospital should be a completely black-controlled and -administered institution. An unyielding Williams left Provident in 1894 to launch the Freedmen's Hospital nurse training program in Washington, D.C. When he returned, years later, to Chicago, his authority at Provident had all but disappeared. In 1910 Williams resigned from Provident, and his nemesis, physician George Cleveland Hall, assumed control.

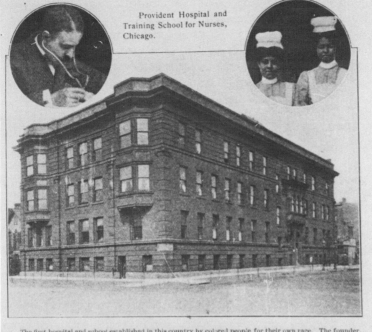

Provident Hospital and School of Nursing, on the south side of Chicago during the 1920s, was founded, in 1891, by black physician Daniel Hale Williams (*upper left corner*). It was the first such institution established by Afro-Americans. Courtesy of the Schomburg Center for Research in Black Culture, New York Public Library.

Clearly ambivalent on certain racial matters, Williams throughout the 1890s preached the need for blacks to establish separate hospitals and training schools. As long as racial discrimination and exclusion existed as the dominant fact of black life, Williams urged parallel development of health and educational institutions. Yet he also appreciated that without white financial support, many such institutions foundered. Therefore, as a racial pragmatist, he publicly embraced an integrationist posture as an essential strategy to ensure the growth and survival of Provident. Accordingly, Williams had little patience with those who argued that the existence of a reputable black facility enabled white leaders in Chicago to justify continued exclusion of blacks from all other hospitals and training schools.

Throughout Provident's formative years, donations from major white Chicago philanthropists and industrial capitalists facilitated the purchase of critical equipment and supplies and the land upon which a nurses' home was constructed. To be sure, many of the white contributors gave to the hospital out of enlightened self-interest. Among the white supporters were George M. Pullman, J. Ogden Armour, Phillip D. Armour, Marshall Field, Cyrus H. McCormick, and Potter Palmer. Some of these men gave money to Provident in order to make sure that a facility existed for the treatment of their injured black employees, especially those who worked at the stockyards and on the railways.

In a lengthy letter to William C. Graves, an officer of Sears, Roebuck and Company, attorney Robert McMurdy detailed the contributions of Chicago's white elite capitalists. According to McMurdy,

> H. H. Kohlsaat, who was a large employer of colored labor, contributed the ground upon which the present hospital stands. Mr. Armour bought the lot north of the original lot and Mr. [Nathan C.] Freer the two lots upon which the Training School and play ground for the nurses are located. . . . It was $25,000, which amount includes land and all. . . . The land and building of our present plant and properties [are worth] $100,000 of which Mr. Armour contributed about $40,000. George M. Pullman, Marshall Field, and others were among the original contributors.[5]

In spite of this support from both the white and black communities, Provident functioned always on the brink of financial collapse. Few of the patients could pay for services. The student nurses endured unending hardships. McMurdy, remarking on conditions during this early phase in Provident's history, recalled, "At one time the nurses were living on bread and molasses. Later a judgement was rendered against the hospital and the place was only saved by contributions of some white people."[6]

George Cleveland Hall, following Williams's departure to Washington, D.C., became the new chief of staff of Provident Hospital and directed its development over the next forty years. Hall had migrated to Chicago from Michigan in the 1880s. He completed his medical training at Bennett College, a school operated by the Eclectics, a somewhat questionable medical sect. Hall belonged to and supported a number of black-advancement organizations, including the National Negro Business League, the National Association for the Advancement of Colored People, and the National Urban League. He also, in 1916, joined Carter G. Woodson to found the Association for the Study of Negro Life and History.

A shrewd, ambitious man, Hall fit well into the two major ideological camps within the black community. When necessary he supported the accommodationist philosophy, accepting racial segregation as but a temporary trade-off, one of many in the continuous struggle for full equality and integration. Like Williams, Hall therefore adopted a racially pragmatic strategy. During the early 1920s he invested considerable time appealing to white philanthropists in an attempt to raise a million-dollar endowment for the hospital. Under Hall's administration, by 1928 Provident had trained 220 nurses and was moving into a new sixty-five-bed facility. Both the American College of Surgeons and the American Medical Association approved the institution as appropriate for providing internships.[7]

The Rosenwald Fund proved especially responsive to Hall's entreaties for endowment contributions. Edwin R. Embree, the new president of the fund, developed its official policy governing contributions to any black hospital and training school. He declared, "There is no crying need for additional beds for sick Negroes, but there is the greatest need for facilities by which to train nurses, internes and medical students both in Chicago and elsewhere. It is on these features that the emphasis has been placed in the hospitals aided as it must be on any others which are favorably considered by the Fund."[8]

While Embree imagined there to be little need for more hospital beds for Negroes, actual conditions at Provident Hospital and in the training school over the years revealed the opposite. Not only did demand exceed supply of beds, but the old hospital needed massive repairs and upgrading. Still, most white philanthropists were primarily interested in training the professionals. There were exceptions.

Some white benefactors threatened a discontinuation of funds as internal conditions within the hospital deteriorated. Armour and Company, for one, said that it would send its sick and injured black employees elsewhere if Provident did not improve. By 1929 even Embree asserted, "It's fair to say that the work and standards of the hospital recently are not as good as they were a decade or two ago."[9]

Most of the factors contributing to Provident's decline in the mid-twenties were beyond the control of the black physician leaders. The health-care needs of Chicago's black population had exploded in the wake of the great migrations before and after World War I. In 1900 the black population numbered 30,000, but by the mid-1930s it stood at more than 235,000, the majority living in a comparatively narrow and restricted ghetto on Chicago's south side.[10] Provident Hospital was expected somehow to provide medical care for the thousands of new black migrants. It was an unreasonable expectation.

In 1929, as the need for more beds and better clinical facilities for black health-care personnel grew more urgent, the managers of the Julius Rosenwald Fund and the General Education Board joined forces to underwrite a short-lived Provident Hospital–University of Chicago affiliation plan. The foundations promised the university $1 million toward its endowment if it would agree to "use the [Provident] hospital not only for care of the sick but also for training of nurses and interns and—most important of all—educating Negro medical students during the latter two years of their courses."[11] Provident was assured a new physical plant. The Rosenwald Fund and other donors agreed to contribute $750,000 toward the $1.5 million desired in order to rebuild and maintain the hospital. The university was attracted to the proposed affiliation because it offered a reasonable solution to the problem of providing black medical students with the clinical experience required but denied to them in the university's white clinic.

Rosenwald reassured Frank Billings, former president of the American Medical Association, that "Provident as a teaching hospital under university auspices will mean much for Negro health by offering the highest type of training to colored medical students and physicians and to interns and nurses."[12] Shortly after the agreement was sealed, University of Chicago Medical School dean Basil C. H. Harvey with smug satisfaction announced to the 1930 meeting of the American Medical Association:

> As a result of certain plans now materializing at Chicago, we can continue to admit capable and carefully selected colored students and to give them every facility and opportunity available to any students in the first two years. And we can do it hereafter with more satisfaction than heretofore, because we have had to tell such students in the past that we would be unable to give them adequate training in the third and fourth years, and have had to advise them to seek their clinical training elsewhere. . . . it is a great satisfaction to me to be able to announce on behalf of the University of Chicago that hereafter they can look forward to unrestricted opportunity within the university in the work of the third, fourth and fifth years.[13]

According to the agreement plan, Provident officials had only to maintain a 100-bed facility, an outpatient department, and the nursing school. Most important, they agreed to raise and maintain an endowment of not less than $400,000. Adopting the slogan "Germs Have No Color Line," the Provident leaders launched a major fundraising campaign. Because of the advent of the Great Depression, the fundraising proved only a partial success.[14]

In May 1933, Provident Hospital moved into remodeled larger facilities at Fifty-first Street and Washington Park. The building previously had been the site of the old Chicago Lying-in Hospital. It cost $1,322,785 for Provident officials to refurbish the place. Meanwhile, under the shadow of the Great Depression, the fundraisers continued to encounter great difficulties in collecting on pledges. More portentous, however, was the rise of antisegregation sentiment in the black community.

Members of the black medical community became increasingly disenchanted with the Provident–University of Chicago affiliation. The university's willingness to send its black medical students to Provident was seen by some black Chicagoans as blatant acquiescence to segregation and racial discrimination. For black people themselves to establish separate institutions meant one thing, an adjustment to racial discrimination, and could not be construed an endorsement of the same. When whites, however, arranged and supported separate facilities for blacks, then this was an entirely different matter, one which engendered heated reactions and occasioned much black disquiet. The black membership of the Cook County Physician's Association, on December 17, 1934, publicly protested the affiliation arrangement:

> We are opposed to and hereby make protest against any act or acts on the part of Provident Hospital or the University of Chicago or both of them that will set up or tend to set up at Provident Hospital a segregated unit of the University of Chicago for the clinical training of Negro medical students of the Medical School of the University of Chicago.[15]

The black medical profession, especially northern urban practitioners, seemingly spoke with one voice denouncing the Provident–University of Chicago–Rosenwald Fund experiment. Black physicians of the Manhattan Medical Society in New York authorized the executive committee to draft and distribute a protest letter which appeared in black newspapers across the country. In it they called for Dean Harvey's dismissal and pointedly criticized the Rosenwald Fund.

Turning to the University of Chicago, the Manhattan physicians charged, "In failing to assure him [the Negro student] justice after accepting him the University is akin to the sheriff who tacitly turns his Negro prisoner over to the mob for the exercise of the lynch law."[16] They asserted, "The Negro citizen, for his own advancement, needs no separate institutions. What the Negro physician needs is equal opportunity for training and practice, no more, no less."[17] More pointedly, they declared, "We maintain that a 'Jim Crow' set-up per se produces a sense of servility, suppresses imagination, and creates artificial and dishonest standards. We submit also that the Julius Rosenwald Fund has contributed in no small way to this unsatisfactory state of affairs."[18]

By 1939 the rising racial tensions and growing discord between the leaders of Provident and the University of Chicago convinced General Education Board officers that the experiment had failed. It was clearly time to cut their losses and retreat. Questions of quality notwithstanding, repercussions of this errant experiment and the concomitant controversy for a long time made it difficult for Provident to fill available internship slots with black graduates of Meharry and Howard medical schools. On the other hand, perhaps not all was lost, for at least one philanthropic officer, Robert Lambert, learned a valuable lesson about the limits of foundation power. He observed, "It has again demonstrated the fact that while backward or underprivileged people may want material help, they do not always welcome guidance and direction." But then Lambert went on to suggest that "to have converted Provident into a first-rate teaching

hospital would have required as heads of the major services able white
men, there being no negroes with the necessary qualifications."[19] Obviously, Lambert's education remained incomplete. Of course qualified
black physicians existed. More to the point, they were perhaps unwilling
to join this doomed experiment.

By the 1940s all ties between Provident and Chicago were severed. In
a fairly reasoned assessment of the several factors contributing to this
"progressive disappointment and defeat," the president of the General
Education Board, Raymond B. Fosdick, in a postmortem concluded, "The
faculty of the medical school of the University of Chicago seemed to show
little interest in the project; some elements in the Chicago Negro community saw in the plan an attempt to foster segregation; the Negro management of Provident Hospital was unquestionably inefficient."[20]

While the black male physician founders and leaders debated with
white philanthropists on the efficacy of integration versus segregation,
Provident's training school continued for two more decades to attract and
train black nurses. These graduates became prominent members of their
profession. Several of them became head nurses and superintendents of
the numerous small black hospitals and nursing schools sprouting up
across the South. Others served as leaders of the struggling black nurses'
professional organization, the National Association of Colored Graduate
Nurses, while some distinguished themselves in public-health nursing in
the northern cities, where they had access to employment opportunities
in settlement houses and at municipal departments of health.

The policies and practices of institutionalized racial exclusion of blacks
from nurse training that motivated Williams to found Provident similarly inspired Nathan Francis Mossell of Philadelphia. Born in Hamilton,
Ontario, Canada, on July 27, 1856, Mossell was the son of Aaron and
Eliza Bowers Mossell, free black natives of Baltimore who migrated to
Ontario to establish a brick-manufacturing business. Young Mossell received his A.B. degree from Lincoln University in 1879 and went on to
attend the University of Pennsylvania Medical School. He pursued postgraduate work at Guy's and St. Thomas's hospitals in London.

A proud man, Mossell chafed under the denial of hospital privileges to
black physicians in Philadelphia. He issued a call to his medical colleagues and to several of the city's leading black ministers and businessmen to join him on June 25, 1895, to discuss launching a separate hospital where black doctors could enjoy staff, consulting, and admitting
privileges, black patients could receive care, and black women could
enter nursing training. At the meeting, leaders of black Philadelphia
vented their concern and disgust with the inadequacies of health care and
the lack of suitable opportunities for the development of black professionals.

With alacrity, Mossell and his supporters rented a three-story house, and on October 31, 1895, opened the Frederick Douglass Memorial Hospital and Nurse Training School. After a long but ultimately successful fundraising drive in 1908, a new Douglass Hospital costing $118,000 opened at 1512 Lombard Street.[21]

Mossell insisted from the outset that Douglass adhere to a color-blind policy of open patient admission. He declared, "Maintenance of such an institution teaches the lesson of self-help in the care of our own sick, yet no one is excluded because of race or color." The open-door policy no doubt enabled Mossell to secure an annual appropriation of $6,000 from the state. In actuality, nearly all of the facility's patients were black. As to the composition of the staff, Mossell proudly proclaimed that "leading white and colored physicians are on the staff of the hospital both as active and consulting members."[22]

Mossell hired Minnie Clemens, a graduate of the University of Pennsylvania, as head nurse and matron. By the second year, 1896, the school had five women enrolled. As with any new hospital and training-school venture, more attention was paid to basic survival issues than to providing substantial instruction. Of course, the student nurses constituted an indispensable, loyal, and obedient unpaid labor force. Without their services the whole undertaking would have collapsed. Each student was required to complete courses in massage and "invalid cooking" before graduation. Meanwhile the hospital had use of their cooking services. During its thirty-two years of existence, 1895 to 1927, the Douglass training school produced approximately two hundred nurses. In 1927 a new nursing home was constructed.[23]

Although it received some state aid, Mossell's Douglass depended heavily—perhaps even more than Williams's Provident—upon the generosity of black citizens to pay essential operating expenses. Black community women played a leading role in providing the resources the hospital needed. Indeed, in order to procure enough funds to purchase linen, foods, equipment, and supplies and to repair a dilapidated physical plant, Mossell's wife organized three separate women's groups. The Douglass Ladies' Auxiliaries #1, #2, and #3 engaged in numerous imaginative community fundraising drives. In addition to raising money, they sponsored cultural and social events to help strengthen relations between the institution and the city's black population.

During one fundraising drive, in 1905, an elderly black woman, unable to contribute money, simply gave what she could, "a mince pie, 1 leg of lamb, 3 cakes of hard soap, and 4 pounds of grits." Fortunately there were other residents in the community capable of giving cash! During the first year, $4,656.31 was raised, of which white Philadelphians contributed less than $700. But even this amount, regardless of how much it was appreciated, failed to meet operating costs.

Douglass officials occasionally admitted embarrassment over the defi-

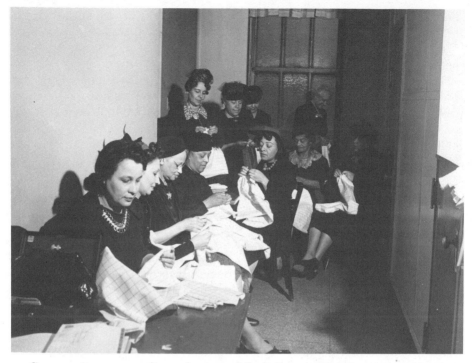

Community women often volunteered their time and services to provide essentials for the hospitals. These women were members of a sewing group making linens for Provident Hospital in Chicago. Courtesy of the Library of Congress.

ciencies of the physical plant and the heavy burden of upkeep thus placed on the student nurses, who were expected to create an atmosphere of order and efficiency. Yet even the student nurses proved incapable of performing some miracles. They could not overcome the structural inadequacies of the old building. Nor could they camouflage the fact that the hospital was inconveniently located and that the basement in which the outpatient department was operated was dark and poorly ventilated, reached only by a narrow, steep stairway.[24]

It was only a matter of time before the chronic shortage of supplies, the deteriorating facilities, and Mossell's increasingly autocratic administrative style provoked mutiny among the junior staff physicians. As early as 1905, dissident doctors, led by E. C. Howard, began publicly to criticize Mossell, charging him with being limited and reactionary. Apparently Mossell had denied, and perhaps too frequently, younger physicians the opportunity to perform certain operations in the hospital. He, after all, was the head of the enterprise and enjoyed enormous prestige and public esteem for his skill as a surgeon and founder of the much-needed institution. Soon the criticism and disaffection reached the boiling point.

Following months of simmering controversy, in September 1905 the board of directors of Douglass Hospital temporarily ousted Mossell and named E. C. Howard the new director. Leading the oust-Mossell movement was Dr. Eugene Theodore Hinson, born in Philadelphia in 1873. Hinson was educated at the Institute for Colored Youth, a Quaker institution, and in 1898 was graduated with honors from the University of Pennsylvania School of Medicine. He served as a member of the board at Douglass from 1900 to 1905.

Mossell's fall from the throne proved short-lived. A wily and adept political manipulator, he quickly marshaled his supporters, and within one month the board reinstated him. The reason given for the reinstatement was that the previous action had been illegal. In short, the board maintained that when the vote was taken to oust Mossell, several members had not been notified of the called meeting. Thus when the new vote was taken, the majority of the board members clearly favored his reinstatement.[25]

Frustrated in his efforts to remove Mossell, and perhaps desiring to further his own ambition, Hinson resigned from the Douglass board. The question he posed to his supporters presaged his subsequent actions. Could black Philadelphia support two hospitals and nurse training schools? Actually the question was rhetorical. After great effort Hinson and a group of like-minded physicians, equally as frustrated with the autocratic Mossell, purchased for $9,900 a private home on the corner of Seventeenth and Fitzwater streets and opened the Mercy Hospital and nurse training school. Fifteen of the twenty-four practicing physicians in Philadelphia participated in this "progressive venture," as it was called.

The first year of operation found Mercy experiencing many of the same problems which plagued the other black hospitals of this era. As one observer noted, "During the first years, there was a shortage of supplies, and on many occasions there were no sheets in the closets. Often there was no money to pay the hospital employees, and several notes fell due with no money to meet them, or even to pay the interest on them."[26]

Within a decade of the founding of Douglass and Mercy, relations between their administrators grew less tense. Of course, the fragile veneer of harmony and peaceful coexistence was easily shattered, especially during competitive fundraising drives. As was often the case with these types of institutions, raising money with which to construct new buildings proved easier than securing funds to upgrade the actual quality of health-care delivery and nursing education. In 1912, Mercy's board purchased the former Episcopal Divinity School, built in 1881, for $125,000 and converted it into a new 100-bed hospital. The conversion took several years, and in 1919 the group moved into its new quarters. Over a period of several years thereafter, Mercy collected enough money to build a $100,000 nursing residence adjacent to the hospital.

The black press, always a useful and potent ally in fundraising, became even more involved in the ideological controversies of northern black hospital administrators and physicians. Through the press, the hospital officials communicated their needs and accomplishments to the black community. During the 1930s, when some race leaders questioned the wisdom of maintaining poor black institutions, the black press provided a forum for the ensuing debates.

At least one publication, the NAACP's *Crisis*, expressed some ambivalence on this critical issue. In one *Crisis* editorial, editor W. E. B. Du Bois made it clear that white racism had caused the black hospital dilemma in Philadelphia. "Negroes are not primarily responsible for the existence of Mercy or Douglass Hospital," he declared. Du Bois then pointed out that "the Philadelphia General Hospital, a city-owned institution, does not train Negro nurses nor Negro physicians."[27] Yet the *Crisis* editor recognized the need for developing separate hospitals and nursing schools, deeming it "wise counsel and wise leadership for Negroes to develop their own hospitals, and theatres, and other social and welfare enterprises, just as they have successfully developed and maintained their own churches."[28] Du Bois declared, "When white people close the doors of every hospital to Negro nurses and physicians there isn't anything left for them to do but establish hospitals of their own. It certainly does not prove that they want to be segregated."[29]

Whether they embraced or objected to segregation, black and white Philadelphians were being asked to support two qualitatively different hospitals and training schools. In 1929 the Pennsylvania State Accreditation Board dropped Douglass from its list of approved institutions. Dr. Haven Emerson's 1928 survey revealed the extent of the hospital's desperate straits. Not only were medical supplies inadequate, but "electric lights were turned off in wards unless nurses or doctors were caring for patients, and only the gifts of some canned or other food stuffs had provided a small reserve for immediate use."[30]

Another factor aggravating the institution's financial woes was Mossell's refusal to allow the black students at Philadelphia's white medical schools to serve their internships at Douglass. He justified this position on the grounds that to accommodate these interns implied acceptance of racial segregation and took the pressure off the white medical schools to provide equal training to the few black students enrolled. Mossell resisted turning Douglass into the black dumping ground for white schools even better equipped to train all of their students but unwilling to provide the same training to blacks. Of course, perhaps he also feared loss of control and a lessening of his autonomy over the hospital. His intransigence on this issue contributed to Douglass's loss of financial support from the Philadelphia Federation of Charities.[31]

Mercy Hospital fared slightly better under the able leadership of Henry McKee Minton. Born in 1870 in Columbia, South Carolina, Minton, the grandson of a wealthy Philadelphia restaurateur and caterer, was graduated from Phillips Exeter Academy in New Hampshire in 1891. After a year of law study at the University of Pennsylvania, he transferred to the Philadelphia College of Pharmacy, earning a Ph.D. degree in 1895. For the next seven years he operated the first black drug store in Philadelphia before entering Jefferson Medical College, from which he received the M.D. degree in 1906. Minton served as the first pharmacist for Douglass Hospital and eventually became the secretary of its board of directors. He did not become affiliated with Mercy until 1920, when Dr. Eugene Hinson recommended him for the position of superintendent of the hospital. Three years later he organized Mercy's first social-service department in an effort to address more effectively the health needs of the growing black community.[32]

An adept fundraiser, Minton correctly understood that the officers of the major philanthropic foundations were most interested in providing training to black health-care professionals. Minton appears to have seen little contradiction between his dreams for Mercy and the white foundations' emphases. A strong, educationally sound nursing program would strengthen the hospital. Thus, he expended considerable effort upgrading the nursing training program at Mercy. He raised admission requirements and increased the enrollment. In 1930 a new modern nursing school costing $100,000 was constructed with aid received from white philanthropists, especially the Julius Rosenwald Fund.

Minton's agreeable personality was his most valuable asset in dealing with the philanthropists. Edwin R. Embree described him as "a splendid person" who possessed "high ideals." Embree added, perhaps in a thinly veiled comparison with Mossell, that Minton was "remarkably free from selfish motives and from personal ambition."[33] Equally as important, in contrast to Mossell, Minton welcomed the opportunity to train black interns at Mercy. He willingly accepted Rosenwald largesse, even though other black physicians asserted that "in the North the Julius Rosenwald Fund had stimulated the segregation of Negroes particularly with respect to health and education."[34]

During the Depression, conditions steadily deteriorated at both Douglass and Mercy. By 1939 influential white and black citizens, long since impatient with the tensions and endless competition for funds, complained that something had to be done to effect a merger. Predictably, the rising pressure for consolidation aroused fear and suspicion among those black professionals with vested interests in preserving the auton-

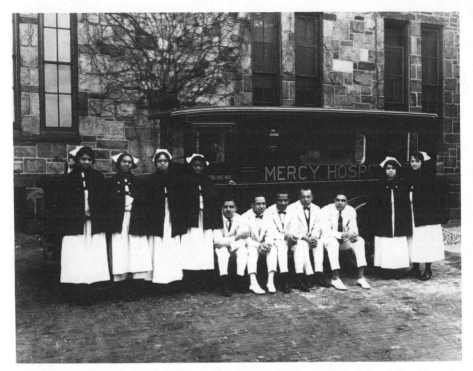

Nurses and house staff of Mercy Hospital. Collection of the Mercy-Douglass
Alumnae Association. Courtesy of the Center for the Study of the History
of Nursing, University of Pennsylvania.

omy and distinct identity of each hospital and nursing school. The decade-
old schisms proved difficult to mend. When the Douglass staff came
around to approving the merger and key administrators threw their support behind the idea, the Mercy camp objected.

The Mercy board of directors resisted the proposed merger, deeming
Douglass an inferior institution. They argued that the hospital lacked
certification by the major professional nursing and medical agencies, including the American Medical Association and the Pennsylvania State
Board of Medical Education and Licensure. To be sure, the Douglass
camp did not deny the hospital's low standing in the nursing and medical
communities. Rather, Douglass officials countered that the health-care
needs of the black population would be better served by one strong, well-
equipped, and generously supported hospital. In 1947, both boards, after
considerable discussion and study, agreed to implement the recommendations of a special investigation committee composed of representatives
from Mercy and Douglass and from the city's Community Chest. The
committee's findings and recommendations created some alarm.[35]

Not surprisingly, the committee recommended that the two hospitals and training schools merge. By this point no one objected to this idea. Black physicians, however, took issue with the suggestion that the single institution thus created should affiliate with the white medical schools in the city. Perhaps it was the wording of the resolution which triggered the ensuing outcry. On the other hand, the sentiments articulated by Mossell years before may have resonated much deeper among black medical men in the City of Brotherly Love than first imagined. In any event, the offending resolution suggested that

> the merged institution should consummate an arrangement with the University of Pennsylvania, Temple University, and Jefferson Medical College and Hospital (or the hospital conducted by them) under which these three medical training centers of Philadelphia through a board of medical consultants will have such control of the administration and staff and give such technical and training assistance in the hospital as may be necessary to assure the accomplishment of the objectives.[36]

Once the offending resolution was scrapped, the leaders of the institutions agreed to the merger. A newly constituted board then commenced to work on raising funds for the construction of a new, larger, 200- to 250-bed Mercy-Douglass Hospital. In 1948 Dr. Wilbur H. Strickland was named the first medical director of Mercy-Douglass, the position he had held at Douglass.

The consolidated board established a committee charged with the responsibility of selecting only the most capable young women for admission to the nursing school. By June 1949, thirty-seven students had been admitted to Mercy-Douglass. Although Strickland occupied the top position only one year, he introduced innovative and progressive measures such as the establishment of a minimum wage and the adoption of higher academic standards in the nursing school. On October 1, 1949, Russell F. Minton, a nephew of Henry M. Minton, was appointed superintendent and medical director. On February 28, 1954, the old Mercy-Douglass Hospital was closed to make way for a new hospital. The school of nursing continued training black women for twelve years. In 1966 white nursing schools in Pennsylvania lifted the racial bar.[37]

Of all the early black nursing institutions, Lincoln Hospital in New York, founded in 1839 by a charitable society of wealthy white women, was deemed superior by managers of philanthropic foundations and by many black nurses themselves. The school had the highest student enrollment and possessed the largest endowment of any of its sister institutions. The fact that Lincoln operated entirely under white management perhaps also influenced the perception of its excellence. Lincoln originated out of the work of the Society for the Relief of Worthy, Aged, Indigent Colored Persons, which had organized a fundraising drive to pay for the construction of a home to alleviate the destitution and suffering of escaped slaves living in New York City. Between 1845 and 1884 the Colored Home and Hospital, as it became known, provided care for over twenty thousands blacks. Support for the institution came from private donations, subscriptions, and bequests, and from the Alms House Department of the city. In 1897 the board of trustees of the Colored Home decided that the time had come to add a nursing training school in order to provide a steady source of students to care for the sick residents of the facility. The board also moved to develop an adjacent hospital to serve the white community of the Bronx. All administrative officers of this combination home, hospital, and nursing school remained white. Only black women were admitted into the training program.[38]

In May 1898 the first class of six student nurses entered the Lincoln Hospital school. In September the Colored Home moved into more substantial quarters at East 141st Street and Southern Boulevard in the Bronx. One of the early graduates of the nursing school, Adah B. Thoms, in describing the physical plant of the hospital section, wrote,

> The buildings were plain but substantial, thoroughly modern and sanitary. A separate building for tuberculosis patients and another for maternity pa-

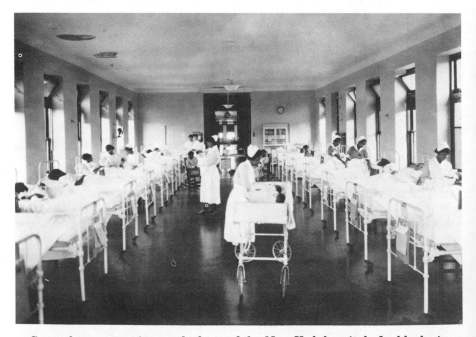

Scene from maternity ward of one of the New York hospitals for blacks in the early twentieth century. Courtesy of the Schomburg Center for Research in Black Culture, New York Public Library.

tients connected with the main building by a covered corridor, an isolated cottage for contagious diseases, a laundry, a power house, and a laboratory and morgue completed the new, yet old, institution. In 1902 the institution was renamed the Lincoln Hospital and Home, School of Nursing. By 1924 the Lincoln Hospital had an endowment of $1,000,000 and the plant site was valued at a half-million dollars.[39]

Lincoln, soon to be the largest black nursing school in the country, grew from the 6 members in the first class into a 134-member student body by 1924. The students provided all of the nursing care both for the home and in the hospital. Thoms recalled her training experiences at Lincoln: "The work was very exacting, there were many duties for the nurses other than caring for the sick patients." She continued, "Most of the classes were conducted in the evenings with a group of tired nurses. A few lectures by the attending physicians and surgeons were given in the afternoon to the senior class, which meant that those nurses had to remain on duty late at night to finish up the work of the day, to write their reports, and relieve the night nurses for classes."[40]

In response to repeated appeals for financial assistance, in 1924 Rockefeller Foundation officers visited and inspected the training school. Edwin R. Embree and Richard Pearce described Lincoln as an "excellent school, probably the best in the country for negro nurses." They noted, "The requirement of high school graduation and other high standards resulted in a picked group of pupils of unusual quality."[41] The Rockefeller Foundation officers approved making small appropriations to Lincoln but rejected requests for substantial funds to repair and remodel the facilities. The student nurses lived in the hospital building in large common dormitories which were formerly wards of the Old Folks' Home. During the course of their inspection the officers noted that "the living quarters are entirely inadequate, no provisions for individual privacy, little opportunity for reading or study; fair light and ventilation."[42] Embree proposed to the board of trustees that Lincoln be closed and its nursing-school operation be transferred to Harlem Hospital, with its newer and superior facilities. He asked, perhaps rhetorically, "Might it be feasible to establish the Lincoln School of Nursing at Harlem Hospital, the trustees of the Lincoln Hospital and the present funds maintaining the home and being responsible for the educational features and general training of pupil nurses?"[43]

The Harlem Hospital School of Nursing, with which Embree appeared to have been so impressed, had opened on January 3, 1923, following years of protest and fighting with black health-care professionals. Black physicians had organized into the North Harlem Medical Association and joined forces with the NAACP to protest racial discrimination and especially Harlem's hiring policies. Harlem Hospital had originated out of the

Harlem Dispensary, founded in 1868 as the first organized effort to provide medical care for the Harlem region's poor. In 1887 the dispensary gave way to Harlem Hospital, a twenty-bed municipal institution occupying a rented three-story wooden building on 120th Street and the East River. Increased patient demand soon overtaxed the resources of the facility, and in 1902 the hospital was placed under the administrative direction of Bellevue and Allied hospitals. A new building was constructed in 1907 with a bed capacity of 150.

By 1910 the area's racial complexion had changed from white to predominantly black, and the black patient load at Harlem Hospital soon exceeded 50 percent. An adjacent wing, expanding the bed capacity to 390, was added in 1915. Prior to 1923, most nursing services at Harlem were provided by white nurses. After the black patient population grew to dominate the facility and in the wake of rising racial tension and controversy, the white nurses were transferred to other municipal institutions. To staff the hospital and to ameliorate racial animosities, Harlem became an essentially all-black nursing school. In the 1924 class there were thirty-eight regular pupil nurses, twelve probationers, and approximately twenty-five black graduate nurses. Administrative control of the hospital and the school remained firmly in white hands.[44]

Controversy continued to plague Harlem Hospital's nursing school during the 1920s. Its transformation into an all-black school resulted in a host of new problems concerning the treatment student nurses received from white administrators and white physicians. At least one of the early black nursing students at Harlem, Birdie E. Brown, although aware of the difficulties, nevertheless managed to develop a positive perspective on her training. She confided in her autobiography, "In all activities, I was always mindful of learning all that I could and utilizing that knowledge whenever needed. Rendering a needed service to mankind in the best possible manner was my aim. There were days when I wondered if this aim was not more than I could hope for.... I weathered the storm."[45]

One black physician, Aubre de L. Maynard, offers a more critical and specific commentary on the difficulties student nurses endured. Maynard reported that "all was not sweetness and light for the girls enrolled in the early period of the school." He described incidents and practices that "sullied the professional atmosphere and wounded the sensibilities of the defenseless girls." According to Maynard, "When a nurse was ill, particularly if she complained of an abdominal pain, she was first seen by a house officer, who subjected the young girl to a pelvic examination, whether or not it was necessary." In every case a smear was taken from the urethra, vagina, and cervix, "with the implication that, as a black girl, she was likely to have a gonorrheal infection." In Maynard's opinion such pelvic examinations were rarely justified. He added, "Even if they were, professional consideration and discretion should have dictated that these procedures be carried out by a mature attending physician and not by a young house doctor in training, with whom the young nurse would have to work in a close relationship."[46]

It is uncertain whether the Lincoln officials knew of the internal personnel problems and tensions at Harlem Hospital. Regardless, the Lincoln board refused to consider affiliation and consolidation with Harlem and relinquish institutional autonomy. The women managers were not without an array of social, political, and financial contacts. They explored other avenues for funding, while Embree, having second thoughts, relented, intimating that the possibility of a small Rockefeller contribution would be considered if Lincoln could be placed in good financial shape "with reasonable expectation of self-support in the future."[47] Privately, Embree doubted that Lincoln would survive. He was proved wrong.

The white female board members of Lincoln Hospital exploited their contacts with political leaders in New York City and worked out an arrangement which saved the school. In 1925 the city agreed to assume responsibility for the school and the hospital, and for the selection of the student nurses. It then purchased the hospital buildings for $750,000, and appointed a joint committee to study ways to improve the nursing school. The board and city officials argued that the Lincoln board of managers should retain control over the school's endowment. Unlike other black nursing schools in the country, Lincoln maintained a separate budget, apart from the hospital budget. That guaranteed the school a measure of independence from the hospital and enhanced the quality of training provided the student nurses by reducing their exploitation as an essentially unpaid labor force. The pupil nurses received their practical experience in the wards of Lincoln Hospital under supervision of a large graduate nursing staff.[48]

By the mid-twenties, black women in New York had the choice of attending one of two nursing schools, Lincoln and Harlem. Although both schools remained under white supervision for several more years, in 1929 Adah Thoms became the first black assistant superintendent of nurses at Lincoln Hospital. In 1945 Alida Cooley Daily, a 1927 graduate of the Harlem school who had received a Red Cross scholarship to do postgraduate study at Columbia University, was appointed the first black director of nursing and superintendent of her alma mater. Actually, she would be the first black woman to hold such a position in all of New York's municipal institutions. Daily brought to the position a wealth of nursing experience. She had worked for ten years as a public-health nurse in Montclair, New Jersey. Five years before assuming the directorship, she became an administrator at the Harlem training school. The last of the diploma nursing programs to do so, Harlem Hospital's nursing school closed its doors on July 5, 1977.[49]

The monetary contributions of northern white elites added to those of the philanthropic foundations made survival possible for most of the major black hospital complexes. The black communities, however, with fewer economic resources but with great determination and committed leaders, bore the responsibility to develop and improve these centers. Without this frequently uneasy and often hostile collaboration between the two groups, black men and women would have had scant access to medical and nursing-training opportunities, and the deplorable health status of many inner-city ghetto residents would have been even worse.

Black leaders never spoke with one voice on the two most important health-care and -training issues of the pre–World War II era. Virtually all of them conceded that integration into the mainstream of American society was blacks' dream. Yet in the opening decades of the century this dream seemed increasingly impossible. By the mid-1930s many blacks, including W. E. B. Du Bois, wanted to give up the elusive quest for integration and instead concentrate more fully on the development of separate black institutions. But to follow this course risked the entrenchment of health-care ghettos and further isolation of black doctors and nurses. This was the crux of the black professional's dilemma.

Some of the physician founders of black hospitals astutely perceived the dangers of all deliberate and even unwitting attempts to create segregated medical ghettos. But were they not themselves engaged in doing what they criticized the philanthropists for? Others, perhaps more pragmatic in outlook, deemed resistance to white philanthropic intervention in the development and maintenance of black hospitals and training schools foolhardy at best. Black people, they correctly reasoned, had not created segregation. Thus the challenge was how best to provide and obtain the health-care education and services for their racial group. If survival and opportunity within a segregated setting meant accepting white philanthropic support, then so be it.

The development of black nursing training in the North is inseparable from the vacillating fortunes of the key hospitals, and the ideological and political disputes of the physicians and administrative overseers. Actually, concentration on these disputes and on the institutional histories of the hospitals threatened to overshadow the steady growth and development of black nursing during the first several decades of the twentieth century. A closer look at the inner workings of nursing training offered at a select number of black hospitals located in the South provides the balance that is often difficult to obtain in the writing of nursing history.

Training Nurses
in Southern Black Hospitals

3 Nowhere in America was there a greater need for the development of black hospitals and nursing training schools than in the South. Yet this region, given its poverty, its racism, and its large black population, offered little chance for the emergence and survival of first-rate black health-care educational institutions. In spite of virtually insurmountable difficulties, however, dozens of such establishments appeared in the period between 1890 and 1930. Writing in 1894, black physician Daniel Hale Williams resolutely proclaimed that "race prejudice in this country is . . . so unrelenting, that our only hope for the next twenty or thirty years . . . is to make opportunities for ourselves by establishing hospitals and training schools."[1] Five of the more resilient of the southern black institutions were Tuskegee Institute's John A. Andrew Hospital (1892–1948), headed by black physician John Kenney; the Hospital and Training School for Nurses in Charleston, South Carolina, founded by Alonzo C. McClennan (1896–1959); the Freedmen's Hospital and Nursing School (1894–1973) in Washington, D.C., founded by Daniel Hale Williams, who had also been responsible for the founding of Provident Hospital School of Nursing in Chicago (1891–1966); the Flint-Goodridge Hospital School of Nursing (originally the Phillis Wheatley Sanitarium and Training School for Nurses in New Orleans (1896–1934); and the Dixie Hospital Training School (1891–1956), soon affiliated with Hampton Institute in Hampton, Virginia.[2]

The founders and administrators of these institutions waged a relentless, often heroic struggle to secure the requisite funds, win community confidence and support, and attract capable young black women into the training programs. While an examination of the internal conditions of these five institutions illuminates the general nature of the training experience, it also provides a glimpse of the range of responsibilities and challenges, and the often exploitative use of the labors, of student nurses. Moreover, it clarifies the relations forged between black health-care

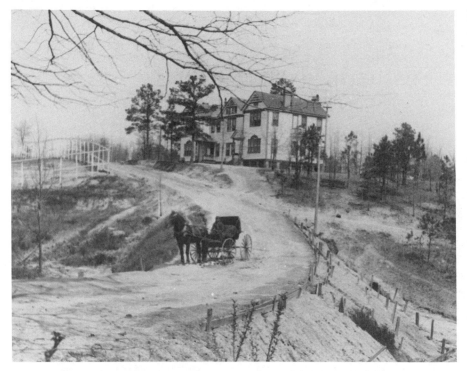

First hospital on campus of Tuskegee Institute. Circa 1895. Courtesy of Tuskegee University Archives.

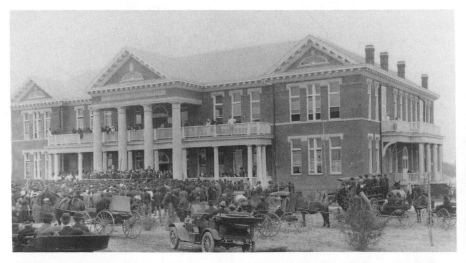

Dedication of the John A. Andrew Hospital, February 21, 1913, on the Tuskegee Institute campus. Courtesy of Tuskegee University Archives.

professionals and the diverse community constituencies which they served.

All of the black nursing schools, whether in the North or South, had similar admission requirements. Students without high-school diplomas had to take rudimentary examinations in reading, writing, and arithmetic. Some were given tutorial courses to make up educational deficiencies. After 1909 Freedmen's nursing pupils were required to have a high-school diploma prior to admission. Married students were not admitted. While students were supposed to be no younger than eighteen or older than forty, in many instances institutional administrators, especially when confronted with a shortage of women, did admit younger women into the program. A Rockefeller Foundation investigator of black nursing schools in the early 1920s lamented that the age requirement was "more honored in the breach than in the observance." At least one employee of a state board of examiners admitted that frequently black graduate nurses applied for registration who were only eighteen, and therefore had to have been no more than fifteen or sixteen when they entered training school. On the whole, hospital administrators displayed a marked preference for younger women, deeming them easier to manage and therefore less "troublesome."[3]

Another prerequisite was that each recruit bring with her a reference letter, preferably two, one from a minister attesting to her good moral character, and the other from a physician affirming sound physical condition. There appeared to be little deviation among white and black schools insofar as this requirement was concerned. Inasmuch as tuberculosis, syphilis, and other communicable diseases were quite prevalent in the early decades of this century, black hospital administrators felt compelled to ensure that the students admitted were not so afflicted. Obviously, this precautionary measure was designed to protect the patients with whom the nurse trainees would come into contact.[4]

Throughout the training period, school administrators paid considerable attention to the student nurses' morality. In part this zealous observance was dictated by the negative perceptions of nurses rampant in the larger society. Stereotypes of nurses as being immoral and sexually promiscuous had acquired currency when hospitals and dispensaries in the early years of their development had had to rely upon untrained, uneducated, and unrefined women to supply nursing and domestic services. At least one prominent late-nineteenth-century white physician and hospital administrator had addressed the issue head-on. John Shaw Billings, of the United States Army Medical Corps, in remarking on the folklore surrounding the nurse's sexual mores, declared, "If a female nurse is a properly organized and healthy woman, she will certainly at times be subject to strong temptation under which occasionally one will fall, and this occurs in all hospitals in which women are employed without any exception whatever."[5]

Superimposed on these negative images of nurses were the widely held views about the alleged immorality of black women in general. Indeed it was the 1895 letter of James W. Jack, president of the Missouri Press Association, in which he had declared that "the Negroes of this country are wholly devoid of morality," and that "the women were prostitutes and all were natural thieves and liars," that had fueled the national mobilization of black women resulting in the formation of the National Association of Colored Women.[6] Black hospital administrators and head nurses therefore appeared especially determined, by the imposition of strict disciplinary rules, to protect the reputations of their students nurses and their institutions.

In 1899, black physician Alonzo C. McClennan proudly submitted in the *Hospital Herald* that "the strict discipline at the Hospital has given the friends of the institution implicit confidence in its management, and the institution has received the hearty endorsement of the Colored Ministers' Union of this city."[7] One agent of the General Education Board of the Rockefeller Foundation in a 1905 report on the Hospital in Charleston approvingly commented on McClennan's militaristic control over the students. "As to discipline Dr. McClennan is doubtless severe, but no more so, it seems to me, than he ought to be. He can hardly be too careful of the young women under his control. And the high regard in which they are held by those in position to know attests to the value of his system."[8] Apparently McClennan and other black educators believed that the severe restrictions of student rights and the strict regulation of virtually every aspect of their lives during training were a small price to pay for high community regard. It did not occur to these proponents of rigid discipline that their actions may, in fact, have fueled negative perceptions of the morality of black women.

The most decisive requirement for admission to the formal training program proved to be the successful completion of a probationary period lasting anywhere from two to six months. During this period the pupil nurse performed a variety of hospital maintenance and domestic chores under the critical and omnipotent eye of the head nurse and hospital superintendent. "It is highly desirable that every nurse have a thorough understanding of domestic duties," Flint-Goodridge authorities maintained, "for to correctly sweep a floor, make a bed or prepare a meal is as necessary as to be able to take a temperature, use a hypodermic or dress a wound."[9] According to the Tuskegee Institute catalogue, probationers had to demonstrate effective multipurpose cleaning skills, including "scrubbing, sweeping, dusting, polishing stoves, washing windows, disinfection of stools and care of vessels." This rigorous probationary period enabled the institute's resident physician and head nurse "to select for pupils only those who have the strongest physique and who have shown some special fitness for the work."[10] Or, as the Flint-Goodridge authorities put it, "much strength of body and good health, together with a patient forbearing and gentle disposition and an unquestioning obedience," were the necessary ingredients for probationary success.[11] Further, the catalogue cautioned that "anyone who does not possess these qualifications, or who is looking for and expecting an easy time should not apply."[12]

Perhaps as a direct consequence of high attrition rates, or maybe as a retention device, Dixie Hospital required that all entering students deposit upon arrival at the school "a sum sufficient for her return traveling expenses." At the end of the probationary period students received a cap, and at Dixie they were given the opportunity to sign an agreement pledging to remain for the duration of the program and to give unswerving obedience to all of the institution's authority figures.[13] The Tuskegee students pledged, after the probationary period, "to remain in this school until the course is completed and during that time to faithfully obey the rules of the school and hospital and to be subordinate to the authority governing the same." The Flint-Goodridge probationer was required to deposit ten dollars upon entering "as assurance that she intends to remain to complete the course and that she will be faithful and loyally abide and be governed by all the rules of the hospital." If the student failed, for whatever reason, to complete the course, she forfeited the ten-dollar deposit. On the other hand, if she survived, the money "minus expense of breakage" was refunded upon graduation.[14]

In two separate but related areas, housing and stipends, wide variation existed among the programs, largely reflecting their financial and spatial resources. While all institutions provided uniforms consisting of white bibbed aprons and collars worn over plain darker-hued gingham dresses and rubber-heeled shoes, few initially were able to provide adequate housing. In the early years Tuskegee student nurses lived in the dormitories with regular students. This particular living arrangement, of course, militated against close scrutiny and supervision. It also hampered the hospital's reliance upon the student nurses' services. Thus as soon as a hospital was established, the founders would launch a fundraising drive to build a separate nurses' residence on hospital grounds. Quite a few of the early black hospitals simply reserved a floor, or part of a ward, for student nurses. The provision of suitable creature comforts in these living arrangements, especially when the students lived in the hospital itself, rarely proved sufficient. Indeed at some of the poorer institutions, students even shared beds, sleeping in shifts.[15]

The institutions' diverse policies regarding the payment of stipends to student nurses revealed both economic imperatives and philosophical ambivalence about the value of the training provided and the status of

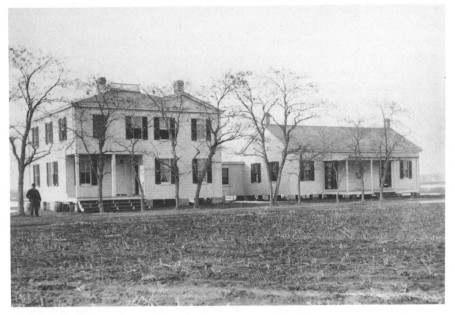

On the left is the nurses' residence, constructed in 1892, next to the Hampton Training School for Nurses, which was built in 1891. Courtesy of the Hampton University Archives, Dixie Hospital Collection.

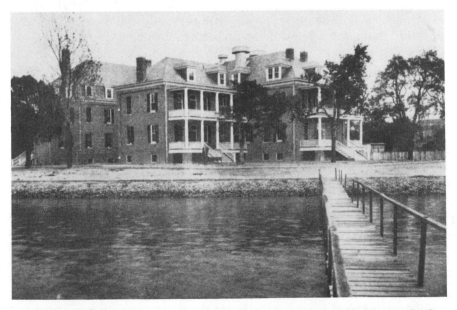

The third building to house the Hampton Training School for Nurses, built in 1913. Courtesy of the Hampton University Archives, Dixie Hospital Collection.

nursing as a profession. Many black and white hospital and training-school authorities viewed nursing as little more than vocational work, while others saw it as a developing learned profession. Medical students did not receive stipends, so why should the student nurses? they mused. Chicago's Provident Hospital did not provide its student nurses with stipends. On the other hand, Freedmen's Hospital, in the early years, paid the student seven dollars per month and furnished her with caps, uniforms, and notebooks. She was also permitted two weeks' vacation, plus one free afternoon a week and a half-day every Sunday. Dixie nurses enjoyed the same vacation time but received a stipend of only four dollars per month. In giving this sum, the school officials emphasized that "neither the allowance nor the final payment is to be regarded as wages," adding, "The education received is full equivalent for the labor given."[16] McClennan's Hospital in Charleston refused to allocate stipends. Indeed, if the superintendent of nurses had had her way, the student would have paid tuition.[17] Of course, few of McClennan's student nurses were in any position to pay fees and tuition for the privilege of attending the school and working in the hospital. The issues of stipends and housing regulations were also hotly debated within the larger nursing profession.

There was remarkable consistency in the various school catalogues' descriptions of course content and instruction. Yet these printed statements tended to be contradicted by some of the reports of investigators and the reminiscences of students and graduates. The catalogues and annual reports of Dixie, Flint-Goodridge, and McClennan's Hospital in Charleston indicated that students received lectures in anatomy, physiology, midwifery, hygiene, bandaging, and wound dressing. They were taught how to care for the patients' rooms, and were instructed in the appropriate methods of rubbing, exercising, and handling the sick. Dixie's annual catalogues contained various descriptions of the training program. In 1896, the school's fourth annual report outlined the instructional component: "The course of instruction includes recitations from text-books, and lectures and demonstrations by the Superintendent, Head Nurse, and members of the Medical Faculty. Examinations by the instructors will be given from time to time. The final test of a nurse's scholarship, however, must lie in her ability to put the instructions received into daily practice in the hospital or at outside cases."[18]

In 1902, in the eleventh annual report, the school's authorities offered further elaboration on the program. "During the course students are sent to the houses of the sick poor to learn by actual practice how to care for the sick in houses where no conveniences can be had." During the second year "the students may be called to cases of any kind at any distance from the hospital." At the end of the two-year courses students were expected to be able to work "in any department of nursing whether in hospitals, among the poor, or in private families of means."[19] The almost identical wording across the catalogues suggests some cross-fertilization. Yet it is well to remember that course catalogues, regardless of the nature of the institution, are notorious for bearing scant resemblance to what is actually taught in any given classroom.

At McClennan's Hospital students heard lectures on the practical aspects of bedside nursing, but were cautioned against overreliance on textbook learning. Black physician Lucy Brown, head of the institution's department of nursing training, advised students that a combination of textbook learning and practical experience was the recipe for success. She added, "Clean hands, well-kept nails, carefully brushed hair, sweet breath, gentle voice are some of the essentials of good nursing."[20] W. T. B. Williams, the black educator who in the 1920s would become field director of the John F. Slater Fund and the Anna T. Jeanes Fund, visited the institution in 1905 and reported to the officers of the General Education Board on conditions there. "The course extends through two years, the first being devoted to lectures and practical work in the hospital, and the second year to practical work in the hospital and to outside cases." He went on to list the textbooks used at the school: "*Practical Points in Nursing*, Emily A. M. Stoney; *Anatomy and Physiology*, Diana C. Kimber; *Surgical Nursing*, Anna M. Fullerton, M.D.; *Materia medica for Nurses*, Lavinia L. Dock; *Pocket Medical Dictionary*, George M. Gould, M.D.,"[21] These texts were the same ones used in the white schools at this time.

At Tuskegee the head nurse delivered demonstration lectures twice per week at a bedside. Second-year students cared for the medical cases, while third-year students were placed in charge of obstetrical and surgical cases in the town. Actually, Tuskegee students often spent their entire senior year assisting white physicians in the town. All fees for these services away from the hospital were paid directly to the institute.[22] Until Freedmen's adopted the three-year course in 1909, the eighteen months were usually divided into two nine-month sequences. In the first session the students served as assistants in the hospital wards, working in twelve-hour shifts. During the final nine months they served as nurses in the hospital and as private-duty nurses in the city.[23]

In reality, as far as nursing instruction was concerned, each school developed its own mix of coursework and field or practical work. Initially all programs adhered to the standard length of eighteen to twenty-four months. Of course there were exceptions, as previously noted in the case of the nursing program inaugurated at Spelman College in 1886. As early as the first decade of the twentieth century, many black nursing schools expanded their courses to three-year terms. A few did so in order to meet new basic licensing and state accreditation laws. For the most part, administrators favored the longer terms, and in many instances the reasons had little to do with accreditation and licensing. Black physician

Austin M. Curtis of Freedmen's supported the longer course. He argued, "It is now universally recognized to be desirable to extend the courses of training for pupil nurses from two to three years, in order to provide women better equipped by knowledge and experience for nursing, to secure a more efficient service to the hospital by nurses in the third year and to obliviate the breakdown of health of nurses attempting to crowd the work training into two short years."[24]

Thus, even when a training program enjoyed reasonable proximity to, if not outright affiliation with, a college, neither hospital authorities nor college administrators viewed student nurses as more than captive workers. As late as the 1930s, Nina Gage (1883–1946), a white nurse educator at Dixie, complained bitterly about the long-standing practice common to both white and black hospitals of sending unsupervised trainees out on assignment. While lucrative to the hospital, this hiring-out practice, she pointed out, endangered the health of the student nurses and the lives of the patients. She argued that the nurses developed bad habits and practiced poor techniques while engaged in this unsupervised work. Gage alleged further that an occasional student was known to extract money from patients by asking for larger fees than required and pocketing the difference. But this extortion was the least of the damage done. She maintained that too many trainees physically broke down under the strain of working often from twelve to fifteen hours without food or rest. A deeply concerned Gage elaborated on the injustice of having student nurses walk long distances back to hospitals from cases in the community, loaded down with heavy equipment bags. Gage did not doubt, and reasonably so, that these young women were in little condition to absorb classroom lectures when they were often so physically exhausted.[25]

Harsh and exacting working conditions at Tuskegee and at Freedmen's, more than anything else, tested the students' emotional resilience and physical capacity to continue in the programs, and sorely tested the depth of their love for and commitment to their chosen profession. A granddaughter of one of the members of the first nursing class at Freedmen's recalled conditions experienced by her relative: "Theirs was a life of hardship," she wrote, "long hours of toil, filling mattresses with straw, scrubbing, dusting, sweeping, chopping ice from the pails and basins, attending fires, as there was only one orderly." As if this were not bad enough, "often times the gas would freeze, they would have to warm food over the coals in the stove, by sticking a pan inside the stove." And then "she would pull her beds around the fires to keep her patients warm, when she herself would be so cold and chilled that she could hardly work."[26]

Many Tuskegee student nurses required periodic leaves of absence simply to recover from the damage done to their health while working in the hospital. Again, Tuskegee was hardly unique in this respect. What is revealing about Tuskegee, however, is that shortly after John Kenney, the superintendent of John A. Andrew, arrived on the scene, the student nurses made known their displeasure with the prevailing working conditions. They resented the interminable toil, the long hours, the stringent regulations, the constant surveillance, and most of all the exploitation inherent in the hiring-out practice.[27] Kenney's response was to suspend a few students. Others simply resigned rather than endure the conditions they complained about. But these were not satisfactory resolutions of student grievances. Nor did they help the embattled administrator who had to confront repeatedly the challenge of attracting bright, energetic, and committed young women into the nursing training program. After all, without them, the existence of the hospital stood in jeopardy.

Eventually, as the dissatisfaction of Tuskegee student nurses mounted, Kenney urged the school's executive council and Booker T. Washington to reduce demands made on the students. Specifically, he suggested relaxing the excessive scrubbing obligations. Confronted with the prospect of disruptions in hospital care caused by a student strike or walkout, the council and Washington capitulated. Kenney, in a follow-up memorandum to Washington, offered a rather subjective and perhaps self-serving explanation that "much of the unrest and instability on the part of the nurses is due to the fact that the great majority of them are not prepared for the serious study of nurses." On the other hand, Kenney remained committed to the practice of hiring out. On May 24, 1910, he informed the executive council, "We have places for several [student nurses] in the town and school community for this summer and I think that everything possible should be done to encourage the use of these girls in the homes and town rather than to place restrictions."[28]

The records are disappointingly silent concerning the extent of this student unrest. It is reasonable to assume that the students' accounts of the origins and nature of their dissatisfaction would have differed substantially from Kenney's observations. Perhaps their records would have described what was really involved in the hiring-out process, and the treatment they received in the black and white families to which they were assigned. Perhaps the accounts also would have revealed how the nurses felt about the payment to the hospital of the "one to four dollars per day" that they had earned on the outside cases.

Although students at McClennan's Hospital in Charleston probably had equally as strong reasons to protest their working conditions as the Tuskegee students, few did so, at least not in public. McClennan ran the hospital like a military outpost. He demanded total institutional loyalty from all involved in the struggling enterprise. Some members of the community, including one disgruntled black physician, criticized McClennan for his "rigid discipline of the nurses."[29] But these criticisms appeared to have mattered little. It is interesting to note, nevertheless, that in the very first issue of the institution's official newsletter, the *Hospital Herald*, McClennan made it crystal clear that it would be "injurious to the success of the work for any of its members to bring before the public any adverse criticism of its management before said criticism has been presented to the executive committee for adjustment."

Perhaps another reason for the apparent harmony and absence of disquiet at McClennan's Hospital was that prominent leaders in the black community served as members of the hospital association. Thus the hospital, in the broadest sense, was seen as a black institution created, sustained, and controlled by black medical men and women and the business elites. Again W. T. B. Williams's observations are revealing. He pointed out admiringly that "the immediate control of the property is vested in an executive committee composed of members of the corporation. It is composed of seven men, all property owners, and in several cases, substantial business men." According to Williams, of these black leaders, one was "a barber with good trade, one a boss drayman, one an insurance agent reputed 'to carry the largest book' in Charleston, and one a wholesale and retail fish and game merchant with considerable real estate holding." With obvious relish Williams concluded, "Altogether they are

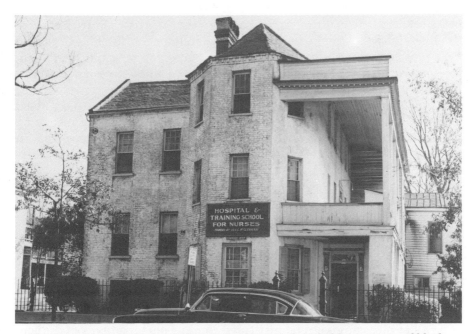

The Hospital and Training School for Nurses, founded by a group of black physicians under the leadership of Dr. Alonzo C. McClennan in 1897 in Charleston, South Carolina. Courtesy of the Waring Historical Library, Medical University of South Carolina.

well qualified for the trust in hand." One notable characteristic of an additional advisory board was its interracial makeup. Williams had noted, as if in passing, "There is also an advisory board composed of prominent white and colored citizens including white lawyers, bankers, ministers and merchants and a colored bishop."[30]

Unarguably the work load and broad responsibilities borne by McClennan's student nurses left little time for protest. As was true of virtually every southern black nursing school, the students were hired out to white and black families in Charleston and the fees collected by the hospital. But in addition to these arrangements, each group of students at the Charleston institution was encouraged to give to the school a class gift upon graduation. Moreover, all student nurses had to participate in the fundraising fairs, the chief moneymaking activity, sponsored by the hospital association. The first class of student nurses (1898) formed a club named the Gatling Guns and performed at the fairs. They perfected a dance routine which proved so successful that they were able to present to the hospital a class gift of an operating table. Subsequent classes, in addition to maintaining the hospital, caring for patients, cooking, and washing, had also to manage a poultry-farm operation and tend the vegetable gardens.[31] In spite of all their labors and sacrifices, the students could always depend on Lucy Brown to remind them that in addition to sweet breath, brushed hair, and gentle voices, all they really needed to be successful was "great adaptability, good judgement, the ability to hold one's tongue and a willingness to do work outside the usual line," and, finally, a willingness to "take for their services what their patients can afford to pay."[32]

Hiring out was much too important a component of the southern black hospitals' overall operation to be viewed as little more than a means by which student nurses were exploited. These institutions were trying, in one sense, to bear too great a responsibility for black health-care delivery, and with too few resources to accomplish it. This is not to deny that some of them were indeed managed by unscrupulous individuals more concerned with making money than training good nurses or caring for the black sick. Too many impartial observers remarked on the deplorable and exploitative conditions black student nurses endured in the weaker schools for their comments to be entirely dismissed or rationalized. As late as the 1930s, black social scientist and Fisk University educator Charles S. Johnson, after studying some of these institutions, concluded that "the conditions under which Negro nurses are trained in Negro hospitals are deplorable." In one of his many reports, Johnson recommended that "a definite campaign be instituted to have each state adopt legislation requiring hospitals to obtain a license before operating a training school for nurses."[33] Only in the 1930s and 1940s would the pressure to upgrade the quality of instruction in black nursing schools and to construct better and integrated hospitals gain momentum. Moreover, the sustained and successful attack launched by black protest organizations such as the National Association for the Advancement of Colored People and the National Medical Association against the entire edifice of separate but unequal education and segregated health-care delivery helped to pave the way for the dismantling of the network of the more impoverished hospitals and nursing schools.[34]

The organized body of the black medical establishment, the National Medical Association, became alarmed over the quality of health care provided in the smaller black hospitals and the treatment of student nurses in the 1920s. After much discussion the NMA on August 27, 1923, formed the National Hospital Association, electing black physician H. M. Green as president. Green's successful private practice and position as the assistant health officer in the Department of Public Welfare in Knoxville, Tennessee, the only black physician in the South to occupy such a position, made him a sensitive and knowledgeable student of the problems plaguing the burgeoning network of southern and northern black hospitals and nursing schools. After reviewing "the character of the actual work being done both in their training schools and practical nursing departments," Green reported that the majority of the 210 black hospitals were small ventures, seldom exceeding more than a couple dozen beds with a half-dozen or so student nurses. He concluded the obvious. The quality of training suffered in such limited settings.[35] A more comprehensive investigation sponsored by the Julius Rosenwald Fund echoed Green's observations. The Rosenwald report indicated that over 70 percent of all black hospitals by the late 1920s possessed fewer than 50 beds. All of the 210 black hospitals collectively possessed a total bed capacity of 6,870, or an average of 1 bed for each 1,941 black Americans. This compared unfavorably to the 6,807 hospitals of all kinds with a total bed capacity of 853,318, or 1 bed for each 139 of the general population. Green calculated that in 1927, "each white citizen of the United States has fourteen times as good a chance at proper hospital care as has the Negro."[36]

Discouraged by much of what he had personally observed, Green conceded that most of the small proprietary hospitals had developed nursing training schools as a means of easing economic burdens. He observed, "For economic reasons many of these small institutions operate training schools, and it is just here that the tragic side of the question presents itself—injustice to the nurse."[37] At the Hale Infirmary, founded in 1889 in Montgomery, Alabama, it was a matter of record that "the maintenance of the Institution is dependent upon a nominal charge for services and revenue derived from the nurses." One description of Hale clearly underscored the importance of the student nurses: "The nurses are trained in a three year course and during their training are frequently called upon to render service outside of the infirmary, and the revenue derived from their services is a valuable asset to the Institution."[38] Green concluded, "With limited bed space and a small variety of cases in such hospitals, the lack of opportunity for well-rounded, practical training is apparent."[39] But perhaps his conclusions are a bit too bleak and critical.

That southern black hospital administrators required student nurses to work outside of the hospital on private cases as part of the training program can be interpreted as a response to the pressures of competing needs. From the administrators' and founders' perspective, hiring out was the most useful means by which they could demonstrate to leading black and white members of the local communities the value of the hospital and nursing school. The student nurses, exploited as they unquestionably were, served as the vehicle through which the heads of these institutions appealed for financial contributions from individuals, foundations, and city, state, and federal governments. McClennan's Hospital in Charleston is the most representative example of the struggle these institutions waged simply to keep going from year to year. At best it was a hand-to-mouth operation, even when its record of good service to the black poor was readily apparent. From its inception through 1905, the city of Charleston repeatedly refused the institution's applications for aid. As the Rockefeller Foundation investigator noted, "The city, however, maintains a training school for white nurses at an annual expenditure . . . of $4,000. This was established after the colored hospital was organized."[40]

The hired-out student nurse, whether she worked among poor blacks or rich whites, was the hospital's goodwill ambassador and front-line attack on morbidity and diseases associated with poverty, unsanitary water and food, and overcrowded living conditions. Again, the comments of white Charlestonians substantiate the good work of the student nurses and hospital, and the positive regard in which they were held in the community. In 1905 the white assistant secretary of Associate Charities enthused about one black angel of mercy:

> It is with sincere feeling I speak of the work of Charleston's Colored Hospital, it is sending forth women who are not only capable, but tender and faithful. . . . I particularly mention Gussie Davis who during an epidemic of typhoid fever, at our Episcopal Church Home, fought hard often night as well as day for the lives of those children and through the Master's blessing many were saved.[41]

The students too, gained, perhaps indirectly, educational and experiential benefits from the hiring-out practice, which at some level offset the deficiencies in the training programs. They encountered a wider range of cases and confronted challenges, and in the process of serving under difficult conditions they became necessarily more autonomous, resourceful, and skilled professionals. To be sure, this "ordeal by fire" for many proved daunting, especially when they were forced to improvise techniques and treatments in the absence of a physician. The student nurses were the first black health-care professionals ever to appear in many of the small black enclaves, settlements, and communities in the South. More often than not, they quickly had to develop and hone communication skills and abilities to win confidence and allay suspicions. Few course catalogues indicated that instruction was provided in these areas.

For a variety of reasons, there existed no arena more conducive to the mastery of practical private-duty nursing skills than hiring out. Once on a private case, until the physician arrived and the ingrained patterns of nursing subordination surfaced, the nurse was, for better or worse, in charge. Her views were the voice of authority, heard and respected, for patients' lives depended upon the manner in which she performed. The practice of hiring out, while institutionally remunerative, nevertheless prepared the student nurses well for future jobs in private duty or as head and staff nurses in the scores of small black hospitals and sanitariums springing up across the country. Not until the 1930s would large numbers of black nurses find official positions in the most autonomous of all nursing practices, public-health nursing. It is nevertheless intriguing that a look at the early decades of the history of the best black hospital nursing schools suggests that black nurses, whether student or graduate, often engaged in public-health nursing from the moment they passed probation. Attending to black health-care needs in a segregated society meant going physically and mentally beyond the whitewashed walls of those structures called hospitals.

The career pattern, spanning the years 1906–1928, of one black nurse, Petra Pinn, a 1906 graduate of the Tuskegee Institute training school and founder of its alumni association, reflects the range of work in which these women professionals engaged. After receiving her diploma, Pinn worked for three years as the head nurse at Hale Infirmary in Montgomery, Alabama, before becoming the superintendent of nurses of the Red Cross Sanitarium and Training School in Louisville, Kentucky. Two years later she joined the city's metropolitan nursing service but, discovering that she preferred institutional work, she sought assistance from John A. Kenney and was able to receive the appointment of superintendent of nurses of Pine Ridge Hospital at West Palm Beach, Florida. She remained in this position for ten years, "making friends for the hospital, raising money and doing most of the work as she was often without any assistant." Eventually the accumulated toil forced her to retire for a year to regain her health. During that period Pinn made two decisions: first, that she would work only in managerial positions in small hospitals, and second, that she would always "serve in small southern communities" in spite of repeated offers to relocate to other regions of the country. In the late 1920s she accepted the position of manager and superintendent of the working Benevolent Society Hospital at Greenville, South Carolina.[42] For Petra Pinn nursing was a route to personal prestige and administrative autonomy, and a means to serve her people. In a society which offered most women, especially black females, scant opportunity for higher education and lucrative employment, nursing was a godsend. Pinn survived the training-school experience and internalized the values of rigid discipline, respect for authority, responsibility for patients, and dedication to her chosen profession.

Pinn's experiences are reflective of the lives of a significant percentage of the approximately three thousand nurses who were graduated from the top black hospital and nursing training schools in the opening decades of the twentieth century. Most black graduate nurses moved from private-duty work after finishing their training, on to hospital work, and finally achieved the highest degree of professional autonomy as public-health nurses. While disparaged by their white nurse counterparts, black nurses were revered and respected by the black communities. These women were more than angels of mercy, they had survived the rigors of training and represented, next to the teacher, the highest ideal of black womanhood.

Black Collegiate Nursing Education: A Case Study

4 In the 1930s, nursing leaders achieved a major breakthrough in their long and arduous struggle to reduce the number of hospital diploma nursing schools. Against staunch opposition from male hospital administrators and physicians, they labored to promote the establishment of more collegiate programs, founding in 1935 the Association of Collegiate Schools of Nursing (ACSN). The thirty-five-member organization endeavored "to develop nursing education on a professional and collegiate level; to promote and strengthen the relationship between nursing and institutions of higher education; and to promote study and experimentation in nursing service and nursing education."[1]

White nurse leaders justified the transition from hospital diplomas to college degrees as essential to liberating nursing education from the service demands of hospitals. They argued that university affiliation would result in a higher standard of nursing care, greater public respectability for the field, and the production of better-prepared nurses. Isabel M. Stewart, director of nursing education at Teachers College, Columbia University, in her essay "Next Step in the Education of Nurses" asserted that "many schools don't know whether they are primarily educational institutions or service departments of hospitals." Stewart further prophesied that "in nursing as in home economics, teaching, library work, and many other similar fields, a bachelor's degree will become in the near future a commonly accepted basic qualification for professional practice."[2]

Black nurse leaders witnessed the growth of collegiate nursing programs with justifiable concern. By 1935 there were seventy undergraduate programs in the country. Rheva A. Speaks, superintendent of nurses at Freedmen's Hospital in Washington, D.C., agreed with the thrust of Stewart's remarks. She wrote, "In fact, hospitals should not be expected to finance nursing schools—since the two have separate and distinct purposes: the one, that of caring for the sick; the other that of educating nurses." Speaks applauded the move to locate schools of nursing at educational institutions where the emphasis was placed on education and col-

lege affiliation. She predicted that the trend toward developing endowed
schools and the charging of fees, along with the elimination of stipends,
would spur the separation of the nursing students from the hospitals.
Speaks encouraged black nurses to adopt the goal and accept the position
that training schools should be independent divisions with control of
their own budgets, and that nurse educators and administrators should
control the selection of students.[3] Few black nurses quarreled with these
lofty objectives, for they as much as their white colleagues desired the
growth of nursing as a profession.

Nevertheless, black nurse leaders were quick to point out that nursing
advances often held adverse consequences for the black women in white.
They anticipated that as collegiate programs acquired dominance and a
bachelor's degree became the standard credential, black women, because
of discrimination and exclusion, would find themselves occupying an
even more acutely marginal status within the profession. In the same
year in which the ACSN was founded, Estelle Riddle, president of the National Association of Colored Graduate Nurses, founded in 1908, lamented,

> While the profession of nursing has advanced to the point that both Yale
> and Western Reserve raised their admission standards to the nursing
> schools to four years of college, as a minimum, this fall, the Negro nursing
> schools apparently have not reached the point where they can uniformly
> raise their minimum above four years of high school.[4]

In a 1937 article Riddle declared, "More Negro nurses should be encouraged through scholarship aid, leaves of absence, etc., to prepare for
the higher positions in hospitals and nursing schools." She concluded,
"There is a dearth of well prepared administrators and instructors."[5] In
yet another article Riddle cut to the heart of the matter: "A college of
nursing, as part of a university, is an urgent need for the education of
Negro nurses."[6]

The urgency of Riddle's plea for the founding of black collegiate nursing departments as autonomous components of institutions of higher education reflected her apprehension about the rigid occupational stratification developing within the profession along racial lines. In the early
years of professional nursing, virtually every nurse, regardless of race,
entered into private-duty work. Now, white nurses armed with bachelor's
and master's degrees would be able to command even higher wages, and
fill important leadership positions, while those black nurses equipped
only with diplomas would be relegated to the lower-status jobs. She observed that as late as 1937 fully "one-third of the schools for Negro nurses
[were] supervised by white superintendents and administrators."[7]

If black women were to become competitive for the top positions in
nursing and maintain a viable presence within the profession, it was in-

cumbent that they have greater access to collegiate nursing education. The persistent and virulent racism effectively prevented their admission to the few white colleges and universities that offered nursing degrees. So as the movement to develop more collegiate nursing-education programs gathered steam, black nurse leaders began to pressure black colleges and universities.

As late as the mid-1930s only one black college, Florida A & M in Tallahassee, boasted a baccalaureate nursing department. Howard University had established a baccalaureate program as early as 1922, but it lasted only three years. Although short-lived, this was truly an amazing feat considering that at the time only a handful of bachelor's-degree programs existed for white women. Thus Florida A & M had the longest continuous bachelor's-degree program in nursing among the black institutions. The situation was soon to change. In 1942, Dillard University in New Orleans established a baccalaureate-degree program. Following Dillard's lead, Hampton Institute in Hampton, Virginia, launched its baccalaureate program in 1944. Meharry Medical College in Nashville, Tennessee, began offering bachelor's degrees in 1947. A year later Tuskegee Institute in Alabama converted its hospital diploma school into a baccalaureate program.[8]

The 1950s witnessed a flurry of activity as several black colleges and universities created new baccalaureate nursing programs. The rising specter of integration propelled southern state governments to increase allocation for the development of separate black programs. Even more important, however, was the rise of massive federally funded health-care and education programs launched during the World War II emergency. In 1952 Prairie View College in Texas initiated a baccalaureate program, followed the next year by North Carolina A & T State University in Greensboro, and in 1954 by Winston-Salem State University in North Carolina.[9] The major white philanthropic foundations, the General Education Board and the Julius Rosenwald Fund, played a critical role in the black collegiate nursing-education movement. The intersection between white philanthropy, federal intervention, black self-determination, and the nursing profession is most graphically illustrated in what became by far the most highly acclaimed program in nursing at the collegiate level, at Dillard University during the 1940s.

When in 1896 the black clubwomen of New Orleans launched the Phillis Wheatley Sanitarium, it marked the first organized attempt by the city's black population to improve health-care delivery to the most oppressed and needy members of the race. The women acted fully cognizant that raising adequate funds to operate the institution would entail continuous and often frustrating effort. Within a few years of its founding, the New Orleans Board of Health condemned the old, dilapidated frame building in which the sanitarium was housed. Fortunately, the president of New Orleans University, a black school supported by the Board of Education of the Methodist Episcopal Church and chartered in 1873, rescued the institution from imminent failure. As a consequence the sanitarium became a practice facility providing clinical experience for the black students enrolled in the university's medical department. A timely grant from a white Bostonian, Caroline W. Mudge, secured, for the time being, the future of the hospital. To express gratitude, the name was changed to the Sarah Goodridge Hospital in honor of Mudge's mother, Sarah Tannot Goodridge. Similarly, a subsequent donation from John D. Flint of Fall River, Massachusetts, to the university's medical unit resulted in its rechristening as Flint Medical College.

As helpful as these sums proved, they were not enough to improve the medical school along the lines called for by the reform-driven American Medical Association. Flint Medical College's inability to provide adequate facilities, modern laboratories, and appropriately trained faculty forced leaders of the Methodist Episcopal church to recommend to the Flint heirs that they close the medical department but permit the remaining funds to be deployed to support and strengthen Goodridge Hospital and the nursing school. The Flint heirs agreed. This money, added to the sums from the Freedmen's Aid Society of the ME church, enabled New Orleans University officials to construct a new fifty-six-bed hospital and to remodel the old structure into a nurses' home. Thereupon they changed the name to the Flint-Goodridge Hospital and School of Nursing.[10]

Throughout the 1920s Flint-Goodridge continued to suffer financial hardships. Help was on the way, however. Fortuitously, the managers of the giant philanthropic foundations the General Education Board and the Julius Rosenwald Fund indicated interest in the hospital. To be more specific, they became intrigued by the possibility of developing in New Orleans a third major higher-education center for blacks in much the same way they had done with the Atlanta University system, and the Fisk University–Meharry Medical College complex in Nashville.[11]

New Orleans held pregnant possibilities for the development of such an educational complex because of the existence of two small black colleges, Straight University, founded in 1869 with the support of the Congregationalists, and New Orleans University. Housed in cramped and antiquated buildings, these two schools struggled to stay afloat. It was obvious that the black population, even with white missionary largesse, could ill afford to maintain two quality institutions. Of course most observers readily acknowledge that the designation "university" reflected more hope than reality. The combined enrollment of Straight and New Orleans for 1926 was 1,366, of whom 438 were in the college departments, 629 in the high-school department, and 188 in the primary grades, while 111 were listed as special students.[12]

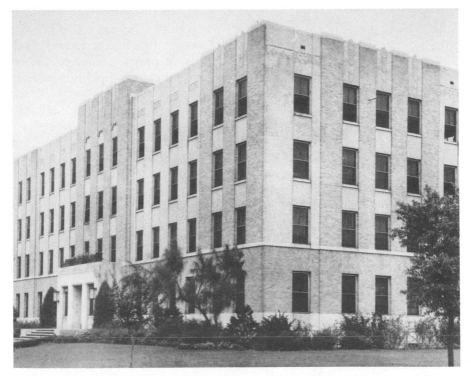

Flint-Goodridge Hospital, New Orleans, circa 1950s. Courtesy of the Amistad Research Center, Tulane University.

The General Education Board and Rosenwald Fund managers had but to await the opportune moment to become molders of the higher-educational future of black New Orleans. When both Straight and New Orleans applied for assistance in the mid-1920s, GEB and Rosenwald Fund officers jointly agreed to deny support unless the two schools merged into a single institution. Actually, as early as 1916 white educators had suggested that the two schools be combined. Strong individual personalities, institutional loyalties, and denominational interests prevented serious and sustained consideration of a merger.[13]

By the mid-1920s, however, both institutions were in dire need of additional financial support. Even more significant, leaders of the white business community in the city began to take an active interest in the two schools. Edgar B. Stern, the son-in-law of Julius Rosenwald and an influential member of the white community, took the lead in organizing a major meeting attended by the trustees of both colleges, representatives of the two denominations, and members of the business community. In February 1929, the group submitted a plan for union to the GEB and to the Rosenwald Fund. They proposed that the Flint-Goodridge Hospital and nursing school form the core of a new university created from the merger of Straight and New Orleans. After months of haggling over financial details, the religious representatives and foundation officers agreed that of the $2 million needed for land purchases and building construction, "the two missionary boards were to pledge $500,000 each, the General Education Board $500,000, and the Rosenwald Fund $250,000. The citizens of New Orleans were to be asked for the final $250,000."[14]

The decision to make Flint-Goodridge Hospital the nucleus of the new institution named in honor of James Hardy Dillard proved a masterful stroke. Dillard, a highly respected, prominent southern white educator, had served as a trustee of both black schools, was a dean at Tulane University, and was a former president and director of the Jeanes and Slater funds. Black and white New Orleans responded with generous enthusiasm to the fundraising drive. As one GEB field agent explained, Flint-Goodridge was "probably better known to the New Orleans people than the academic work of New Orleans University and Straight College." He elaborated, "There is no question about the need of such a hospital and nursing school in such a large city as New Orleans."[15] Indeed, enthusiasm ran so high during the campaign that both black and white residents of the city exceeded their pledge goals. One GEB agent concluded that "sympathetic interest . . . in the hospital rather than in the higher education institution for Negroes" accounted for the successful fundraising.[16] Of course the advent of the Great Depression severely limited the amount actually collected from the people of New Orleans. As a consequence the GEB ended up contributing far more toward the actual construction cost than any other group.[17]

The management of Dillard University was placed in the hands of seventeen trustees, six each from the religious denominations, who in turn chose the remaining five. Edgar B. Stern was named president of the board of trustees. Other members included Alvin P. Howard, local newspaper editor; Monte M. Lemann, a lawyer; and Warren Kearney, a businessman and leader of the Episcopal church. At least five of the members of the board were black.[18] The experiment evoked widespread acclaim as the best example of interracial cooperation in the South. Leo Favrot enthused, "In its establishment are blended the devoted missionary spirit of the North, the kindly benevolence of an awakened South and the laudable aspirations of the Negro people. Dillard University will stand as a symbol of interdenominational, interracial and intersectional cooperation and goodwill."[19] Mordecai Johnson, the black president of Howard University, later declared,

Mark what we have here: an institution for the highest development of the children of slaves; under the leadership of a southern white man; with the

Chairman of the Board of Trustees a southern white man; three or four of the ablest members of the Board southern white men, associating themselves at the same time on the Board of Trustees with Negroes—southern Negroes and northern Negroes.[20]

One cloud loomed over the proclamations of the dawn of a new day of black-white, North-South cooperation. By the time the university opened in 1935, the "important nurse-training program" had ended.

Credit for the success of Flint-Goodridge Hospital and for the development of a collegiate department of nursing at Dillard University belongs to the young, black, talented, and ambitious Albert W. Dent. Born in Atlanta, Georgia, and educated at Morehouse College, the twenty-seven-year-old Dent assumed the superintendency of the newly constructed hospital in February 1932. He was soon heralded as the best black hospital administrator in the country. His successful tenure as superintendent of Flint-Goodridge propelled him in 1942, at age thirty-seven, into the presidency of Dillard University. It was while thus situated that he played his major role in black nursing history by subsequently establishing the baccalaureate degree in nursing at the university. Prior to coming to New Orleans, Dent had served as branch-office auditor for the Atlanta

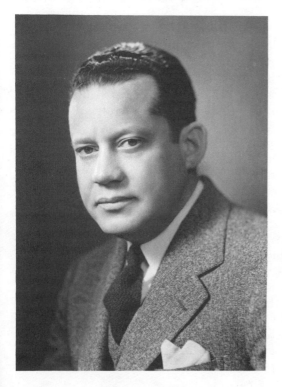

Albert W. Dent, superintendent of Flint-Goodridge Hospital during the 1930s and 1940s. He subsequently became president of Dillard University. This photo was taken in 1945. Courtesy of the Amistad Research Center, Tulane University.

Life Insurance Company, and as vice-president of a real-estate and con-struction company in Houston, Texas. In 1928 he had returned to Morehouse College to organize the school's alumni and to direct an en-dowment campaign to raise $300,000 to match a like sum offered by the General Education Board. In this, too, he had proved successful.[21] Dent was a personally imposing, fair-skinned man, equally at home among blacks and whites. His own personal philosophy was best reflected in an old adage he seemed fond of quoting: "Do what you can with what you have."

Dent had not immediately accepted the superintendency of Flint-Goodridge when approached. With no previous medical education, he was understandably daunted, although he well imagined the problems he would encounter. The self-doubt was not the source of his pause. The 100-bed modern hospital had an annual budget of $60,000, but it needed more. There were in New Orleans thirty-five licensed black doctors, only two of whom had served an internship. A significant proportion of the black population suffered the effects of severe poverty and unsanitary and inadequate housing; they were haunted by rampant tuberculosis and syphilis, and appallingly high infant and maternal morbidity and mor-tality. Compounding these difficulties was the historic black abhorrence of hospitalization. Dent, albeit briefly, hesitated before taking up the gauntlet.[22]

In part, the history of the revitalization of Flint-Goodridge is the story of Dent's attempt to make real a particular social vision.[23] Credit for the reestablishment of the nursing program as an official department of Dillard University belongs to the administrative genius of Dent and the unrelenting efforts of a determined black nurse, Rita E. Miller, who served as the director of the nursing division throughout the 1940s.

The year 1932 was a propitious one for black New Orleans. On the heels of the celebration of the opening of the new Flint-Goodridge Hospi-tal came Dent's announcement of the closing of the hospital's nurse-training program. He had invited representatives of the National League of Nursing Education, the National Organization for Public Health Nurs-ing, and the Louisiana Board of Nurse Examiners to investigate the nurs-ing school for accreditation purposes. In late February, the representa-tives unanimously judged the facilities inadequate for accreditation. The training program lacked proper professional instructors; the hospital did not have the daily requirement of fifty patients or an ameliorating affilia-tion agreement with a larger hospital.

Hospitalization, what little there had been, had dropped precipitously as the large-scale unemployment occasioned by the Great Depression dec-imated black earnings. Dent had no alternative but to close the nursing-school operation after the last of the thirty-nine students had been gradu-ated. Thus in May 1934, the forty-year-old Flint-Goodridge Hospital went out of the nurse-training business. The hospital hired a staff of black graduate nurses supervised by Eola V. Lyons.[24]

Between 1934 and 1940, Dent pursued a number of strategies and programs to boost black hospital use and to persuade the board of trustees and philanthropic leaders to open a new school of nursing offering a baccalaureate degree. Indeed, establishing a high-quality nursing school became an all-consuming quest as much for his own ego satisfaction as for the good of the black community. Fortunately Dent never exhausted his store of innovative ideas designed to increase hospital occupancy. He remained ever alert to opportunities to expand and maintain health-care delivery to black New Orleans, and to secure the hospital's financial solvency. Dent quickly defined the hospital as more than "just buildings and equipment."[25] He now had to persuade poor blacks that it was more than a place where the sick came to receive treatment and scientific medical care prior to death. To the well-known black fear of and hostility to hospitals, Dent added two other factors which determined blacks' reluctance to use them: the general inadequacy of facilities, and the basic inability to pay for private services.[26]

Acting upon his expanded vision of what a hospital should be, Dent resolved that if black patients refused to come to the hospital or were unable to pay for the services, then, quite simply, the hospital must go to them. He employed a few additional trained nurses and dispatched them to the surrounding communities with one primary objective, to allay blacks' fears of hospitalization. To facilitate their mission he established special mobile clinics operated by nurses and social workers. Dent's strategy of bringing the hospital to the people proved, in many respects, to be of limited success. However, the health-care workers successfully identified a number of health problems amenable to correction with satisfactory care.

Among the most vexing medical problems plaguing black communities in the 1930s (and today) was the high incidence of black infant and maternal mortality. There were approximately 149,000 blacks in New Orleans out of a total population of 458,762. New Orleans bore the regrettable distinction of having the highest black death rate of the major southern cities, including Atlanta, Birmingham, Louisville, and Memphis. Indeed, its black infant and maternal death rate was the highest in the country.[27]

During the first six months of operation, only fourteen babies were born at Flint-Goodridge Hospital, while midwives delivered 25 percent of all black babies. Actually, midwives, especially in the rural parishes, delivered as many as ten times more black babies than did black doctors. Dent avoided attacking midwives directly and instead focused on persuading expectant mothers to come to the hospital for pre- and postnatal care. With monies provided by the Rosenwald Fund, he hired a social worker in 1933 to organize mothers' clubs in various sections of the city. To complement the mothers' clubs he established a well-baby clinic at the hospital. New mothers were urged to bring their babies to the clinic once a month for one year for general observation and for instruction as to the proper care of the infant.

The mothers' clubs met twice per month. At one of the meetings the social worker arranged for a speaker, usually a Flint-Goodridge employee, staff doctor, nurse, or dietitian, to address the group of expectant mothers on rudimentary prenatal care and to impress upon them the value of hospital birth. At alternate meetings, the mothers-to-be learned how to make baby clothing and received instruction in embroidery, basket weaving, hand painting, and gardening, thus creating a relaxed atmosphere in which to discuss health problems and prevention.[28] The strategy worked, and by 1939, the hospital delivery rates had improved. Indeed, the number of hospital births at Flint-Goodridge reflected a 400 percent increase over the 1932 figure.[29]

Yet this increase was not enough, for in the rural areas surrounding the city, poor black women continued to rely on the services of midwives. A white physician, L. C. Spencer, director of the Health Unit of Catahoula Parish in Harrisonburg, Louisiana, voiced many of the complaints local doctors had about the midwives. With no attempt to conceal his disdain, Spencer wrote to Dent, "The midwifery among our negro population is in the hands of old granny women, and to the best of my knowledge and belief, none of these women can read or write." He continued, "Many of them are actually decrepit with old age, almost blind, crippled with rheumatism, and embarrassed with heart lesions." There is, of course, a possibility that Spencer may have exaggerated, though it is curious to note that Dent avoided wholesale denunciation of black midwives. Nevertheless, Spencer assured Dent that he spoke "with definite authority."[30]

To lessen the influence of midwives and promote the status of Flint-Goodridge, Dent developed two new strategies. Endeavoring to provide pregnant women with services and conveniences identical to those offered by the midwives, he introduced a "home delivery service" which was cheaper and more convenient for the mothers—especially for those already with small children who could not afford a lengthy hospital confinement. This approach proved somewhat successful, and the hospital's obstetrical service increased by two hundred cases per year. But even this tactic did not completely resolve the problem. Fortuitously, the availability of government grants in the early 1940s motivated Dent to take advantage of midwives' seemingly entrenched position by training nurses in midwifery. With funds provided by the United States Children's Bureau of the United States Public Health Service and additional grants from the Rosenwald Fund in 1942, he developed a six-month course for graduate nurses. The program lasted only one year, producing two black nurse-midwives. A similar venture was begun earlier at Tuskegee Institute. In 1941, under the guidance of Margaret Thomas and F. Carrington Owens and with federal, state, and philanthropic funds, the Tuskegee Nurse-Midwifery School opened in Alabama. By the time it closed in 1946, it had graduated twenty-five black nurse-midwives. Both the Dillard and the Tuskegee schools throughout their existence worked in close cooperation with the Maternity Center Association in New York.[31]

Even as Dent contemplated and devised ways to circumvent the midwifery problem, he continued to take advantage of any opportunity to extend the hospital's hegemony and add to its coffers. When the National Youth Administration, established as part of the New Deal machinery, offered funds to institutions willing to provide vocational training to unemployed black youths, Dent initiated courses to train black teenagers and young adults for work as nursemaids and orderlies. The hospital's nursemaid course, taught to over four hundred young black women between 1936 and 1942, was designed to prepare them for work in hospitals and private homes. The program consisted of classroom and practical instruction in such matters as personal hygiene, dishwashing, housecleaning, and proper care of iceboxes, baby bottles, clothing, and bedding. Students' learning ranged from the proper way to answer the telephone to the preparation of surgical dressings. Dent maintained that the course basically was intended to "improve their usefulness to themselves and the families which they may later acquire."[32] The National Youth Administration also subsidized the hospital's course for orderlies. Forty young black men took the course, which qualified them for jobs in the city hospitals. They were given instruction in ideal patient service. Most of the time, however, was spent learning manual tasks such as operating elevators, painting and repairing furniture, general cleaning of floors, walls, and windows, and the proper disposal of waste and garbage.[33]

To be sure, this training project was essentially a formal version and more lucrative extension of a program in which the hospital was already engaged. Each year since its inception, Flint-Goodridge had cooperated with a summer playground program sponsored by the Council of Social Agencies. The hospital released its staff physicians and nurses to speak to the children who were brought into the institution. During the summer of 1935, a motor corps of black women was organized in order to bring black teenage girls from playgrounds to the hospital, where staff nurses lectured to them and gave demonstrations on the fundamentals of personal hygiene.[34]

In 1935, as a further manifestation of Dent's community-outreach strategy, he organized a women's auxiliary to serve as liaison between the hospital and the community. Dent viewed the formation of the auxiliary as "an additional means of creating good will." Its two hundred members, representing a cross section of black community life, were divided

into four groups—"sewing, educational, social service and beautification
of lawn and building." Each year the auxiliary hosted an open-house tea
at the hospital, sponsored Christmas parties for clinic children, and conducted special activities to convey the institution's programs, interests,
and needs to the broader community. Dent shrewdly observed that "two
hundred women talking about the good work of Flint-Goodridge Hospital
is a tremendous asset."[35]

Dent attracted nationwide attention and increased black esteem for
Flint-Goodridge Hospital when he launched a pioneering hospitalization
insurance program which catapulted the institution and its able young
administrator into the limelight as had nothing else. By the fall of 1932,
Dent had effected an agreement with the black public schoolteachers of
New Orleans whereby they would be furnished hospital services for a
fixed annual premium. A few years later he extended the service to other
groups, eventually including Pullman car porters, post office employees,
department store workers, hotel employees, nurses' associations, and
members of churches and the black medical society. To reach the people
in the lower income brackets, Dent devised in 1936 the "penny-a-day"
plan. This arrangement allowed groups of employed individuals to contract to pay $3.65 a year per person in exchange for complete hospital
services. A $4,500 Julius Rosenwald Fund grant underwrote the program
until Dent had accumulated a sufficient number of subscribers to make
it profitable. The Rosenwald grant was extra insurance, for by 1943, approximately five thousand people were signed up.

The plan's success had several important ramifications. It extended
hospital services to a much larger group of people while measurably increasing the institution's earnings. More than this, it further strengthened black support for and identification with the hospital. The plan was
discontinued in 1943 when Flint-Goodridge joined the Hospital Service
Association of New Orleans, a city-wide hospitalization plan.[36]

In attempting to counter the high infant and maternal morbidity and
mortality prevalent at the time in the black community, Dent gained increased recognition for the hospital. He established three clinics for
the treatment of syphilis, tuberculosis, and obstetrics and pediatrics. A
$22,000 grant from the Rosenwald Fund paid the salaries of three black
public-health nurses, one for each clinic. The nurse in the syphilis clinic
emphasized the need for more education concerning venereal disease and
the value of early detection. She lectured at public schools, colleges, and
industrial plants and before parent-teachers associations and ministerial
groups on the importance of seeking immediate assistance for a suspected
infection. The nurse encouraged those who thought they might have the
disease to come to the clinic to take the Wassermann and Hinton test
for syphilis. The hospital established a special Monday- and Thursday-
night clinic for the black poor and provided examination and treatment

at a nominal fee of twenty-five cents. In 1940, the state and federal governments assumed complete financial responsibility for the syphilis clinic.

The tuberculosis clinic operated in much the same manner. Convinced that early detection checked the spread of disease, the clinic made available to black New Orleans free blood-testing services. In 1941 Dent wrote, "We have assumed some responsibility for the control of tuberculosis in New Orleans through early diagnosis and ambulatory treatment." Dent was particularly proud of the fact that Flint-Goodridge established the first pneumothorax (chest x-ray) clinic in the city. The obstetrics and pediatrics clinic continued the work of encouraging mothers-to-be to have their babies in the hospital. Dent instructed the black public-health nurses to go to black women and "tell them that we will take any maternity case that comes to us for a flat rate of ten dollars, to include doctors, medicine, and hospitalization for as long as seven days."[37]

There was yet another dimension to Dent's vision of a black hospital. In addition to everything else, the hospital was an educational institution. Dent was determined that Flint-Goodridge would excel in providing opportunities for internships, residencies, and postgraduate study to the city's black physicians. Therefore, each summer, beginning in 1936, the hospital operated a two-week postgraduate course which attracted dozens of black physicians from neighboring states. White professors from the Tulane and Louisiana State University medical schools taught the subjects, demonstrating the latest medical and surgical techniques and procedures. Thirty-two of the thirty-seven black physicians in New Orleans served on the active staff or were in some way affiliated with the hospital. Between October and May of each year, Flint-Goodridge hosted a series of thirty-six Tuesday-night seminars, to which all physicians in New Orleans and those living within a radius of 150 miles were invited. Heads of departments at the hospital and white professors in the local medical schools conducted the weekly seminars, which usually had an attendance of approximately fifteen black physicians.[38]

Dent used his considerable influence with the officers of the General Education Board and Rosenwald Fund administrators to secure fellowships for those black doctors desiring to pursue intensive study at other institutions in the North or abroad. For example, Dr. Logan W. Horton spent a year in Vienna, London, and Paris, and upon his return to New Orleans was elevated to chief of the departments of eye and ear, nose, and throat. Dr. C. H. D. Bowers, after studying a year at Bellevue Hospital and the School of Medicine of New York University, was given complete charge of the hospital's syphilis work at the end of 1940. In the beginning, distinguished white physicians served as senior consultants and headed all but one of the nine medical services at the hospital. After four years, however, most of these positions had been turned over to black physicians. In this way Flint-Goodridge fostered a greater degree of inter-racial contact between doctors than did any other institution of its kind.[39] It also, and this is important, became a strong force in building black pro-fessional self-confidence.

Yet all of these plans and efforts to strengthen the hospital and to forge links between black health-care personnel and the black communities did not satisfy the ambitious young superintendent. In his view, one critical component of the black hospital complex was missing. As early as 1935, Dent had begun making plans to reopen the Flint-Goodridge school of nursing. Each successful program had elevated the institution's national stature and had pushed Dent closer to realization of this objective. Dent fervently believed that Flint-Goodridge Hospital would be incomplete, and his mission unfulfilled, until he had reopened the nursing school. As far as he was concerned, his work amounted to little "until we are able to broaden our influence by sending forth a group of thoroughly trained nurses each year to meet the health needs of the community."[40]

As an enlightened hospital administrator, Dent placed high value on the centrality of the black nurses' role in the smooth operation of the plant and in the care of the patients. His reflections on their importance were devoid of melodramatic stereotypes. He did not subscribe to the "angel" or "saint" model which viewed the nurse as the eternally suffer-ing, meek, inarticulate, selfless, almost bloodless figure.[41] Dent recog-nized the fact that quite often the black nurse bore the primary responsi-bility for black survival in many parts of the South. His own experience and observations convinced him that she was a major factor in lowering the high death rate among blacks. He deemed the nurse to be as much if not more of an asset to the community in which she lived than was the average college graduate. Dent wrote, "The nurses are community workers extending the service of the hospital to every corner of the city." He pointed out that the nurse also served as an interpreter between doc-tor and patients, particularly when social differences threatened to inter-fere with the treatment. He asserted that, indeed, success in treating ill-ness depended largely "on the use of adequate interpretation as an effective method for keeping patients under treatment."[42] His perceptions endeared him to the nurses who served with him.

These progressive views undoubtedly placed Dent in the company of a minority of hospital administrators and physicians. At least one promi-nent black doctor concurred in this assessment. Louis T. Wright, of Har-lem Hospital in New York City, observed that "by and large, the public health nurse has done more for health education than the doctors practic-ing in the same communities."[43] Of course not all physicians, black or white, shared these perceptions. From the perspective of the nurse, too many hospital administrators and physicians seemed unable to divorce themselves from the "submissive programmed robot" conception of the nurse. Significantly, then, in Dent's view the nurse was as important as the physician and the hospital, for without her, the other two units could never effectively minister to the total health care–delivery needs of black communities. Possessed of this fundamental belief in the "worth of the nurse," Dent increasingly focused on the reestablishment of the Flint-Goodridge program.

As early as 1936, Dent had approached the General Education Board officers for a grant with which to reopen the nursing school. The officers denied his request, explaining that the hospital's deficiencies still over-shadowed its positive attributes, and thus it did not warrant funds to re-open the school. To be sure, Flint-Goodridge possessed good housing facil-ities for student nurses, and was winning the confidence and support of all segments of the city's population. The GEB officers agreed that the hospital's greatest asset, Albert Dent, had demonstrated considerable talent and had proved that he possessed the social vision required to con-duct a high-caliber nursing school "which would place emphasis on the value of community service." One GEB official who had voted to fund the reopening wrote, "My admiration for Superintendent Dent . . . and for the way in which the hospital is conducted is so great that I would not have any doubt about his employing the right kind of instructors and setting up the instruction on a high plane."[44]

In spite of the advantages of good housing, community confidence, and sound management, Flint-Goodridge remained seriously handicapped by the persistently low daily number of patients. Dent attempted to address this problem by working out an affiliation agreement with Charity Hos-pital, a much larger, white-managed municipal institution. The proposed agreement stipulated that student nurses from Flint-Goodridge would re-ceive clinical experience in Charity Hospital's segregated black wards. At this juncture, Mary Beard, the GEB nursing consultant, vetoed the plan, pointing out to her colleagues Charity's notorious inadequacies. She observed that "only recently a visitor there reported finding two patients in one bed, and not one but several of these."[45]

Undaunted by the foundation's rejection, Dent continued to expand the hospital's operations and increased his efforts to turn the insurance plans into a higher-profit–making enterprise. To be sure, he never completely relinquished hopes of foundation subvention. Meanwhile he proposed to use the funds generated from the insurance plan to finance the reopening of the nursing school, asserting that "with the continued increase in pay patients in addition to the increased revenue from these hospital insur-ance plans, the hospital will be able financially . . . to carry the school of nursing in its regular budget." But in 1940 Dent abandoned the plan to reopen the school, devising a different strategy. Although the hospital had by now reached the minimum daily patient requirement needed for accreditation, Dent decided to push for the establishment of a collegiate nursing school. Repeating the general arguments advanced by nurse leaders, he declared that "a nursing division in Dillard University should develop better persons as well as better nurses; persons who will provide leadership in an increasingly important profession."[46]

When Dent visited the GEB headquarters in 1942, he was accompanied by Rita E. Miller, an especially able black nurse who had earned an M.A. degree from Teacher's College, Columbia University. Dent introduced Miller as "one of the best qualified nursing educators" in the country "from the standpoint of educational background, experience and temperament." Together they made a well-rehearsed and persuasive argument for the establishment of a black collegiate school of nursing. Apparently Miller made "a very favorable impression," as one GEB official remarked. She shared with them her plans to select personally a nursing faculty and to employ a well-qualified black public-health nurse who would provide thorough basic instruction in the preventive and social aspects of nursing.[47] Foundation officers found the presentations provocative and decided to give the plan further consideration.

To aid their deliberations, GEB president Robert Lambert dispatched Mary Elizabeth Tennant, nursing adviser on the staff of the International Health Division of the Rockefeller Foundation, to visit Dillard University

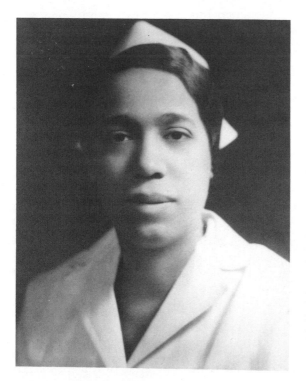

Rita E. Miller received her diploma in 1924 from Mercy Hospital School of Nursing. She served briefly as the educational director at Mercy Hospital before launching the collegiate nursing education division at Dillard University in New Orleans. Collection of the Mercy-Douglass Alumnae Association. Courtesy of the Center for the Study of the History of Nursing, University of Pennsylvania.

and make recommendations. As expected, Tennant reported favorably on both the physical plant and the quality of leadership. Significantly, she also pointed out that Dillard held "real promise" for the development of a good basic professional course in nursing. She made numerous recommendations, beginning with the suggestion that Rita Miller be appointed director of the division of nursing and given a regular faculty rank.[48] Tennant recommended that the GEB contribute $4,000 for the first year to augment the $5,000 pledged by the Julius Rosenwald Fund and the $10,500 promised by the United States Public Health Service. In all the Rosenwald Fund granted more than $1 million to Dillard University, and in addition "provided $54,475 for improvements to the Flint-Goodridge staff and the establishment of a nurses' training program."[49] These funds were all that Dent needed to make his dream a reality. The nursing division subsequently opened for classes in September 1942 with thirty students and Miller serving as director and professor of nursing.

After a successful first year, Dent again approached the GEB, this time requesting a more substantial five-year appropriation to defray the school's expenses. While Lambert approved the grant, he cautioned Dent not to think of the board as the chief financial support of the school. Lambert further advised that the demand for more and better-trained Negro nurses would increase once the war ended. He meanwhile expressed hope that the government would enter into the business of providing proper medical care "for the masses—white and colored." Lambert was ambivalent. He remained convinced that because "good schools cannot be created overnight," the GEB should not pass up the opportunity to finance the Dillard program.

Lambert's misgiving were undoubtedly relaxed by Tennant's enthusiastic pronouncement that the Dillard University Division of Nursing was "one of the most interesting developments in nursing education in the country, irrespective of race," and was, she insisted, "the best there is in the South."[50] Federal government officials apparently concurred with this assessment, and Dillard benefited greatly from government largesse. Dent applied for virtually every grant available. In 1949 he announced, for example, receipt of a $125,000 appropriation from the National Foundation for Infantile Paralysis, payable in installments of $25,000 per year.[51]

Once the school's financial status was secure, Dent and Miller stepped up efforts to develop a first-rate collegiate division of nursing at Dillard. Miller was convinced that this effort would become a model for the development of programs at other black colleges and universities. Shortly after classes began, the GEB arranged for Miller to take a study tour of various nursing schools throughout the country. Beginning with a week-long stop at the University of Toronto School of Nursing, she visited black, white, integrated, and segregated nursing schools, including some of the best and worst of them. Miller also conferred with leaders of the National Association of Colored Graduate Nurses, the National League of Nursing Education, the National Organization for Public Health Nursing, and the American Nurses' Association.[52] Upon her return, she completed a report outlining the problems generally confronting black nursing schools—inadequate, underprepared faculty, poor curriculum, and weak administrative management. Miller then designed, with Tennant's and Dent's assistance, a plan in which she methodically addressed each problem ranging from the securing of outstanding faculty and better students to the development of a well-constructed, scientifically sound curriculum.

Miller pointed out that the black nursing schools in the South suffered severe handicaps, stemming in part from the fact that too many accepted graduates from nonaccredited high schools. All of the schools experienced tremendous problems obtaining an educational staff sufficiently qualified to teach science and the nursing arts. Consequently, underprepared instructors carried exceptionally heavy teaching loads, and overworked clinical instructors often were on duty in excess of forty-eight hours per week. On the whole, the preparation of the supervisors and head nurses, of which there was an acute shortage, was deemed inferior to that of the instructors in science and nursing arts. Insofar as rational management was concerned, Miller found it disconcerting that instructors frequently lacked proper titles, thus making it difficult to determine the functions and responsibilities of each individual. More frequently than not, the schools were without adequate science laboratories and good libraries. The majority of the schools languished under ineffective and uninspired administrators, and Miller observed that where two training programs existed, one for blacks and the other for whites, under a single all-white administration, relationships between the two races were decidedly strained.[53]

To avoid many of the pitfalls encountered in other black nursing schools, Dent, now the new president of the university, immediately placed the Division of Nursing at Dillard on a level equal to the other divisions within the university. Nursing instructors were accorded professional rank, tenure, and commensurate salaries. The shortage of a large, viable pool of specially trained personnel dictated that the division initially employ nursing instructors possessed of minimum qualifications. All faculty members in the university were required to have at least a master's degree, while most of the nursing faculty had bachelor's degrees only. This did not cause Dent or Miller concern. In a well-conceived hiring plan, they selected only instructors who were young, college graduates, ambitious, and professionally aggressive, and who had high potential for further growth and development. Dent and Miller shared the conviction that it was advisable to retain their outstanding graduates and to encourage them to remain in the nursing service at Flint-Goodridge Hospital. While this latter practice risked accusations of favoritism, it also provided continuity and consistency in the nurses' devotion to the hospital, resulting in less problematic management.

After she selected her faculty, Miller arranged for GEB fellowships for each nursing instructor to pursue additional specialized training. During the first few years of operation, it was not unusual for one-fourth to one-half of the instructors in the nursing division to be on leave. For example, Juliette Lee had a Bachelor of Arts degree in education from Loyola University in Chicago and served as the division's nursing-arts instructor. She attended Teachers College, Columbia University, during the 1943–44 term and earned an M.A. degree. The clinical instructor, Jurhetta Coleman, a graduate of Harlem Hospital and holder of a Bachelor of Arts degree from West Virginia State College, was sent to the University of Chicago to work on her M.A. degree. By 1948, all of the nursing instructors, with one exception, had M.A. degrees. Tennant applauded Miller's efforts, noting that she had "assembled an unusually fine nursing staff, probably one of the best in the colored schools of nursing in the country."[54]

Miller also designed a curriculum to better prepare the students for the general practice of nursing. She focused on five areas—biological and physical sciences, social sciences, humanities, medical science, and nursing. The program was a five-year course leading to a Bachelor of Science degree. The student spent her first eighteen months at the university taking general academic subjects, including courses in the history of nursing. In the second summer quarter she was introduced to nursing arts, applied physics, and nutrition. The final three years were spent in Flint-Goodridge or in the affiliated institution, Charity Hospital. Flint-Goodridge provided nursing experience in surgery, operating room, diet kitchen, and outpatient services, while Charity gave experience and instruction in medicine, communicable disease, tuberculosis, obstetrics, and pediatrics.[55]

After the first five years, Miller revised the curriculum considerably—anatomy and physiology replaced general biology. She introduced a course in the nursing applications of physics, which was taught by the science and nursing-arts instructor. She arranged, at the students' insistence, a seminar for the fourth- and fifth-year students to provide opportunity for discussion of current trends, developments, and problems in nursing and related health professions. Finally, she sought to expand the program to offer courses for graduate nurses employed in hospitals and other agencies in the state in order to raise the level of practice among persons already in the field. By 1948, the school had graduated twenty nursing students; all except four of them remained in the South, ten found employment in New Orleans, and seven worked at Flint-Goodridge

---

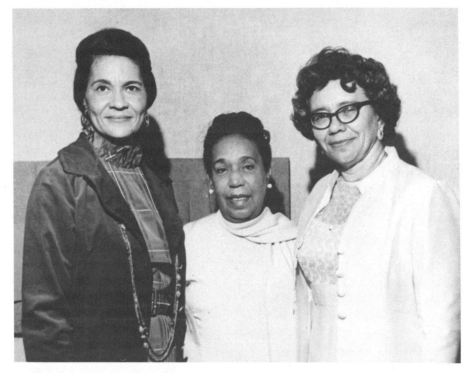

Rita E. Miller (*middle*), first chair of the Division of Nursing at Dillard University, with two of her former students, Marguerite Hartman Rucker (*left*) and Stella Telcot Robinson (*right*), both of whom were students in the 1948 nursing class. Miller was also the black consultant to the Cadet Nurse Corps during World War II. Courtesy of the Amistad Research Center, Tulane University.

Hospital. Eight of the twenty were married shortly after graduation, but as was usual for black women, they continued to work.[56]

Flint-Goodridge Hospital and the Dillard University School of Nursing represent a black success story in nursing education, community health service, and hospital management. Under Dent's guidance, the concept of a black hospital was transformed, at least insofar as black New Orleans was concerned, from a dreaded place denoting sickness and death into an educational force concerned with the total physical and mental well-being of the black community. The mixture of public-health activities with the lay involvement of a broad spectrum of women on the auxiliary board; the provision of professional postgraduate courses; and the implementation of the "penny-a-day" insurance plan enabled Dent to enlarge the scope and purview of the hospital. Flint-Goodridge conse-

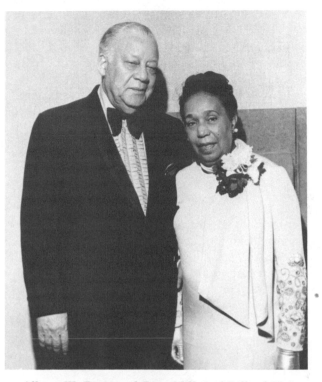

Albert W. Dent and Rita Miller of Dillard University, New Orleans, after decades of service. Photo taken circa 1970s. Courtesy of the Amistad Research Center, Tulane University.

quently shared an esteem more commonly conferred only upon black colleges and the black church.

Dillard University was a modern black educational institution created and endowed by white philanthropists but administered and guided primarily by blacks. It came into existence during the worst economic depression Americans had experienced, and the Division of Nursing Education was established at the beginning of the worldwide calamity of war. The Fascist threat and Hitler's master-race ideology represented the extreme manifestation of racism. Yet the Division of Nursing Education at Dillard flourished during the World War II years as it attracted significant government funds and also witnessed the enrollment of a new type of student, described by John Procope, the new superintendent of Flint-Goodridge Hospital, as "earnest and conscientious" and "eager and optimistic." The new black nursing students desired to play an active role in hospital care services and demanded a higher quality of instruction.

In early 1943, on their own initiative, the students arranged and paid expenses for special lectures on ward management and other subjects not covered in their curriculum. They also organized an in-training program of in-house seminars. The black nurse students' attitudes and perceptions were undoubtedly conditioned by national and international events. The rising visibility of the National Association of Colored Graduate Nurses and the relentless struggle of black nurse leaders to obliterate the barriers of professional exclusion and to win for black nurses the right to serve in the United States Army and Navy Nurse Corps during World War II fanned the flame of an increased awareness among the young students.[57]

As all black nurses, to varying degrees, became more aware of and less willing to tolerate their subordinate status in the profession, the major white nurse leaders took note. Thus the second phase of black nursing history spans the decade of the Great Depression and World War II. This phase witnessed the emergence of a determined, more resourceful cadre of black nurse leaders. The walls of segregation were destined to collapse under their relentless assault.

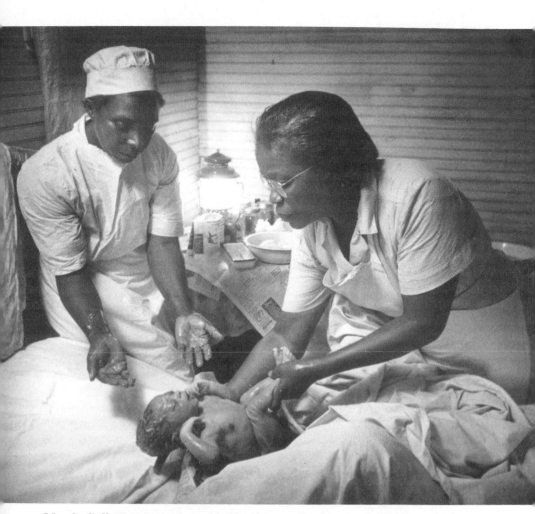

Maude Callen was a nurse-midwife who practiced in rural North Carolina during the 1940s and 1950s. She and hundreds like her helped to bring generations of southern blacks into the world. Photo by W. Eugene Smith, 1951. Courtesy of the Black Star Agency, New York.

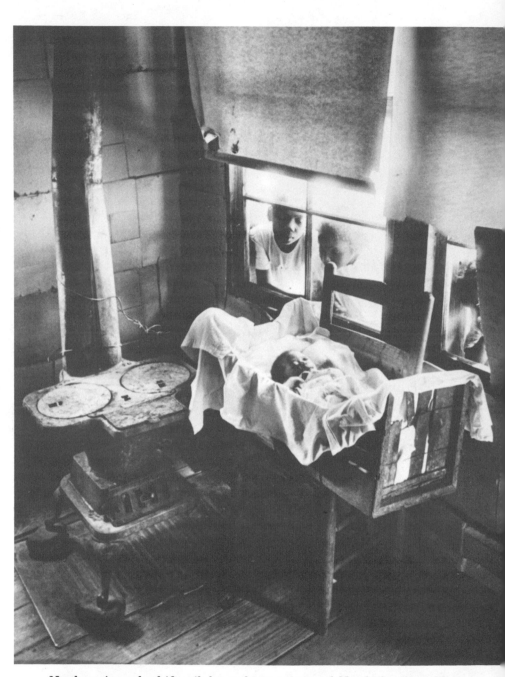

Newborn in makeshift crib by cook stove in rural North Carolina. Photo by W. Eugene Smith. Courtesy of the Black Star Agency, New York.

PART TWO

More Than Angels of Mercy

Racism, Status, and the Professionalization of Black Nursing

5 The evolution of nursing from a low-status occupation too frequently associated with domestic drudgery and with uneducated and unrefined women into a profession—that is, an occupational group appropriating unto its members an "altruistic guardianship over the ethics and performance standards of a vital social service"— occurred during the same period, 1890–1925, which witnessed the solidification of racial segregation and discrimination in America. The professionalization of American nursing and its concomitant subordination of and discrimination against black nurses shed light on the intersection of race conflict and quests for status within the profession.

By the late 1890s an elite cadre of white nurse leaders had emerged to give shape and guidance to the professionalization of nursing. They founded professional organizations, launched journals, created a special body of scholarship, agitated for standardized curriculum, demanded more autonomy for administrators and supervisors, and criticized the gross overproduction of nurses resulting from the proliferation of schools of dubious quality. In addition, they pressed for the implementation of higher admission standards, better working conditions, and higher wages. At every step in the professionalization process the nurse leaders had to contend with hostile physicians and hospital superintendents who feared loss of control over nursing-student labor and education as nurses achieved greater control and professional autonomy.

Throughout these unsettling, turbulent decades, the approximately six thousand trained black nurses and physicians continued the work begun in the 1890s. They had no choice. They founded new hospitals and nurse training schools and launched new organizations and journals to promote their professional advance and to extend health-care information to lay men and women. At Tuskegee Institute, black health-care givers and educators spearheaded, with the aid of black businesses such as the North Carolina Mutual Life Insurance Company of Durham, the National Negro Health movement. The movement focused the country's attention on the excessively high incidence of black maternal and infant mortality, tuberculosis, venereal disease, and other manifestations of the poor health status of Afro-Americans born of poverty, oppression, and despair.

Yet as the first post–Civil War generation of black health-care providers could have attested, precious little progress toward good health, decent housing, equal educational opportunities, and political freedom was possible without adequate financial resources and interracial cooperation. For decade after frustrating decade, professionals armed with the least amount of social, economic, and political capital struggled to do for themselves, and for an entire race of over eleven million people, those things generously provided to other groups by virtue of their skin color. Through the agency of national organizations—the Society of Superintendents of Training Schools for Nurses in the United States and Canada, founded in 1894 and renamed in 1912 the National League of Nursing Education (NLNE); the Nurses' Associated Alumnae of the United States and Canada, founded in 1896 and renamed in 1911 the American Nurses' Association (ANA); and the National Organization for Public Health Nursing (NOPHN), created in 1912—white nurse leaders worked to promote the educational, economic, and social interests of nursing.

The Society of Superintendents originated during the June 1893 meeting of the International Congress of Charities, Corrections, and Philanthropy held in conjunction with the Chicago World's Fair. Key supporters of the founding of this organization included Ethel Gordon Fenwick, founder of the British Nurses' Association; Isabel Hampton Robb, superintendent of the training school at Johns Hopkins Hospital in Baltimore; Lavinia L. Dock, assistant superintendent of nurses at Johns Hopkins; Louise Darche, superintendent of the New York City Training School; and Mary Adelaide Nutting, also an assistant superintendent of nurses at Johns Hopkins and destined to become in 1907 the first nurse to hold a university chair, professor of hospital economics and institutional administration at Teachers College, Columbia University. These women, led by Robb, became the architects chiefly responsible for the subsequent evolution of the nursing profession.

The participants at the meeting discussed the critical issues concerning nursing education and practice, and the conflict between training-school needs and hospital demands, and they identified the objectives to be addressed by the new organization. Among the initial roster of issues were whether stipends should be paid to pupil nurses, justifications for demanding the inauguration of three-year training programs, development of postgraduate courses to prepare future nurse educators, and means by which the role of the female superintendents in hospitals could be enhanced, especially with regard to the selection of applicants and the disciplining of students. They also deliberated on the importance of training-school alumnae groups. In 1894 the members of the society adopted a constitution defining as its objective "to further the best interest of the nursing profession by establishing and maintaining a universal standard of training and by promoting fellowship among its members." At succeeding meetings the society assumed responsibility for the operation of registries and the organization of an all-inclusive association.[1]

When the society became the NLNE in 1912, the membership expanded to include all nursing-school instructors and supervisors, public-health nurses engaged in teaching, and nurses serving on state boards of nurse examiners. Still there existed a need for a broadly based organization to attend to the interests and issues of concern to all practicing nurses. Thus one of the deliberately executed accomplishments of the Society of Superintendents was the laying of the foundation for the creation of the Nurses' Associated Alumnae, which endeavored "to establish and maintain a code of ethics; to elevate the standard of nursing education; to promote the usefulness and honor, the financial and other interests of the nursing profession."[2]

In 1897 the Associated Alumnae decreed that membership was open to alumnae associations of schools of nursing connected with general hospitals offering not less than two years of hospital training. By 1910 approximately fifteen thousand nurses representing 135 alumnae associations belonged. When the group became the American Nurses' Association in 1911, membership eligibility was also amended: "Any state, county or city association or one of national charter which shall be approved by the Eligibility Committee shall be eligible for membership. Any Alumnae Association from a school which gives its pupil three years training in a hospital or in one or more hospitals shall be eligible for membership." By 1913 there were thirty-eight state nurses' associations of the ANA, and within five years the alumnae groups were essentially historical relics.[3]

One major objective, as a means to achieve greater autonomy or the power of self-regulation, was persuading state legislators to enact mandatory laws for registration and licensing of nurses. By the turn of the century it became apparent that a system of state registration that would impose order and uniformity could best be achieved through the organized action of nurses working through state nurses' societies. In 1901 the first such groups were organized, and within a few years fifteen state nurses' associations had secured the enactment of state legislation establishing guidelines for nursing education and practice. In 1903 North Carolina adopted a "nurse practice act," and by 1914 forty states had passed similar laws. The 1903 nurse registration law passed by the New York state legislature created a board of examiners invested with the power to determine the level of preliminary training of entering students, the scope and evaluation of the qualifying examinations, and the issuance of registration certificates to licensed professional nurses. Most state boards also formulated the rules and regulations governing reciprocity arrangements with other states. It should be noted that these state nurse-practice laws "prohibited no one from nursing for hire, whatever his or her qualifications." They merely guaranteed that those practitioners identifying themselves as "registered" nurses had met the states' standards.[4]

In 1912 the third-largest organization of American nurses, the National Organization for Public Health Nursing, was created. This new body defined as its primary objective the stimulation of "the general public and the visiting nurse association to the extension and support of public health nursing services, to facilitate harmonious cooperation among the workers and supporters, and develop a standard of ethics and techniques, and also to act as a clearing house for information for those interested in such work." Within three years of its founding, the organization counted fifteen thousand members, which included, unlike the ANA or the NLNE, lay members.

From the very beginning black nurses were able to belong to the NOPHN, inasmuch as members joined the national body directly. The organization extended membership to nonnurses because private citizens often provided much-needed financial support for the visiting nurses' associations and programs employing public-health nurses. Actually, the NOPHN muted the potential power of lay persons by assigning them to associate nonvoting membership categories. This latter policy enabled the NOPHN to retain its corporate membership in the ANA. Significantly, the broader membership base enlarged the financial resources at the disposal of the organization. In keeping with its public concern and broadly based humanitarian support, the NOPHN soon took on pressure-group characteristics, pushing for health-care reform, and cajoling nursing to adapt to changing social and health-care conditions within American society.[5] The NOPHN introduced into professionalization discussions the whole concept of specialization within nursing and was the one organization early to evidence concern for the status and development of black nurses.

The professionalization process raised the overall status of nursing, but in so doing it created a number of problems for black practitioners. Although black nurses supported the adoption of legislative measures and applauded attempts to elevate standards of education and practice, they quickly discovered that the application of these new laws and requirements erected additional barriers to their own professional advance. Most southern states either barred black nurses from taking registration examinations or administered to them separate examinations.

The founder and first superintendent of nurses at the Grady Hospital Municipal Training School for Colored Nurses in Atlanta, Ludie C. Andrews, a 1906 graduate of the Spelman College nursing program, engaged in a ten-year legal battle against the Georgia State Board of Nurse Examiners in order to win, in 1920, the right of black nurses to take the same examinations as did whites to become licensed to practice nursing, and for a fair appraisal of the examinations when taken. According to Andrews, the board's policy of issuing certificates to black nurses based upon different standards and procedures from those applied to white examinees diminished their chances for employment by in effect branding them as inferior members of the profession. Andrews maintained that the special Negro certification granted to the state's black nurses made it difficult for them to secure postgraduate education and employment in other states. When the state of Georgia offered to give her a license, she refused to accept it unless other black nurses were accorded the same recognition. Not until 1920 did the board permit black nurses who were graduated from Georgia state-approved schools of nursing to take the same licensure examinations as did whites.[6]

In 1929 Adda Eldredge, director of nursing education for the Wisconsin State Board of Health, surveyed employment opportunities available to black nurses in thirteen southern states. State board examiners responded to a variety of questions ranging from the wages paid, to the professional status of black nurses. Their comments provided additional substantiation to black nurses' claims of unequal and discriminatory treatment. The Virginia Board of Nurse Examiners conceded that the status of black nurses was lower than that of white nurses but rationalized that "two years were required of white nurses and four years required for colored nurses because colored high schools were not equal to white high schools."[7] Across the South, black graduate nurses performing identical duties received lower salaries than whites when employed by the same agencies and municipal health departments. The Virginia State Board of Health employed thirty-seven nurses, only one of whom was black. The state paid the white nurses $125 per month, while the black nurse received only $100. In Richmond, the Instructive Visiting Nurse Association, a voluntary organization for public-health nursing, paid its thirteen white nurses $110 per month but gave the six black nurses a mere $80. The association's director declared that such a discrepancy was "unavoidable in the South."[8]

White health-care authorities in Alabama and Tennessee reported similar race-based wage discrepancies. The board of health for Jefferson County and the city of Birmingham employed twelve white and nine black nurses, paying them monthly salaries of $110 and $65 respectively. Zoe La Forge, the county director of the public-health nursing services, admitted that the two groups of nurses performed the same duties but that the agency restricted black nurses to practice only among the black population. La Forge went on to offer a highly subjective and biased estimation of the quality of the work performed by black nurses, perhaps to justify the discrimination in salaries. She acknowledged that although the black nurses performed satisfactory bedside work, their chief defects, in her opinion, were "poor judgement," "irresponsibility," and "limited intellectual capacity." In sum, she asserted that the black nurses "seem incapable of abstract thinking."[9]

In a parallel manner, Ivah Uffelman of the Public Health Nursing Council in Nashville, Tennessee, confided that while she preferred not to hire black nurses in any capacity, the eight who were employed earned a minimum salary of $80 per month, while all of the white nurses received $100. Like La Forge, Uffelman considered the black graduate nurses "inferior in intelligence, in judgement, and in stability." Southern white health-care officials justified paying black nurses lower salaries in part because, as they insisted, it cost less for them to live than it did for white nurses.[10]

The denial of membership in the national professional nursing associations was the most blatant affront to black nurses' self-esteem. Furthermore, this lack of membership reflected, as perhaps nothing else did, their marginal position in the larger profession. The only significant group of black nurses belonging to the ANA prior to the First World War was the alumnae association of Freedmen's Hospital in Washington, D.C. This group continued to be a part of the larger body because it had obtained membership before the reorganization of the old Nurses' Associated Alumnae. Inasmuch as the vast majority of black nurses lived and worked in southern states, they were unable to secure membership in state associations and thus could not join the parent organizations. Excluded from membership in the NLNE and the ANA, black nurses for the most part eschewed any involvement in professional associations. A few, however, never quite acquiesced to this exclusion. Left with no other alternative, they simply went their separate ways.

The convergence of the twin processes of professionalization and the institutionalization of black subordination within nursing impelled the founding, in 1908, of the National Association of Colored Graduate Nurses (NACGN), and indirectly underlay the subsequent creation of the short-lived, but nevertheless significant, Blue Circle Nurses of the Circle for Negro Relief.[11] These two organizations represented black nurses' determination to achieve a modicum of status as professionals while embracing responsibility and gaining authority for their own personal and professional advance. An equally important impetus for their founding was the desire to band together in order to hold annual conventions, and to keep abreast of developments in the profession to improve career mobility. Though the notion was never overtly articulated by black nurse leaders, they undoubtedly used these organizations as shields from the excessive racism, hostility, and denigration of their white colleagues, behind which they developed and honed leadership skills essential to attaining the ultimate objective of integration and acceptance into the mainstream of American nursing.

Beginning in 1906, Martha Minerva Franklin (1870–1968), a black graduate (1897) of the Woman's Hospital Training School for Nurses in Philadelphia, mailed over fifteen hundred letters to black graduate nurses, superintendents of nursing schools, and nursing alumnae associations in order to determine whether interest or need existed for the founding of a separate black nursing organization. The letters struck a responsive chord among the members and leaders of the Lincoln School for Nurses Alumnae Association. Adah Belle Thoms (1870–1943), a 1905 graduate of Lincoln and president of the association, agreed to arrange a meeting. Members of the Lincoln Alumnae Association, organized in 1903, like those of the Freedmen's Hospital School of Nursing Alumni Association, organized in 1897, were eligible for membership in the American Nurses' Association.

Thoms was born in Virginia and had taught school in Richmond before migrating to New York in the 1890s, where she entered the Women's Infirmary and School of Therapeutic Massage. She worked for a time as head nurse at St. Agnes Hospital in Raleigh, North Carolina, but soon returned to New York to earn her nursing diploma at Lincoln Hospital. In August 1908, fifty-two nurses convened at St. Mark's Episcopal Church in New York City to found the NACGN and elected Franklin president. They decided to accept all black nurses for the time being, but to reserve full membership privileges for registered nurses who had been graduated from three-year hospital-based nursing schools. Three other classes of membership were associate nurses, for those who had not completed training at registered schools; lay membership, for those who were interested in the promotion of nursing in general and black nurses in particular; and honorary membership, accorded to those individuals recommended by the NACGN board of directors. In 1912 the NACGN members numbered 125, and by 1920, 500.[12]

The NACGN leadership defined a number of objectives for the new organization, some of which differed markedly from those of the white nursing associations. Like the NLNE and the ANA, black nurse leaders expressed a strong desire to improve the quality of nursing training and to exert more influence on the selection of "superior women" into the schools. They resolved to urge schools to raise admission standards, encourage black nurses to seek advanced training to qualify for positions in public-health nursing, promote interracial cooperation with white nursing groups, and attack job discrimination, salary discrepancies, and the racial exclusion practiced by the professional nursing organizations. Moreover, the NACGN leaders vowed to combat the unfair system of "dual" state registration practiced in southern states. During the forma-

Adah Belle Samuels Thoms (1870–1943), a major force in the founding and early years of the National Association of Colored Graduate Nurses (1908–1951). She served as acting director of the Lincoln Hospital School for Nurses from 1906 through 1923, and was the first recipient of the Mary Mahoney Award (1936). She authored *Pathfinders* in 1929, the first book on the history of the black nursing profession. Mabel K. Staupers Papers. Courtesy of the Moorland-Spingarn Research Center, Howard University.

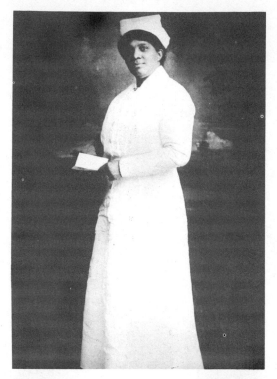

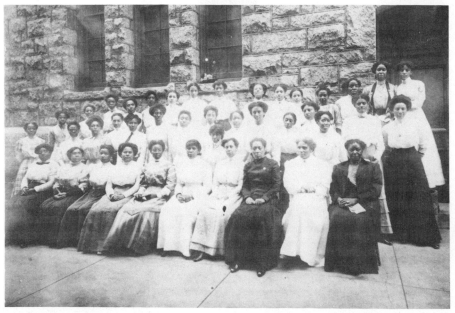

Twenty-six of the fifty-two nurses who attended the organizing meeting of the National Association of Colored Graduate Nurses participated in its first convention, held in Boston, 1909. Courtesy of the Schomburg Center for Research in Black Culture, New York Public Library.

tive years, the organization was handicapped by a lack of an official organ and headquarters. To communicate with members, leaders depended upon the black press to disseminate information about state board examinations and other pertinent activities and issues. They encouraged local affiliates to organize "coaching classes" to help black nurses better prepare for the board examinations.[13]

The process of professionalization of black nursing was littered with obstacles. Nevertheless, under the leadership of two forceful personalities, presidents Adah B. Thoms (1915–1920) and Carrie E. Bullock (1927–1930), the association did make some strides. During Thoms's presidency the NACGN secured for temporary headquarters a room in New York City in the Young Women's Christian Association's Thirty-seventh Street branch. In an address on the significance of a permanent headquarters, Thoms declared, "If we wish to keep alive the fire that now burns within us . . . we need such a place where we can come together and discuss our problems and from which to direct the affairs of the association." By 1920 the NACGN counted approximately five hundred black nurses as members. In that year, Thoms filed the NACGN incorporation papers and then established a national registry of black graduate nurses to assist them in finding employment.[14] Although most white nursing organizations maintained registries, few included black nurses.

A 1909 graduate of Provident Hospital, Bullock was born in Laurens, South Carolina, and reared by her grandparents, Thomas and Myra Crisp, who were ex-slaves. She spent two years at the Presbyterian Missionary School at Aiken, South Carolina, and in 1904 was graduated from Scotia Seminary. She taught school in a rural area at Cross Hill in South Carolina before entering the training school at Dixie Hospital in Hampton, Virginia, in 1906. A few months after entering Dixie, Bullock transferred to Provident Hospital, where she completed her nursing training. She joined the staff of the Chicago Visiting Nurses Association in 1909 and ten years later was promoted to supervisor of black nurses.[15]

Bullock focused on two key issues during her presidency. To open lines of communication between and to foster a greater sense of professional and organizational involvement among black nurses, she founded and edited, in 1928, the first issue of the NACGN's official organ, the *National News Bulletin*. Second, to encourage black women nurses to pursue postgraduate education, she initiated contact with managers of the Julius Rosenwald Fund, which subsequently led to the establishment of a special fellowship program for black graduate nurses.[16] The first recipient of the Rosenwald Fellowship was Estelle Massey Riddle Osborne, who became the first black to earn a Master of Arts degree at Teachers College, Columbia University, and who was destined to play a leading role in the history of the NACGN.

In August 1927 the NACGN held its twentieth annual session at Tuskegee Institute. The meeting was attended by more than one hundred delegates and was considered "the most successful from the point of attendance and constructive work in the history of the organization." The general program included Bullock's presidential address and various papers focused on public-health nursing, on the training of black nurses, and on one of the major health issues of the day, tuberculosis. One paper dealt with "The Art and Value of X-Ray as Anesthesia."[17] In spite of the NACGN's accomplishments in advancing the cause of black nurses by holding conventions, establishing a headquarters and registry, founding a journal, and securing a fellowship program, the deeply entrenched racism and segregation in the nursing profession and in the broader American society defied eradication.

Try as they might, black nurses found it impossible to change white nurses' negative opinions of their professional competence. Moreover, the fact that blacks as a group occupied a subordinate position in American society influenced the negative assessments of their overall leadership and intellectual abilities. In training schools and on the job, wherever black nurses encountered white nurses, such interactions appeared to reinforce mutual suspicions and, on occasion, deep loathing. There was no sorority of consciousness across the color line. Ethel Johns, in a report prepared under the aegis of the Rockefeller Foundation in 1925, pointedly opined that "if the influence of race conflict could be eliminated from the situation, the problem of the negro nurse would not differ greatly from that of the relatively inferior type of white nurse, and a common solution might possibly be found for both."[18] Indeed Johns, during a tour of twenty-three black nursing schools and interviews with white nurse supervisors, educators, and administrators of public-health agencies, was so struck by the prevalence of racism and the accompanying discrimination against black nurses that at one point in her written report she apologized: "It has not been the intention to make too much of these, but they exist and they cannot be ignored." Later, she recalled her experience of hearing the Fisk University choir sing the song "My Lord, What Shall I Do?" and declared, "That one poignant phrase expresses as nothing else could the blind groping of negro nurses towards the light they feel to be denied them."[19]

The racial attitudes, practices, and policies of northern white nurses and hospital and health-department administrators greatly circumscribed the career advancement and professional development of black nurses. Yet white nurse administrators consistently failed to assume culpability for the impediments their racism placed before black nurses, preferring instead to blame the victim for any and all alleged shortcomings. In attempting to account for the absence of black women in top-level supervisory or administrative positions at Lincoln Hospital in New York, the white superintendent alleged that the "colored nurses" did not possess the capacity to fill positions which entailed very heavy responsibility and that discipline could not be maintained without "firm and competent white direction."[20] Even Johns, a usually sensitive and impartial commentator, was prone to declare, "My observations lead me to believe that the negro woman is temperamentally unsuited for the constant unremitting grind of a hospital superintendent's life. She finds it difficult to discipline her staff and yet to remain on friendly terms with them."[21] The assistant superintendent of nursing at Harlem Hospital asserted that although "colored graduate nurses were acutely sensitive to anything that even savored of segregation," white nurses adhered to the customary practice of eating at racially separate tables in the dining room only because "the superior rank of the white nursing staff justified the segregation."[22]

In response to queries as to why black nurses were not well represented in administrative positions at the New York Board of Health, the director of nursing service, Welhelmina Rothermund, explained that white nurses would strongly resent any arrangement which would "entail a colored woman being given direction of white nurses." Rothermund unapologetically insisted that any alteration of the composition of the city's public-health staff, which was composed of 375 nurses, 40 of whom were black, was impossible because "too large a proportion of negro women might have the unfortunate effect of preventing desirable white nurses from joining the staff."[23]

White nurse administrators in Chicago were equally as blind to the effects of their racial attitudes on the professional aspirations of black nurses. Convinced of the so-called inferiority of black nurses, Margaret Butler, chief nurse of the Chicago City Health Department, which employed 10 black and 158 white nurses frankly admitted a preference for hiring only whites. She contended that black nurses' techniques were "inferior to that of the white nurses, they are not punctual, and are incapable of analyzing a social situation." Butler added that, in her opinion, black nurses did poor clerical work and were able to be used only among the black population. Moreover, she declared that even "the colored group," if presented a choice, preferred the services of a white nurse. Without elaborating on the specifics of the racial friction between black and white nurses, Butler asserted that black nurses created problems because of their marked tendency "to organize against authority" and "to engage in political intrigue."[24] Such assertions obviously reflect the fact that black nurses resented the negative perceptions of their abilities and used whatever means they could to protect their tenuous positions.

Margaret Hanrahan, director of nursing service at the Chicago Municipal Tuberculosis Service, echoed Butler's contentions. She indicated that the 16 black nurses were segregated from their 140 white counterparts and were completely "kept away from white patients." Like Butler, Hanrahan charged that the black nurses "worked well with their hands but know nothing of social problems and are unable to handle the situation." She too expressed dismay mixed with contempt in asserting that black nurses "do not hesitate to use political influence in connection with their appointments." The director thereupon lamented the great difficulty she experienced in trying to dismiss black nurses without "stirring up trouble."[25]

By the mid-twenties more than two-thirds of the approximately twenty-five hundred black graduate nurses, as was the case with white nurses, worked in institutional settings or in private duty.[26] Economic exigencies and racism compelled many of them to act in ways which reinforced existing negative images of them in the minds of their white colleagues. Undoubtedly many white private-duty or bedside nurses feared that any increase in the number of black private-duty nurses would exacerbate their own economically depressed condition. Such fears only fed tensions and widened the gulf between the two groups situated at the bottom of the nursing-profession hierarchy.

To be sure, white nurses may have had just reason to resent the black nurses, yet few accepted the fact that their own attitudes contributed to the behavior of their black fellow professionals. For example, many black nurses charged lower prices for their services and worked longer hours. They were frequently expected to, and often did, perform household and child-care chores in addition to tending to the sick members of a family. Indeed, the fact that many white physicians, especially in the South, spoke in glowing terms of the submissive and accommodating black nurses who adapted "well to the needs of the household" and who were "willing to render the small personal services only grudgingly performed by white nurses," did not endear them to white nurses.[27]

During the 1920s and 1930s, as hospitals attracted more paying patients, the demand for and status of all private-duty nurses declined. Historian Susan Reverby has argued that "by the mid-1930s, the old system of staffing hospitals primarily with nursing students began to crack." The decline of private duty added to the unchecked proliferation of nurses, perhaps encouraging white perceptions of black nurses as those least committed to advancing the profession and more willing to compromise on salary and working conditions. Thus among practically all groups of white nurses, whether involved in hospital work, private practice, educational institutions, public-health associations, or professional organizations, located in the North or South, the predominant image of the black nurse was that of a professional, moral, and social inferior.[28] The white superintendent of nurses for both the white and black divisions of Henry Grady Hospital in Atlanta, Anne Bess Feeback, confessed "a frank contempt for 'niggers.'" She declared, "They can't direct one another, a negro cannot work a negro," adding that "most of them haven't any morals." Feeback went on to share her opinion of the black student nurses under her charge: "They are such liars. . . . They shift responsibility whenever they can. . . . They quarrel constantly among themselves and will cut up each other's clothes for spite. . . . Unless they are constantly watched, they will steal anything in sight."[29]

White nurse educator Margaret Bruesche bore responsibility for instructing the black student nurses at the Tennessee Coal and Iron Company Employees' Hospital located in Fairfield, Alabama. Her opinions of black students were virtually identical to, and equally as hostile as, those expressed by Feeback. Bruesche believed that "the negro woman has no place as a graduate nurse." On the other hand, she advised that the black woman could "fill a great need in the South as a trained attendant, who would work for a lower wage than the fully trained woman." Bruesche claimed that black women simply lacked the intelligence and educational background to become good graduate nurses. She asserted that only about one-sixth of the black nursing students could be compared to even "the most mediocre white student." She elaborated, "They are fit only for the practical side of things," inasmuch as "they lack judgement, they are not conscientious and their sense of responsibility is very weak."[30]

To be sure, not all white nurses held disparaging and hostile opinions of black nurses. Several directors of visiting nursing services did comment favorably on the role of the small number of black nurses doing public-health work. Lillian Wald, founder of the Henry Street Settlement and a staunch friend of black nurses, employed 25 black and 150 white nurses, paid them equal salaries, and accorded them identical professional courtesies and recognition. Even here, however, black and white nurses were treated differently in two respects: black nurses were never sent to white homes, nor were they promoted to supervisory positions.[31]

In short, as far as white nurse educators, administrators, supervisors, and leaders were concerned, black nurses' low status in the profession was a result of their allegedly inferior training, lack of executive skills, limited intelligence, weak character, and inability to withstand pressure. Only when she dealt with black patients did the black nurse stand a chance of being referred to as a competent and adept professional. Only to the extent that she remained stationed within the black community, caring only for black patients, could she earn praise and respect from her white counterparts. Ethel Johns embodied the crux of the race and status dilemma of black nursing when she argued:

> It is quite apparent that the negro nurse cannot be utilized successfully in public health work except among her own people. Even among them she has not the same authority as the white nurse although she has a better psychological approach. She has been very successful in overcoming their

superstitious fears regarding immunization, vaccination and other preventative measures. The social and economic problems involved in case work are commonly too much for her but she can ferret out information and interpret domestic complications which would baffle a white nurse who lacks her intuitive understanding of racial characteristics.[32]

When even such an enlightened white nurse as Ethel Johns embraced such an unfounded notion of the inherent limited abilities of black nurses, is there little wonder that their status on the nursing ladder remained firmly on the bottom rung?

White nurses were joined in their discrimination against and low estimation of black nurses by various federal agencies, specifically the Armed Forces Nurse Corps and the American Red Cross. The leaders of these organizations shattered many a black nurse's dream of achieving acceptance, recognition, higher status, and increased public esteem during and after World War I. The racially exclusionary practices and policies of the federal government had a dual impact. While they reinforced some black nurses' sense of professional marginality and alienation, they simultaneously strengthened others' resistance to being regarded as outcasts.

In spite of the dismal record of the Woodrow Wilson presidential administration on racial issues, the advent of World War I momentarily encouraged black nurses and the leaders of the NACGN to intensify their quest for professional recognition and acceptance. In his first term in office, Wilson had issued an executive order establishing racially separate eating and restroom facilities in government buildings. Additional laws receiving his approval segregated and eliminated numbers of blacks from civil service jobs.[33] Nevertheless, black nurses looked to the war emergency and the ensuing call for nurses to make available to them as well as their white colleagues the opportunity to serve their country, and to demonstrate, once and for all, their skill and competency.[34]

Undaunted by the past record of exclusion, a number of black nurses immediately attempted to enlist in the Armed Forces Nurse Corps, then managed by the American Red Cross. The Red Cross had been incorporated in 1900 and was reorganized and recognized by the U.S. Congress on January 5, 1905, as an official auxiliary of the Army Nurse Corps. It assumed full responsibility for identifying, recruiting, and enrolling nurses, plus establishing a pool from which the Army Nurse Corps selected personnel as the need arose.[35] Under the leadership of the former superintendent of the Army Nurse Corps and chairman of the National Red Cross, Jane Delano, a graduate of Bellevue Hospital Nursing School, the first group of 120 American Red Cross Nurses was organized and sent overseas.[36] In 1912 the Red Cross was again reorganized. Delano crafted a voluntary affiliation between the organization and the American

Nurses' Association in which the ANA agreed to supply the Red Cross with nurses required for military service. The Red Cross classified into First and Second reserves the nurses who possessed the educational, moral, and personal qualifications required by the military nurse corps. The Second Reserve consisted of nurses who were available for critical civilian nursing but who were not eligible for service in the First Reserve.[37]

Black nurses quickly volunteered but waited in vain for calls from the Army Nurse Corps and the Red Cross. Several wrote Jane Delano and even the surgeon general seeking some explanation for their exclusion. Delano responded to all queries as to why so few black nurses were called or enrolled into either the First or Second Reserve: "We are enrolling colored nurses at the present time and shall continue to do so in order that they may be available if at any time there is an opportunity to assign them to duty in military hospitals."[38] The time and opportunity, however, never came.

When the Red Cross was criticized for its failure to call and assign black nurses, its leaders first insisted that few of the black nurses who volunteered met the prerequisite of having been graduated from a hospital maintaining at least a fifty-bed occupancy. In the face of further black protest, the Red Cross reluctantly agreed to give some black women provisional enrollment until they were registered or had acquired additional training in larger hospital training schools.[39]

Throughout the war, leaders of the army had been ambivalent as to whether to tap black nursing service. The navy, however, refused even to consider the matter. Actually, a month before the war ended with the signing of the armistice on November 11, 1918, the Red Cross called a couple of dozen black nurses to serve at three army camps, Sherman in Ohio, Grant in Illinois, and Sevier in South Carolina. During the war, twenty-two thousand nurses were enrolled in the Army Nurse Corps. Of these, eleven thousand served in government hospitals and installations in the United States, and approximately ten thousand were sent overseas. The Red Cross nurses numbered about eleven thousand. Thus, approximately thirty-three thousand nurses served in the war effort. One black nurse leader, commenting on the fact that only thirty or so black nurses were called to duty, and that at the end of World War I, bitterly proclaimed, "We were left out."[40]

As the war drew to an end, the American Red Cross received increasingly sharp criticism, and not only from black nurses. In spite of the explanation and reassurances its officials proffered, black nurses, educators, and civil rights leaders relentlessly challenged the organization's apparent reluctance to call black nurses into active war service. Robert R. Moton, successor to Booker T. Washington as president of Tuskegee Institute, and Emmett J. Scott, black special assistant in the War Department, raised the issue time after time with government officials. Black leaders wrote to the secretary of war and the surgeon general informing them of the widespread black disillusionment with the American Red Cross. Moton declared that the Red Cross's "exclusion of colored nurses . . . reacts in a certain sort of indifference on the part of colored people which ought not to be when the country needs every ounce of effort along every available line."[41]

Although they agitated for the right to serve in the Army Nurse Corps, black nurse leaders of the NACGN, sensing the futility of this quest, resolved to work on other fronts to demonstrate their value. In 1917, Adah Thoms led the way by helping to set up an organization of visiting nurses associated with the recently founded Circle for Negro War Relief. The board of directors of this new service organization comprised some of the country's most prominent and influential white and black, male and female, citizens. Editor of the NAACP's *Crisis*, W. E. B. Du Bois; Tuskegee's president, Robert R. Moton; former New York governor Charles Young; writer Ray Stannard Baker; Grace Neil Johnson (wife of NAACP Executive Secretary James Weldon Johnson); white philanthropist George Foster Peabody; and Captain Arthur B. Spingarn (future head of the NAACP's legal council) were a few of the prominent members.[42] The Circle's objective, defined in a manner strikingly similar to that of the American Red Cross, was to promote the interests and improve the conditions of black soldiers and sailors at home and abroad.

In order to carry out an important feature of the Circle's envisioned national public-health work, and especially to provide care and assistance to needy black families of disabled servicemen, Adah Thoms helped to establish a new order of black war nurses, called the Blue Circle Nurses. The Circle for Negro War Relief recruited these nurses and paid them to work in local communities, instructing poor rural blacks on the importance of sanitation, proper diet, and appropriate clothing. In several communities they virtually functioned as visiting or public-health nurses, maintaining contact with county and state health officials in order to alert them to serious health problems among black residents. In many respects the Blue Circle Nurses administered to that black constituency infrequently or inadequately served by the American Red Cross. When the war ended, the Circle for Negro War Relief leaders dropped *War* from the name and assumed the new appellation the Circle for Negro Relief Incorporated. By 1919 the Circle leaders had drafted a new peacetime program focused primarily on providing health and welfare assistance to impoverished rural black southern communities.[43] Circle officials sought in vain, however, to raise all of the money necessary to train and pay portions of the salaries of the Blue Circle Nurses, to create day nurseries and kindergartens, and to provide financial assistance to small, struggling community hospitals.

As she became more involved with the Circle, Thoms, along with Etnah R. Boutté, the Circle's executive secretary, dreamed of transforming it into a "clearing house" for black nurses. They convinced themselves that it could become a national institution or a central organization capable of standardizing and coordinating the black public-health work done by all black organizations across the country. Thoms and Boutté believed that the cooperation and endorsement of the American Red Cross and substantial financial contributions from philanthropic foundations would ensure the success of the envisioned program.

Thereupon, to raise funds to pay the Blue Circle Nurses' salaries and to operate the organization, Boutté and Thoms appealed to the managers of the major white philanthropic foundations. Edwin Embree of the Rockefeller Foundation assured the Circle of the foundation's sympathy and commitment to improving black health care but denied the request for funds. Embree, however, did elaborate on the rejection in a private interoffice memorandum to the extent that, as far as he could determine, most of the Circle's meager resources were used to cover overhead expenses. Moreover, he reiterated that it was contrary to the foundation's policy to contribute to private voluntary health-care agencies.[44]

Undaunted by the failure to secure foundation funding, Boutté and Thoms proceeded with plans (dreams may be a more apt description) to work out an affiliation with the American Red Cross. The Circle board organized a committee in cooperation with the Red Cross and named white attorney and NAACP official Arthur B. Spingarn as chair. From 1920 to 1923 Boutté and Thoms, conducting the actual negotiations, met with Red Cross leaders and representatives of the U.S. Public Health Service.[45]

Thoms and Boutté greatly desired the affiliation but were equally as determined to preserve a separate and distinct identity for the Blue Circle Nurses. They insisted that Circle nurses did not want to become carbon Red Cross nurses but preferred to retain their distinct identities, and to wear their own emblems and uniforms. They supported the suggestion that all Blue Circle Nurses should be required to meet the same requirements for qualification as established by the American Red Cross. Thoms and Boutté also agreed to place the Circle nursing service under the authority of the supervising nurse of each state department of health or to have the director of the local Red Cross division of nursing monitor their work. Thoms even went so far as to volunteer to serve a half-day each week in the Circle's headquarters, to assume responsibility for the recruitment of black nurses, and to write a monthly report describing Circle nursing activities to the Red Cross director of nursing. In return for all these concessions, Thoms and Boutté asked only that the Circle remain a distinctly identifiable entity and that local Red Cross chapters assist in paying the salaries of the Blue Circle Nurses.[46]

In their internal deliberations, the Red Cross leadership conceded that their organization had failed to address adequately the needs of blacks. They admitted that the appointing of only six black nurses in the entire South under the aegis of the Bureau of Public Health Nursing of the Red Cross was a gross underrepresentation and underutilization of available black nursing talent.[47] Although many white public-health nurses were employed in the South, much of their work had been restricted by the local customs and laws prohibiting white women from nursing black people, especially black men. One interoffice Red Cross memorandum noted that "many towns and counties made up almost entirely of colored people have been given no nursing service whatsoever." Clearly, then, any arrangement whereby Circle nurses could undertake some of the public-health work in the South would have improved the Red Cross's efforts. Red Cross leaders were not unmindful of the opportunity affiliation would provide to encourage larger numbers of black women to enter the field of public-health nursing. The memorandum continued: "It would seem to be sound policy to stimulate moral and financial responsibility among the colored for work among their own people and to give them an opportunity for service according to recognized standards."[48]

Still, compelling reasons notwithstanding, the Red Cross leaders were extremely skeptical and reluctant to endorse the proposed plan. One memorandum delineated the five arguments against cooperation. Red Cross leaders accused the Circle officers of being ignorant: "The National Officers of the Circle appear to have little knowledge of the scope, standards or practice of public health nursing." The organization was then criticized for being unprepared to conduct its part of the plan: "The Circle has no public health nurse in its national headquarters or in the field to direct the organization of such work, to secure qualified personnel and to supervise the work." This point led to the assertion that there were in fact few black nurses prepared to do public-health nursing: "There is at present no body of colored nurses trained for this work and the tendency would be to use untrained workers." Given the above, the conclusion drawn was that black nurses were simply not capable: "Experience has shown that while colored women make good bedside nurses, they have little initiative, executive ability or organizing ability." The fifth argument reflected a pragmatic assessment of and capitulation to southern racial mores and a closing justification for eschewing cooperation with the Circle: "Prejudice is so great in the South that white nurses will refuse to take up public health nursing if colored nurses are employed on the same status. It would be necessary in all cases to place the colored nurse under a white nurse."[49]

It was only a matter of time before all recognized the futility of further discussion. Black and white nurses had a long way to go before they could agree to cooperate on anything. In the mid- to late twenties, the Circle, now the National Health Circle for Colored People, concentrated on providing scholarships to black nurses to take postgraduate courses in public-health nursing.[50]

Black nurses, excluded from membership in the white professional nursing organization, founded and worked with alternative structures. Yet the NACGN and the Blue Circle for Negro Relief never denied their yearning to be accepted and recognized as competent professionals by the larger organizations. Further advance in the status of black nurses awaited change in the larger society's racial attitudes and practices. It was up to black nurses, however, to transform themselves into effective agents for social and professional change. After all, progress never is achieved by those who sit and wait. As Thoms probably would have put it, black nurses had to create their own paths to equality.

The Politics of Agency
and the Revitalization of the NACGN

The 1930s and the advent of the Great Depression spelled disaster for the vast majority of Americans. Black nurses were no more immune to the ravages of this greatest period of economic dislocation than anyone else in American society. They already had been relegated to the bottom of the nursing profession, and the Depression merely deepened their economic woes. The persistence of racial discrimination and exclusion as practiced by white nurses and the institutional infrastructure of the profession—schools, hospitals, associations, and public-health agencies—exacerbated feelings of frustration. To be sure, many black nurses continued to work for reduced wages, when they could get them, and turned their attention inward, toward helping their families and the communities in which they resided. These nurses, though deeply affected by racial discrimination and professional exclusion, focused on doing the best they could to get by. During this period the median salary for Negro nurses was approximately one thousand two hundred dollars per year. Those employed in private duty were especially susceptible to economic fluctuations and often earned significantly less than this amount.[1]

Yet there were always a few black nurses possessed of tremendous energy, optimism, and leadership potential who refused to accept the second-class status to which they had been assigned within the profession. These women chafed under the denial of educational opportunities and discriminatory hiring and wages. They objected to the prevalent attitude that the color of their skin and the texture of their hair meant that they were inferior human beings and therefore inferior nurses, unworthy of fair and equitable treatment and respect.

The few black women who emerged as leaders and spokespersons for the majority of the nation's approximately four thousand black nurses were determined to break the shackles of their oppression. As one black physician described them, "These hard-headed, practical women have no misconception as to nurses being 'angels of mercy.'" To launch a major, sustained assault against the structure of oppression erected over the previous five to six decades, however, required more than sheer grit, will, and determination. For over three generations, white nurses and the structures in which they were trained and worked had solidified and institutionalized negative attitudes and actions toward black nurses. Segregation and separation of the races within the profession seemed the natural order of things. Seventeen southern state affiliates of the American Nurses' Association and the National League of Nursing Education flatly denied black nurses membership.[2] As always, of course, there were some individual white nurses who despaired over the discrimination black nurses encountered. These women were potential allies of the black nurses, but like their darker-hued colleagues they often possessed neither the power nor the resources to challenge effectively the wall of segregation and separation within their chosen profession.

At the outset of the decade, prospects for improved race relations within nursing appeared bleak indeed. Yet there were small glimmers of hope shining through the thick fog of racism. The black nurses may not have possessed tremendous financial resources, and the number of well-trained leaders may have been few. But what they did have, and this proved significant, was the skeleton of an organization, floundering on the brink of dissolution, to be sure, but not yet expired—the National Association of Colored Graduate Nurses. Thus, they knew, as did some of their potential white allies, that a revitalization of the NACGN was absolutely essential to the success of their quest for full integration into the mainstream of American nursing. But in 1933 the association counted only 175 members.[3]

There were many reasons for the less-than-noteworthy record of success in the struggle against racial discrimination and segregation on the national front. Heading the list were the shortage of funds, the lack of a national headquarters, and the absence of a salaried executive director. A most critical need was for a clearly defined and articulated strategy to achieve integration. To become a force in the world of nursing politics, to win for black nurses respect, fair compensation for their work, and equal access to educational institutions, the NACGN needed funds, friends, leaders, and a strategy, or rather a multiplicity of strategies, operating in concert. Critical to all of these requirements was the need of a healthy dose of patience, for as the black nurse leaders knew, effecting social and attitudinal change within a profession, as within the society at large, was slow, tedious, and frequently frustrating work.

Perhaps it was the existence of such widespread black misery in America in spite of the New Deal reforms of Franklin Roosevelt, or maybe it was the gathering storm on the European front with the rise of German Fascism and Italian Nazism. It could have been the growing militance of blacks such as Marcus Garvey and A. Philip Randolph, or even the threat of an increasingly attractive Communism. Perhaps it was all of these things, and more, that made the bleak 1930s a decade nevertheless fraught with pregnant possibilities for black nurses' advance.[4] After all, blacks were so far down, there was no place to go but up. Just as black nurses possessed no immunity to economic impoverishment, they could not escape being affected by the political currents swirling across the country and the globe. If integration into nursing and destruction of the Jim Crow barriers were to be achieved, then the foundation for the struggle to eradicate the color line had to be laid in this most propitious of decades.

Three elements converged in the mid-thirties to set the course for the transformation of black nursing fortunes. There was a noticeable change in the perspectives of some key white nursing leaders, especially evident in the new advocacy role of white officers of the National Organization for Public Health Nursing. Moreover, the willingness of white philanthropists, notably Frances Payne Bolton of Cleveland, Ohio, the Julius Rosenwald Fund, and the General Education Board, to underwrite all expenses incurred in the NACGN-led struggle for integration proved of no small import. Significantly, the emergence of two talented black nursing leaders, Estelle Massey Riddle and Mabel K. Staupers, who eagerly assumed the reins of the fledgling NACGN and worked assiduously to resuscitate it, proved most critical to the mobilization of the entire black nursing profession. The connections between these factors and the development and evolution of a unique style of black nursing leadership cohered in the mid- to late 1930s to lay the foundation for the achievement of nursing integration in the aftermath of World War II.

On January 27, 1934, the NACGN sponsored its first regional conference to assess the status of black nurses and to lay a course for future development. The conferees met at Lincoln Hospital in New York. In attendance were the white executive secretaries of the American Nurses' Association, the National League of Nursing Education, and the National Organization for Public Health Nursing. Also attending were officials of the Julius Rosenwald Fund, the National Medical Association, and the National Health Circle for Colored People, many of the directors of black schools of nursing in the Northeast, along with members of local affiliates and the board of directors of the NACGN. The official organs of the National Urban League and the NAACP, *Opportunity Magazine: A Journal of Negro Life* and *Crisis*, respectively, also sent representatives to the meeting, which was subsequently dubbed "to be just as important to the future of the Negro nurse as the first historic meeting of the NACGN in 1908."[5]

The conference agenda focused on the following problems: the impact of the economic crisis on the salaries and wages of black nurses; the urgent need to train more black public-health nurses; the continued discrimination against and denial of admission of black nurses to universities offering advanced courses in nursing; the difficulty inherent in improving the black hospital nursing schools; and finally, the need to develop the NACGN "so that it might serve as an instrument for representing the Negro nurse in every area of nursing in communities across the nation." There was some attention devoted to the concern to bring the black nurses' organization closer to the other national nursing organizations. As was later reported, "the most immediate result of the conference was the unanimous decision to establish national headquarters again despite the economic instability of the Negro nurse at that time, and to appoint a nurse executive who could carry forward a program of action."[6]

There was yet another immediate result of the New York NACGN regional conference, the sensitizing of white nurse leaders to the problems of the black nurse. Although white nursing leaders had not devoted a great deal of attention to black nurses and their low status within the profession, even the most distracted of them had to have been aware of this issue. Granted, white nurse leaders had to be, and often were, more concerned with the issues of nurse registration, licensure, the need for quality postgraduate instruction, the proliferation of hospitals and the attendant decline in patient cases available for private-duty nurses, and the development of collegiate departments of nursing. They had to expend considerable energy protecting hard-won gains, and preserving nursing autonomy in the face of an imperialistic and dominating male medical profession. This is merely to point out that there were dozens of major issues and concerns daily confronting and demanding the attention of the elite white nursing leaders.[7] Yet, the problem of black nurses was also important, and not amenable to quick redress. Try as they might to avoid the issue, some white nurse leaders were well aware that the day was near when they would have to confront and revoke policies contributing to the professional ostracism of the black nurse.

The day before the January 27, 1934, black nurses' regional conference, white nurse Alma Haupt, associate director of the National Organization for Public Health Nursing, placed the issue of black nurses and their future relationship to organized white nursing squarely before the members of the board of directors of the American Nurses' Association. In a sharply focused statement, Haupt challenged her colleagues to think creatively and constructively about the future relationship between black nurses and the ANA.[8] That a leader of the NOPHN should have been the one to press the issue and articulate the problems and difficulties of black nurses is not surprising. As historian M. Louise Fitzpatrick argues, the NOPHN leaders could well afford to take risks to advocate unpopular causes, to adopt and express progressive postures regarding race relations. Fitzpatrick posits that, compared to the white leaders of other nursing organizations, the NOPHN leaders usually occupied the vanguard of movements for improved health care.[9]

In a similar vein, historian Barbara Melosh suggests that "by the measures of aspiring professionals, public-health nurses did constitute an elite." Melosh elaborates: "They had more education than their counterparts in private duty and on hospital staffs, and, on the average, they could claim more credentials than even supervisory or administrative nurses in hospitals." She further notes that "many public health nurses were recruited from the more prestigious schools of nursing in larger hospitals—another measure of stature within nursing." Historian Karen Buhler-Wilkerson offers a different perspective on public-health nursing. She argues that the field was actually in decline by the mid-1920s because of the virtual cessation of immigration, the growth in hospital occupancy, the increased difficulty of raising funds for programs and agencies, and the declining significance of infectious diseases among white Americans.[10]

While the relative supremacy of the three nursing groups—private-duty, hospital staff, or public-health—remains open to question, the important fact is that the NOPHN had early evidenced a concern for black nursing, especially black public-health nursing. Indeed, as early as 1930 the organization had played a major role, with financial support from the Julius Rosenwald Fund, in conducting a revealing study of black public-health nursing. In the published report, salary inequalities, job discrimination, and the limited nature of educational opportunities available to black nurses had received candid and judicious treatment.[11] Again, as Fitzpatrick observes, the NOPHN was "in sympathy with the NACGN," and more than any of the other nursing organizations, it took positive steps toward supporting and aiding the black nursing association. The NOPHN was the first white nursing group to "endorse a program of equal salaries and opportunities for employment for all public health nurses, regardless of race, color or creed."[12] In part, to explain these liberal leanings on matters of race, it bears noting also that the NOPHN, among the largely conservative professional organizations, long enjoyed the reputation of being a radical, albeit elite, organization of nurses. This perception was undoubtedly fed by the widely based nature of community support and the active involvement of many influential and wealthy lay patrons in the affairs of the organization.[13]

Alma Haupt's speech to the ANA board of directors underscored a sense of urgency both to deal with the position of black nurses in the profession and to discover ways of improving race relations. She first identified what she perceived to be the most pressing need of black nurses: "I think the immediate objective is to develop leadership among the negro group." In a reflection laden with patronizing overtones, however, Haupt asserted,

"They have still such a long way to go. Few of them ever sat on a committee and only a few know how to preside at a meeting."[14] Of course the comment was unfounded inasmuch as black nurses had been presiding over the meetings of their own organizations and clubs since the turn of the century. But Haupt knew this, so her preliminary remarks were simply designed to buttress her suggestion that white nurses help black nurses develop leadership skills by inviting them to participate in and to serve on special committees within the ANA and the National League of Nursing Education.

Haupt then queried the board members, perhaps rhetorically, "I would like to know if you think that it is sound development to go on encouraging them to raise money for an Executive Secretary and for Headquarters near us?"[15] The question reflected the outside status of black nurses and the fact that the NACGN possessed neither a salaried executive nor office quarters where the other nursing organizations were located. It also hints that from time to time previously, at least some of the white nurses had encouraged and supported black nurses. Whether financial or moral, the nature of that support remained unclear.

Haupt's speech illuminates yet a deeper motive for forging closer professional ties between black and white nurses. Appealing to their need and desire to preserve professional autonomy, Haupt warned white nurses that neglect of and disinterest in black nurses could ultimately result in black nurses' aligning themselves more tightly with black doctors. She explained, "There is another factor about our helping them now. There is a National Medical Association composed of colored physicians and they include nurses and pharmacists; and there is a negro hospital association. They have asked the negro nurses' association to form a joint committee." Haupt cautioned her white colleagues, "I think that unless we keep very close to them they are apt to become a subsidiary group to other negro associations."[16]

White nurse leaders, regardless of their organizational affiliations, were of one mind when it came to the matter of maintaining professional autonomy. They had fought long and hard to draw the boundaries between the nursing and medical professions and desired more than anything to be viewed as a distinct group of professionals complete with their own code of professional ethics, practice, and pedagogy. They yearned to break away from the stereotype of nurse as "physician's hand." Nurses continually insisted that they were equal members in the health care–delivery enterprise. For a group of professional nurses, regardless of racial identity, willingly to become a subsidiary of a group of doctors or hospital administrators constituted a breach of faith and could not be allowed to occur, especially at this stage in nursing's historical development. To allow black nurses to become allies with, and possibly come under the control of, black physicians would establish a potentially damaging precedent. Yet what could the white nurses do to protect the profession and prevent the black nursing organization from embarking upon this course of action? Public-health nurses were especially sensitive to this issue of autonomy and control, and thus, again, it is no surprise that Haupt alerted the ANA leadership. As historian Melosh points out, "The organization of public-health work provided an institutional form within which nurses' independence could flourish. . . . More than either private-duty or hospital nurses, public-health nurses shook off their role as the physician's hand, to set out and act on their own sense of nursing's sphere and missions."[17]

To be sure, Haupt's warnings and fears, whether real or imagined, placed her fellow white nurses in a quandary. None of them questioned the wisdom or necessity to "keep very close" and thus exercise more control over black nurses to prevent them from even exploring the possibility of forming a subsidiary alliance with black physicians and hospital administrators. The problem white nurses had to contend with was one of strategy. There were two options, neither of them satisfactory: They could move to absorb black nurses into the white professional organizations, or they could simply ignore the issue and hope for the best. To integrate black nurses would have been the rational thing to do, but racism is seldom rational. Haupt well understood that the vast majority of white nurses would rather risk assaults to professional autonomy than jeopardize the racial integrity of their professional organizations. Integration would have entailed the effective dismantling of the whole edifice of racial segregation and separatism.

Haupt, deeply mindful of the ambivalence of her white colleagues, addressed both sides of this dilemma. She asked her white colleagues, "Should we look forward in the future to having them in all our organization[s]?" She reiterated, "Is our final objective to bring them in with us?" Taking another tack, perhaps anticipating their objections, Haupt confided that she did not really think that black nurses were ready for full participation in or integration into the organized structure of nursing. She went so far as to muse, "I think they [black nurses] would like to be included and be considered as professional equals—not social but professional—but they realize that is a long time in the future."[18]

It is important to keep in mind that this was 1934, and the country as a whole had rejected the idea of social equality for black people. Haupt, like many Americans, believed that blacks, in this instance black nurses, needed somehow to elevate themselves to a higher level before social equality could be conferred. The burden rested heavily upon the victim, the black outsider. She suggested a way out for the white nurses by recommending that perhaps it was necessary to perpetuate separate black and white nursing organizations until white nurses had a chance "to develop leadership among them [black nurses] and to accustom us to working with them." Meanwhile, Haupt advised that white nursing groups support the development of a stronger NACGN with a nationwide network of state affiliates. A stronger NACGN, she reasoned, would provide black nurses the organizational framework within which to develop more leadership talent. She concluded her remarks with a recommendation implicit in the question, "If you develop separate negro nursing associations in the states, could there be some change in the ANA by-laws by which members of those states' associations could be members of the ANA?"[19]

Haupt's query concerning a future alteration in the ANA's membership process was born of the unique policy the NOPHN had adopted regarding black members. The organization permitted members to join directly through the national body and thus was at structural variance with the ANA's policy, which mandated that prospective members join the national body only through constituent state associations. To have permitted black nurses to become members of the ANA through separate NACGN affiliates would have required a fundamental overhaul of the association's entire structure. The composition of the membership of the two organizations also differed in significant ways. Unlike the NOPHN with its highly educated members, the ANA was basically an association of private-duty nurses, precisely those most threatened by economic competition with black nurses. Historian Susan Reverby, after noting the heavy concentration of private-duty nurses among ANA members, observed, "Those who stayed in private duty, the majority of whom were graduates of the smaller nursing schools, were often less educated and less prepared than nurses in either institutional or public health positions."[20]

While some of the ANA leaders, almost all of whom were public-health nurses, educators, or superintendents, undoubtedly shared most of Haupt's and the NOPHN's views on the necessity of integrating black women into the organization, their less progressive and more economically vulnerable membership thought otherwise. Actively to pursue an integrationist policy would have meant alienating the membership further, and this the leaders were unprepared to do. Moreover, the association's leaders had to be mindful of the fact that the vast majority of graduate nurses were not yet ANA members; thus, to some extent future recruitment, growth, and development of the ANA dictated a careful adherence to the color line. As late as 1928, only three out of every ten active graduate nurses in the United States belonged to the ANA.

As the decade of the 1930s opened, private-duty nurses still constituted the clear plurality of employed nurses, and they jealously guarded their control over state nursing associations.[21] It was upon these white nurses that any burden of achieving integration in the organization would be placed. Under the best of circumstances, then, an attempt to implement a new membership structure so as to accommodate black nurses threat-

ened organizational suicide for the ANA. Thus it is not surprising that
in 1934 the association's leaders offered no official resolution or response
to Haupt's queries or recommendations. Probably none was needed. Yet
the fact that she raised these issues in a formal presentation to the ANA's
board of directors reflects a deepening consciousness among white nursing leaders of the special problems of discrimination and segregation that
shaped and retarded the professional development and careers of black
nurses. These debates concerning the nature of race relations within
nursing continued through the 1930s.

At the same time that white nurse leaders were becoming increasingly
sensitive to the urgent need to raise the status of black nurses, so too
were key white philanthropists, in particular Frances Payne Bolton of
Cleveland, Ohio, and the officers of the Julius Rosenwald Fund. Bolton,
born in 1885, was an heiress. One of her uncles, Oliver Payne, had
cofounded with John D. Rockefeller the Standard Oil Company and had
established a substantial trust for her. From 1918 Bolton remained an
active member of the NOPHN's advisory council, serving on its finance
committee at one point. During this early period, she served as director
of the Cleveland Visiting Nurses Association and apparently developed
a lifelong commitment to the ideal of social service as a way of improving
society. Bolton had accompanied her husband, U.S. Republican Congressman Chester Bolton, to Washington, D.C., in 1929. Ten years later, following his untimely death, she would assume his congressional seat.
From the House of Representatives, and as chief architect of the 1943
Bolton Bill establishing the U.S. Cadet Nurses program, Bolton rendered
invaluable assistance to nurses of every stripe and hue.[22]

Bolton and the Rosenwald Fund were the major white benefactors to
respond to appeals for the financial assistance needed to bring into existence a stronger, revitalized organization of black nurses. To be sure, Bolton had for years given generously of her time and money to promote
nurses' interests. Although she was a long-time friend of nurses and a
strong advocate of their interests, it is not altogether clear why she desired to assist in the transformation of the NACGN into a potent weapon
with which black nurses could mount a sustained attack against the exclusion and discriminatory treatment they suffered. Bolton appeared immune to the racist stereotypes then prevalent throughout America. In
1934 she gave $250 to the NACGN and pledged to match an additional
$1,000 raised from other sources. This was only the beginning of a si-
lent partnership between an elite white woman patron and black nurse
leaders. From 1934 to 1951 Bolton annually contributed $2,000 to the
NACGN, divided into quarterly installments. This sum paid much of
the $2,500 annual salary of the soon-to-be-hired NACGN executive
secretary.

Much of the work, progress, and development of the NACGN could not have been achieved without Bolton's support. Yet Bolton eschewed public acknowledgment or celebration of her giving, seeming to prefer to remain in the background, advising, persuading, pressuring, cajoling those black and white organizations, educational institutions, and leaders to move steadily forward in the struggle to eradicate the racial barriers in nursing. U.S. Senator Margaret Chase Smith of Maine offered a penetrating description of her friend Bolton:

> Frances often is most active on behalf of an issue when she seems to be doing nothing. She approaches a problem with skill and versatility, learning just who should be talked to or won over before she moves. She can subordinate herself to the goal, too, when that seems the best strategy, and she has a great talent for reconciling people and conflicting points of view. One reason for her success is that she has mastered the technique of disagreeing agreeably.[23]

Second only to Bolton's giving was that of the Julius Rosenwald Fund. Black physician M. O. Bousfield, associate director for Negro health of the Rosenwald Fund, developed a close, mutually respectful relationship with the black nurse leaders. In 1934 the fund granted the NACGN $1,250, and it followed up the next year with another $900. Whereas Bolton's money was designated to pay most of the salary of an NACGN executive secretary, the Rosenwald contributions went directly toward the rental of a new headquarters, and paid much of the travel expenses incurred as the executive director traversed the country speaking to and urging black nurses to become members of the NACGN.

Only the adverse effects of the Great Depression curtailed Rosenwald largesse. In 1936 the fund was in no position to grant awards. Fortunately the officers of the General Education Board responded to NACGN appeals with a $500 grant. Actually, this sum was contributed only after Mary Beard, who in 1912 had been an elected member of the first board of directors of the NOPHN and was a trusted and respected adviser and consultant to the Rockefeller Foundation philanthropies, indicated that the black nursing leaders very much needed and would make good use of this support.[24] Armed with the requisite financial aid, the NACGN secured its first executive secretary. Thus, after years of floundering, it is fair to say that in 1934 the organization was about to come into its own. On May 15, 1934, the NACGN moved into offices in the Rockefeller Center, joining the other major nursing organizations.[25]

Philanthropic largesse, coming at this most propitious moment in the history of the NACGN, proved invaluable. Of equal, if not more, importance to the revitalization process was the leadership of two dynamic black nurses: Estelle Massey Riddle and Mabel Keaton Staupers. In 1934 the NACGN members elected Riddle president; she in turn oversaw the hiring of Staupers as the organization's first executive secretary. The membership ratified Staupers's appointment at the convention held in August 1935 in Nashville, Tennessee. Both women were experienced administrators, already well known in white nursing circles. Indeed, Riddle, the best-educated black nurse in the country, had served on an important NOPHN educational committee, and Staupers had served as a member of the NOPHN's Committee on Organization and Administration.[26]

Riddle and Staupers, of course, knew of each other's work. The network of black nurse leaders was small and intimate. Both women evinced an unwavering commitment to the advance of black nurses and were willing to do whatever it took to achieve integration. They understood and accepted the responsibility of strengthening the NACGN while simultaneously building coalitions with sensitive and sympathetic white nursing leaders. One of them working alone could not have provided all of the skills needed to achieve these two objectives. Together, however, they were able to motivate and organize black nurses on local levels while continuing to negotiate and interact with white nurse leaders on the national front.

While Riddle and Staupers may have been ideological clones, in personal style, physical appearance, family background, and political strategy they presented an interesting study in contrasts. Yet their very differences as much as their shared singular vision of the future of black nursing fortified and intensified their collective strength. In other words, both their similarities and their differences made them a formidable force in the struggle for professional empowerment and integration.

Riddle was born on April 3, 1903, in Palestine, Texas. She briefly attended Prairie View College before entering in 1920 the nursing school at Homer G. Phillips Hospital, the old City Hospital No. 2, in St. Louis. She was graduated in 1923 and shortly thereafter passed the Missouri State Board Examination with an average of 93.3%. Although throughout her years as a student the hospital operated under white administrators and supervisors, Riddle was the first black to crack the administrative color barrier when she accepted an appointment as head nurse of one of the largest wards in the hospital. Ambitious and talented, Riddle quickly seized advantage of any new opportunity for professional development. Accordingly, when the Julius Rosenwald Fund established its scholarship program for postgraduate education for black nurses, she moved swiftly to secure the first of the coveted awards.

In 1927 Riddle left Homer G. Phillips and moved to New York City to enroll in Teachers College, Columbia University. She received a Bachelor of Science degree in nursing education in 1930. A year later she became the first black nurse in America to earn a Master of Arts degree in nursing education. She thereupon added another "first" to a growing list by becoming the first black part-time instructor to serve on the staff of the

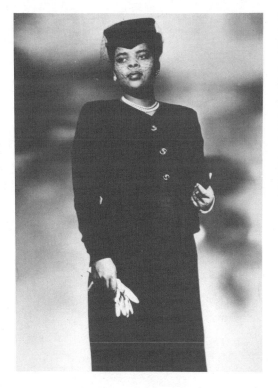

Geneva Estelle Massey Riddle Osborne (1901–1981), the first black nurse in the United States to earn a master's degree, and the first black instructor at New York University and the Harlem Hospital School of Nursing. She served as president of the NACGN from 1934 to 1939. In 1946, Osborne received the Mary Mahoney Award. Courtesy of the Moorland-Spingarn Research Center, Howard University.

Harlem Hospital nursing school. Following a brief stint in this position, Riddle moved again, to assume the even more prestigious position of educational director of Freedmen's Hospital in Washington, D.C. In the midthirties she returned to St. Louis, this time to serve as the first black superintendent of her alma mater, the Homer G. Phillips nurse training school, a position she held throughout her tenure as president of the NACGN.[27]

Staupers was born on February 27, 1890, in Barbados, West Indies. Her parents brought her to New York City in 1903. After completing early education in the city, Staupers won admission to the Freedmen's Hospital nursing school and was graduated in 1917. She returned to New York City to work as a private-duty nurse. While in New York, she played a key role in organizing the Booker T. Washington Sanitarium, one of the earliest institutions in the city permitting black physicians to treat their patients. She became the director of nurses at the new institution.

Equally as determined as Riddle to acquire more administrative nursing experience, Staupers left New York to accept employment at Mudget Hospital in Philadelphia as superintendent of nurses. While in Philadelphia, she also worked with officials of the Pennsylvania state board on

Mabel Keaton Staupers (1898–), the first executive director (1934–1946) and last president (1949–1951) of the NACGN. Staupers led the fight to integrate the Armed Forces Nurse Corps during World War II and presided over the dissolution of the NACGN. In 1951 she received the Spingarn Medal of the National Association for the Advancement of Colored People. Mabel K. Staupers Papers. Courtesy of the Moorland-Spingarn Research Center, Howard University.

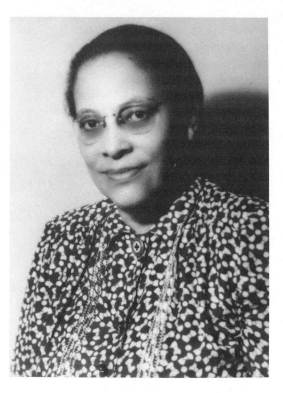

a project designed to standardize the training of nurses. Further, the energetic Staupers also served for a few months as a resident nurse at the city's House of St. Michael and All Angels for Crippled Children.

Staupers's career underwent a major shift when, beginning in 1922, she helped to conduct a survey of the health needs of New York City's Harlem community. The report evaluated the services available to blacks in the city and state tuberculosis facilities. Her work on the project attracted attention and acclaim. The survey became the rationale for the establishment of the Harlem Committee of the New York Tuberculosis and Health Association. She was appointed the association's first executive secretary, a position which enabled her to meet and form close friendships with black political and social elites in the city. For the next twelve years Staupers served in this position, leaving only to assume the post of executive secretary of the NACGN.[28]

That Riddle and Staupers brought to the NACGN a wealth of administrative talent and experience, and wide-ranging contacts with black health-care professionals, is clear. Moreover, these self-confident women moved in and out of integrated and segregated circles with ease.

Staupers's primary base of operation and contacts across professional lines was in the Northeast, while Riddle had strong ties and friendships in the Middle West and in the South. In their personal lives the similarities were again striking. Both women had initially married black physicians, were divorced, and had remarried, and neither bore children.

Possessed of so many similarities, Riddle and Staupers enjoyed an easy friendship and worked together harmoniously. Yet there were those little differences between them which boded well for the future of the NACGN. One obvious minor contrast was seen in their personal style and physical appearance. According to Lillian Harvey, a former dean of nursing at Tuskegee Institute, Staupers made an unforgettable first impression. Harvey recalled that during her senior year at Lincoln Hospital, she attended a lecture given by Staupers. She reminisced that Staupers was "very small, very dynamic," and was "very interested in young nurses." She added that Staupers "talked a mile a minute with a good bit of humor involved." Harvey mused, "I don't see how in the world she had that much energy." She elaborated that Staupers "wasn't afraid of anything or anyone . . . [she] could say whether she thought something was good, bad, or indifferent, worth something or worth nothing and say it in a kind of way with a little tinge of humor that you would not take offense."

According to Harvey, Riddle evoked a different image. She was "tall, had a high sense of fashion, wore exquisite jewelry, was noted for her hats, and her sense of grooming and dress." She added that Riddle always appeared as if she "would have been perfectly at home in *Vogue* or *Harper's Bazaar*." Harvey concluded, "These were flamboyant women."[29] They were not only flamboyant, it must be added, they were also shrewd agents for social change within professional nursing.

The two women were willing to invest themselves totally in the quest for that elusive professional integration. Riddle's personal dignity and elegant bearing led one officer of a philanthropic foundation to extol her as "a superior type person." Riddle could calmly, patiently, and with quiet diplomacy negotiate with white nurse leaders and philanthropic backers for support and funds for the NACGN, while Staupers, drawing upon her inexhaustible store of energy and wit, could ensure that the job of revitalizing the association would be done. While Riddle endured the tedious deliberations and discussions taking place throughout the 1930s at the interracial-relations committees and meetings within the upper echelons of white nursing circles, Staupers played the more active, highly visible role of "interpreting the Negro nurse" to the general public and marshaling the mass support so essential to their short-run struggle for equal education, fair employment opportunities, and professional integration. Thus within a very short time, these strong-willed, politically savvy, committed, hard-headed angels of mercy arrived at a rather comfortable division of labor. To be sure, the spheres were not drawn in cement, but each knew and valued the other's strengths and understood how they complemented each other for maximum effectiveness.

On November 6, 1934, at the first meeting of the board of directors of NACGN headquarters, President Riddle delineated the steps to be taken toward the development of a new program. Thus, as the first order of business, the board and officers had to devise a grand design for revitalizing the NACGN. The strategy had to be grounded upon a candid assessment of existing organizational ills, and a frank appraisal of what it would be possible for them to achieve given the racist proscriptions prevalent both within and without the nursing profession. An extended tour around the country during which Riddle and Staupers spoke with hundreds of black nurses helped them to see more precisely the magnitude of the task before them. They encountered dozens of moribund state affiliates, disillusioned nurses, and a generally uninformed public. They therefore had to do several things before even beginning to tackle the problem of systematic inequality of educational and employment opportunities, and achieving the integration of black nurses into the mainstream of American nursing. The NACGN needed to establish an information service for nurses and the public; publish and disseminate the official organ, the *National News Bulletin*, on a regular schedule; and launch an intensive membership campaign.[30]

The procedures for increasing membership, raising operating expenses, resuscitating moribund state branches, and establishing new ones where warranted were all interrelated. The overwhelming majority of black nurses neither belonged to nor apparently identified with the NACGN. According to the 1930 United States census, there were 5,728 graduate registered nurses in the country, yet when Riddle and Staupers assumed the leadership of the NACGN, the organization had only 380 members. Within three years Staupers would inform an officer of the General Education Board that she and Riddle had increased the number of members to 791, of whom 450 had actually paid their dues. As late as 1943 the NACGN had only 947 active members in spite of intense annual membership campaigns.[31]

How could the organization's leaders justify their assertion of working in behalf of and representing the interests of all black nurses in light of this small number of members? In the end it did not really matter that only a small fraction of eligible black nurses joined, for Riddle and Staupers simply declared the NACGN to be the recognized organization of black nurses, and it was considered as such by the white nursing establishment. Actually, it was to no one's advantage to refute or challenge their claim. For in reality, the white nursing associations, too, could claim only a small percentage of nurses as members.

The reasons eligible white nurses did not become members of the ANA

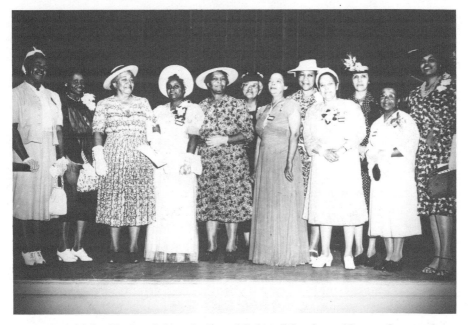

Leaders of the National Association of Colored Graduate Nurses, Inc., gathered at the First Biennial, Los Angeles, 1941. *Far right*, Estelle Massey Riddle; *fourth from right*, Mabel K. Staupers. Mabel K. Staupers Papers. Courtesy of the Moorland- Spingarn Research Center, Howard University.

in large numbers also explain the low number of black nurses in the NACGN. Historian Susan Reverby speculates that loyalties to the "home hospital" and alumnae associations so deeply fostered during training may have militated against the development of a broader sense of professional or occupational loyalty. Furthermore, public indifference and hostility on the part of physicians and hospitals to the efforts and desires of nursing leaders via their associations to control, upgrade, and standardize nursing instruction and practice may have impeded the taking out of professional membership by white and black nurses.[32] To these conjectures one could add that low salaries and the demanding nature of their work may also have played a role. Moreover, many private-duty white and black nurses may simply have failed to perceive any personal or professional advantage to belonging to a nursing organization. Superimposed on all of these explanations is the fact that a significant proportion of nurses still adhered to the traditional altruistic view of nursing as a calling. These nurses rejected the emerging professional ideology and attendant professional organizations no matter how advantageous they might prove in aiding their quest for better salaries or improved working conditions.

Undaunted by the low number of members, Riddle and fellow NACGN board members acknowledged that years of inactivity and the absence of a sustained coherent program fed the gulf between local black nurses and the leaders of the association. As long as black nurses believed the NACGN to be a powerless, formless organization, it remained irrelevant to their daily lives. But these ruminations needed substantiation. To discover what black nurses in fact thought, Riddle joined forces with Eola Lyons Taylor, a member of the NACGN's board of directors living in New Orleans, and called a conference in 1935 of southern black nurses. More than one hundred black nurses from nine southern states (Alabama, Arkansas, Florida, Georgia, Louisiana, Mississippi, Oklahoma, Tennessee, and Texas) responded to the call. They convened at the Flint-Goodridge Hospital in New Orleans, and as later reported in the NACGN's *National News Bulletin*, the spirited discussions touched not only upon the needs for a stronger organization but also upon improving relations between black nurses and black doctors.[33]

In her address before the New Orleans gathering, Riddle concentrated on the two issues then receiving a great deal of attention within the entire nursing profession. As historian Susan Reverby asserts, "During the Depression years, nursing's 'great transformation' from private duty to hospital staffing took place." Whereas in the opening decades of the twentieth century, the vast majority of graduate nurses embarked immediately upon careers in private duty, by the mid-1930s more of them sought staff positions in hospitals. There is a danger in writing nursing history without taking race into account. This "great transformation" did not affect black nurses in the same way. Few white or integrated hospitals sought their services. Many of the black hospitals seemed reluctant to employ graduate nurses when the student nurses could be exploited to take care of patients and the hospital as well. Riddle confronted the problem head-on. She stressed the need for those black hospitals that did exist to employ black graduate nurses. She made the same arguments that the white leadership made to the white hospitals about graduate labor. Riddle maintained that graduate nurses could provide cheaper, more dependable and disciplined, skilled service to the hospital than could the student nurses.

Finally, Riddle spoke to the importance of exercising quality control of nursing recruits. She emphasized, in addition, the need to discourage small southern hospitals from operating nursing schools. As reported in the *National News Bulletin*, the black nurse leaders echoed in the end that the "really important task" was to develop "intelligent propaganda so that public interest is aroused to the possibilities of nursing as a career—not for the high school and college failures but for the superior young woman."[34]

The New Orleans meeting was the precursor of a whole series of conferences arranged by Riddle, Staupers, and black nurses in different regions throughout 1936. Riddle and Staupers logged thousands of miles traveling to the conferences and meeting hundreds of black nurses in Chicago, Tuskegee, Durham, and Washington, D.C. Only a combined total of 154 black nurses paid the registration fees for all four of the conferences. Staupers took pains to report that more than this number actually attended the meetings. In Washington, D.C., for example, only 32 nurses paid the registration fee, but 135 attended the luncheon. In the following year, 1937, the regional conferences were held at Hampton, Virginia; Louisville, Kentucky; Richmond, Virginia; and Nashville, Tennessee.[35]

At each conference Riddle and Staupers delivered the same message. They discussed the necessity of and outlined the means of strengthening local and state NACGN associations; called for closer relations between local nurses and the national headquarters; recommended the organization of regional councils of black nursing-school executives; and underscored the urgency "to improve the economic security of Negro nurses in local, state, and federal nursing services." Staupers and Riddle never failed to impress upon local black nurses the importance of increased understanding and cooperation between white and black nurses. Accordingly, local black nurses invited white ANA state association secretaries to attend each regional NACGN conference. Inasmuch as the philanthropic donors continually expressed their concern with improving interracial relations in nursing, black nursing leaders frequently reassured their benefactors that progress was being made toward integration. Staupers reiterated to one General Education Board official that they were "working earnestly to bring about a better relationship with the American Nurses' Association, and to eliminate the need for a special organization." This could not be achieved overnight, as Staupers reminded: "Before this can be an assured fact there is much education to be done with both groups."[36]

The regional conferences went far beyond calling for greater interaction with white nurses. This was just one aspect of the complex and multi-dimensional agenda. Riddle and Staupers used the conferences effectively to acquaint black nurses with the inner workings of the NACGN headquarters and to disseminate information concerning the organization's financial status. Creating an air of openness, Staupers and Riddle hoped, would engender greater local-level participation, especially among the younger black graduate nurses. For too long a shroud of secrecy had seemingly hung over the association's financial affairs, giving rise to unanswered speculations. Staupers noted at one point, "We are telling nurses everywhere how the money is spent and how it is raised." She preferred full disclosure in order to overcome the reluctance of black nurses to give money to the organization simply for, as she put it, "sentimental reasons."

The dynamic twosome worked assiduously to transform the NACGN into a more democratic organization. To stimulate apathetic older nurses further, Riddle and Staupers inaugurated the Mary Mahoney Award, given annually to recognize outstanding achievement in "nursing and human service." The first recipient was Adah B. Thoms, in 1936. Riddle and Staupers freely admitted that they intended to use the Mahoney Award also as a means "to get this older group again interested in the Association." Subsequent awards were given to black nursing stalwarts Nancy Kemp in 1937, Carrie E. Bullock in 1938, and Ludie Andrews in 1941.[37]

Moreover, the regional conferences served a larger educational and community-outreach function. Riddle and Staupers were well attuned to the value of widespread public support for and understanding of the black nurse and her struggle. Staupers, for one, insisted that black nurses, working through their local NACGN, cultivate close cooperative relationships with local leaders of nonnursing organizations such as the National Association for the Advancement of Colored People and the National Urban League. Under her skillful tutelage, black nurses began to master the art of coalition formation. In order to be in a position to call upon the assistance of the NAACP and the NUL, Riddle and Staupers cajoled local black nurses into demonstrating an interest in all racial-advancement work. Riddle suggested that the black nurses initiate monthly meetings with other groups of black professionals, especially social workers, teachers, school principals, and ministers. Such meetings, she explained, should be used to disseminate information about the work and worth of the black nurse to the entire community.[38]

As the capstone of nurse-community interaction, Staupers advised local black nurses to organize interracial citizens' committees. The New York nurses were the first group to do so. In 1935 they spearheaded the founding of the New York Citizens' Committee. By 1942 twelve different citizens' groups across the country were working diligently to improve the image and perceptions of black nurses and to win for them greater employment opportunities in local hospitals and visiting health agencies. Staupers, in explaining this course of action to a GEB officer, declared, "In doing this we are following the trend in other nursing organizations." She added, "This is valuable, since the nurse needs their help and the layman needs to understand the nurse."[39]

Staupers proved an adept practitioner of coalition-building politics and forged lasting ties between the NACGN and the officers of several national black-rights organizations. She proved equally as competent in generating massive publicity for the black nurse. She persuaded the editors of the NAACP's *Crisis*, the NUL's *Opportunity*, and the National Medical Association's *Journal*, as well as Claude Barnett, founder of the

Associated Negro Press, to publish feature-length articles and stories about black nurses, emphasizing their struggles and their contributions to improved black health-care delivery. From her actions it is clear that Staupers believed that black nurses' claim for equitable treatment and recognition within the profession could receive legitimacy and strength through publicity and propaganda. She performed her publicity duties with consummate skill, as was most notably demonstrated in the publication of the November 1937 issue of *Opportunity*, which was devoted exclusively to black nurses.

Between 1934 and 1940, Staupers worked unrelentingly to improve the quality of the NACGN's own official organ, the *National News Bulletin*. The task of breathing new life into the *Bulletin* was a difficult one. For years it had limped along; issues had appeared irregularly, and subscribers' complaints of sporadic delivery had gone unanswered. For a brief period her efforts bore fruit as the *Bulletin* became the chief mechanism for communication with a steadily growing NACGN membership. During a short-lived revitalization, the *Bulletin* solicited and published articles written by black nurses on a variety of educational issues, highlighted pending congressional legislation of import to the profession, published biographical profiles of significant black nurse leaders, and included news of what was occurring in all of the local, state, and regional branches of the organization. In spite of the remarkable improvement in quality, however, the *Bulletin* eventually succumbed to insurmountable economic pressures. In 1942, in the face of severe financial difficulties, the *Bulletin* committee recommended that the organ reduce publication to twice a year and that the NACGN inaugurate a less expensive monthly newsletter to communicate with its membership.[40]

As Staupers struggled to improve communication and build coalitions between black nurses and other black organizations, Riddle involved herself ever more deeply in the affairs of white nursing organizations. This is not to suggest that Riddle was not active in building bridges with black organizations. Significantly, in 1935 she was elected the second vice-president of the newly founded National Council of Negro Women. Mary McLeod Bethune established the new organization and served as its first president. Mary Church Terrell, one of the leading black clubwomen organizers of her time, assisted her and became the first vice-president. Terrell had been the president of the National Association of Colored Women from 1899 to 1901. Bethune, known nationally, was the founder of Bethune-Cookman College in Daytona, Florida, and was an influential member of Franklin Roosevelt's Black Cabinet. The connection between the black nurses and other black women's organizations would later prove instrumental in helping the nurses to battle segregation and discrimination. The NCNW was destined to become the largest body of organized black women in the country. By the mid-1940s it had 800,000 members distributed among eighteen national organizations and fourteen metropolitan councils.[41]

Riddle shared the NCNW's commitment to winning back lost political rights for black men and women through the overthrow of the poll tax. Yet from the outset, perhaps reflecting her influence, the council declared the development of a viable public-health system in America to be one of its chief objectives. The NACGN, as did the NCNW, participated in and supported all the black protest campaigns against education and employment discrimination, and lobbied for antilynching and anti–poll tax legislation. Moreover, local and state NACGN affiliates raised money for the Scottsboro Defense Committee. Indeed, wherever possible, black nurses pressured for fair trials for the nine black youths unjustly accused of raping two white women in Scottsboro, Alabama. The NACGN also joined with the NMA to press for the inclusion of an antidiscrimination clause in the aborted National Health Act of 1939.[42]

In 1938 Staupers established a National Advisory Council for the NACGN to broaden the organization's community and professional contacts in New York City. She selected as members only the most eminent figures in their respective fields. In so doing she adhered to the model established in the formative years by the founders of the NOPHN. Exercising her keen judgment of character and strength, Staupers invited one of her best friends, Ruth Logan Roberts, a prominent member of the city's black middle class, to serve as chairperson of the council. M. O. Bousfield of Chicago, a former president of the NMA and associate director of Negro health programs for the Julius Rosenwald Fund, was named vice-president.

Ruth Logan Roberts, the daughter of Tuskegee Institute vice-president Warren Logan and suffragist Adella Hunt Logan, was born in 1891. She attended Oberlin College and subsequently received training in physical therapy and physical education, which she put to good use as director of women's physical education at Tuskegee Institute. She left Tuskegee in 1917 to marry black physician Eugene Percy Roberts of New York City. Dr. Roberts was the first black member of the board of education in the city. Ruth Roberts readily adapted to and embraced her roles as community activist, Harlem hostess, and Republican Party stalwart. She served on numerous boards, including that of the Tuberculosis Association, where she developed her close friendship with Staupers. A niece described Roberts as "tall, athletic, big but not fat, looked white, but had a very strong black identity. She possessed a perfect combination of being able to strong arm and charm."[43]

The National Advisory Council played a useful, indeed critical, role in the articulation of the NACGN's "philosophy of integration." At the initial meeting on November 3, 1939, council members deemed most important "the integration of the Negro nurse in all programs and organizations of interest to nurses." Logan summarized what was involved in promoting black nursing integration: "This has meant conferences, correspondence and cooperation with representatives of the other National Nursing organizations, with the agencies of the Federal Government concerned with nursing activities, with private agencies having programs with individuals with interest and influence in this field." She added, "It has also meant observance and scrutiny of proposed national legislation and the preparation and expression of opinion on such legislation."[44]

Staupers and Riddle accomplished a great deal within a very short time, yet their major objective of integrating black nurses into the profession remained as elusive as ever. Beginning in 1934, for ten years, the two NACGN officers appeared, as Staupers informed Bolton, "before the House of Delegates at the Biennial Meetings of the American Nurses' Association and presented to this group the need for complete integration." Staupers confided that "each year although we have not gained our ultimate objective we have gained friends and are in a stronger position than ever before."[45] Staupers's optimism notwithstanding, the struggle for integration was one which both black and white nurse leaders found trying. Although there were many forces exerting behind-the-scenes pressure on professional nursing organizations to integrate black nurses, there remained considerable internal resistance within the profession.

In 1937 Mary Beard and Leo Favrot repeated to Riddle and Staupers their concern about black nurses' finding some way to achieve integration. When Riddle suggested that additional funds from the General Education Board would enable the NACGN to hire someone specifically to "work on Negro participation in the nation's nursing organizations," she met a cool reception. Beard noted in her diary, "I explained that this did not seem to me to be a desirable way to work." Instead she informed Staupers that "if the ANA would add a Negro nurse to its staff, the financing of this would be a suitable request to make of the GEB."[46]

Anxious to improve relations any way she could, Staupers shared this intimation of GEB support with ANA leaders but received no reply. Riddle thereupon contacted ANA leaders and attempted to negotiate an agreement whereby black nurses could enjoy membership in the organization through their own state associations and the NACGN.[47] She also requested that the ANA consider appointing more black nurses to standing committees within the association. The ANA rejected both ideas and took pains to delineate to the black nurses their status within the profession. Riddle was reminded that "as membership in the A.N.A. is based upon State Association Membership, colored nurses are accepted into A.N.A. membership through membership in a State Nurses' Association. Therefore, no colored nurse can be accepted into A.N.A. membership who is not a member in a State Nurses' Association, either through her alumnae or individually." Riddle was likewise informed that only qualified members could be appointed to any of the ANA's standing committees.[48]

In spite of some positive steps toward integration, as the decade of the Great Depression drew to a close, in April 1939, Jim Crow again reared its ugly head in such a way as to assure black nurses of the long path still to be traveled. The occasion was the annual meeting of the Advisory Council of the ANA. Julia Stimson invited Estelle Riddle to attend it in order to continue discussions concerning the status of black nurses in the profession. A delighted and enthusiastic Riddle eagerly looked forward to joining her white colleagues in New Orleans. Soon, however, she would confide to Walter White of the NAACP,

> I have been specially invited to the Advisory Committee meeting of the ANA, which is quite a gain in our striving for recognition from them. The National Organization for Public Health Nursing has been far more liberal than the ANA. This is the first time the latter organization has extended such a courtesy to our organization. I regret so much that Jim Crow is about to spoil it.[49]

Unfortunately the St. Charles Hotel, the site of the meeting, made it clear that blacks were not welcome. Its managers stipulated that all black guests must "use the service entrance and freight elevator." Riddle sent a telegram to Stimson from her home in Akron, Ohio, urging her to use her official position as the ANA's president to protest this discrimination. She also wrote to Claribel Wheeler, executive secretary of the National League of Nursing Education, suggesting that a protest of some sort was in order.[50] Wheeler did not respond. The reply Riddle received from ANA headquarters was unsatisfactory. Instead of protesting the hotel's discriminatory treatment of blacks in general, and of Riddle in particular, Stimson offered to meet Riddle "at the train and enter the hotel's service entrance and elevator" with her.[51] In a follow-up letter Riddle was asked to understand that "neither she [Stimson] personally, nor the A.N.A. can deal with the racial question involved."[52]

Riddle appreciated Stimson's position and did not question her personal interest in black nurses, yet she found the substitute proposal unacceptable. She rejoined that Stimson's offer to meet her at the train and accompany her on the freight elevator "would make neither the ANA nor the hotel management aware of any facing of the problem." Riddle correctly observed, "Then, too, she [Stimson] could not escort me to and from every meeting during the week, and there are other Negro nurses to be considered."[53] The racial discrimination of southern hotels proved a major impediment to almost all black professionals during this period, preventing many from attending conventions and conferences.

Riddle had also sought advice from Walter White and Ruth Logan Roberts as to how best to handle this issue. Both advised her to refuse to attend the meeting. White bluntly declared that he "could not imagine any self-respecting person submitting to the humiliation of using service entrance and elevators." White elaborated, "Since you asked my advice I would strongly urge you both as President of the National Association of Colored Graduate Nurses and as a self-respecting individual to refuse to attend unless you could enter the meeting places on the same bases as anyone else." He continued, "The A.N.A. and the N.L.N.E. should be asked to take an unequivocal stand just as other organizations . . . have taken the stand that they will not go to a city unless all delegates can be treated alike."[54]

Roberts took a more direct approach than White and drafted a chilly letter to Stimson. She chastised Stimson for her handling of the matter and then recommended that "this unfortunate occurrence may be used as an educational experience for your group." Roberts objected to the ANA's "philosophy of defeatism," describing it as "suicidal in this day of growing intolerance." She explained that whenever individuals and organizations "have been clear and positive in their desire to insure the basic civil and human rights of all people they have been able to impress hotel managers and other less enlightened individuals with the importance of this principle."[55] Neither the ANA nor the NLNE wanted any publicity given to this matter. Inasmuch as the whole thing erupted a mere week before the annual meeting, nothing was done. Thus as the 1930s ended, black nurses experienced the continued pain of exclusion and rejection as professional Jim Crow remained impervious to challenges and deaf to the entreaties of the black outsiders.

It would take the cataclysmic events of World War II and an unrelenting struggle waged by Riddle and the indomitable Staupers to turn the white tide of racism and free black nurses completely from their professional prison of discrimination and exclusion. The timing, therefore, of the push for integration was important. After all, the crisis of the Depression wreaked havoc on nurses' economic status. Salaries plummeted, and many private-duty and graduate nurses lost jobs. The specter of integrating with black nurses, recognizing them and providing them the same professional opportunities, may have been simply too threatening for many white nurses to contemplate. All nurses desired better pay and working conditions and more professional autonomy. What they did not want was more competition. The introduction of subsidiary nursing personnel and hospital workers, orderlies and aides, and domestics only exacerbated the nurses' distress and fear that their jobs would be taken away both within and outside of the hospital.[56] Thus the ANA could not have progressed more quickly toward integration, for to do so would have risked further alienation and estrangement of its private-duty and hospital staff nurses.

As the 1930s drew to a close, black nurse leaders Riddle and Staupers, lay supporter Ruth Logan Roberts, and Frances Payne Bolton could have, had they had time to pause and reflect, surveyed the accomplishments with a modicum of pride. In transforming the NACGN, Riddle and Staupers had also grown. They had acquired that elusive yet essential property of agency. Through a revitalized NACGN, these black nurses became forceful agents of social change. Only the most obtuse observer could fail to see their growing personal power, both as individuals and as professional black women.

Riddle and Staupers could now look to the future secure in their conviction that although the struggle was fraught with pain and humiliation, integration into the mainstream of nursing would be theirs. They had engaged in and mastered the art of political empowerment. They not only had deliberately forged important coalitions with eminent and powerful white philanthropists and white nurse leaders, but had simultaneously strengthened their connections with leaders of black-rights groups such as the NAACP, NUL, and NCNW and with the black press. To be sure, their white nurse sympathizers proved reluctant to go public with the struggle for integration. They had much racism and fear of their own to overcome. More important, however, in appealing to and retrieving the lost, or lukewarm, support and involving all black nurses in the process of rebuilding the organization, Riddle and Staupers had planted and nurtured the seed for heightened professional consciousness and intragroup solidarity. These accomplishments would serve them well in the World War II decade as the quest for integration gained new momentum, increased urgency, and more progressive white nurse allies.

Black Women in White

7 The racism, poverty, and myriad other forces that in-fluenced black women's decisions to become nurses all receded once they were actually enrolled in the various training programs. Survival dictated that the student nurses imbibe a sense of the special nature and meaning of their calling. Black nurse supervisors and educators saw to it that their charges measured up to the highest ideals of nursing. If the young novices or probationers failed to be transformed, they were dismissed.

"To make a difference": this desire undergirded the thoughts and actions of most of the leaders and not a few of the practitioners in the black nursing profession. Perhaps Lillian Harvey, dean of the School of Nursing of Tuskegee Institute from 1944 to 1973, summed up best what it meant to be a nurse. At heart, a good nurse controlled the environment of healing and possessed a holistic understanding of patients' needs. Harvey explained:

> The nurse who can look at her patient, for example, and understand what is going on in that patient's body, anticipate some of the things and alert the doctor, the social worker and other persons to what is going on and what might possibly happen and then make herself the facilitator for get-ting the right people there to take care of whatever it is that is coming up. I feel that a nurse is really the patient's advocate. You are supposed to be there for the patient on the patient's side to look after the patient's best interests. You are like the legal advisor is or the lawyer is in a situa-tion with his clients. . . . If her patient needs something she should be able to understand it, see it coming and make provision for it. It might be love—it might be they need to see their grandmother instead of their brother or a sister who might irritate them to death. They might need to get the doc-tor to look at the combination of medications they are getting to see if the results are what he expects or wants or whether the results are what the patient might need. Maybe that is too idealistic for nursing but in my mind and in my opinion that is nursing at its very best and at its highest.[1]

The lives and careers of several nurses, specifically Eunice Rivers Laurie, Lillian Harvey, Frances Elliot Davis, and Salaria Kee O'Reilly, exemplify the striving and measured achievement of black nursing. In conjunction with a concern to develop their skills, these women viewed nursing as the best means of helping victims of poverty, racial oppression, and disease. Each pursued a different path toward these same goals. Yet their lives and experiences hold an even greater significance. They reflect the collective difficulties encountered in the first half of the twentieth century by all black women who aspired simultaneously to nurse and to live up to the altruistic ideals of their profession.

A powerful combination of parental prodding, head-on collisions with racial discrimination, and desire to reduce suffering encouraged not a few black women to consider a nursing career. Eunice Rivers Laurie, born in Early County, Georgia, on November 12, 1899, initially balked when her father suggested that she take up nursing at John A. Andrew Hospital at Tuskegee Institute. Rivers had pleaded, "But Papa, I don't want to be no nurse, I don't want folks dying on me." Undaunted, the father countered, "Well, Eunice, everybody ain't gonna die on you. That's why you should be a nurse. That's what is being a good nurse, so you could help save the people." Mollified, Rivers asserted to an interviewer, "Well, I decided and he influenced me, but I made up my mind myself."[2]

The immediate impact of the racially motivated denial of care to blacks and the unnecessary loss of countless lives haunted Lillian Harvey. Indeed, Harvey's painful remembrances of her father's untimely death suggest that a deep-seated desire to combat racial discrimination lay at the heart of her determination to enter nursing. She recounted, "My father was killed in an accident when I was about six years old. He lost his leg in a mower and he bled to death. He bled to death in Franklin, Virginia because he was a Black man and they did not admit Black men to their hospital even though he was a sandy-haired Black man with gray eyes. It didn't make any difference to them."[3]

Perhaps the lack of sufficient nurturing early in life fostered in Frances Elliott Davis a need and desire to care for others, somehow to provide for the sick and helpless that which she had yearned for as a child. America's first black Red Cross nurse, Davis was born in 1882 in Knoxville, Tennessee. The daughter of an unmarried white plantation heiress and a Cherokee-Negro agricultural worker, she was orphaned at age six and spent the next several years of her life in a succession of foster homes. While still very young, however, she confided to one of her foster mothers her desire to "be a nurse and help little children." Later, when she was befriended by a wealthy white couple who became her patrons, Davis reiterated her desire. Her patron objected, arguing, "You're much too frail to be a nurse, Fannie. Nursing is very hard and menial work. You would have to be very strong to stand up under the training. Mr. Reed and I

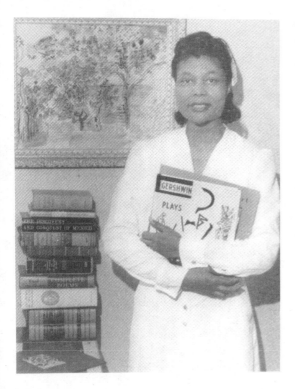

Lillian H. Harvey, a graduate of Lincoln Hospital School for Nurses, New York, arrived in Alabama in 1944 to become the first dean of the School of Nursing of Tuskegee University. This was, in 1948, the first baccalaureate nursing program in the state of Alabama. Photo circa 1950. The Washington Collection. Courtesy of Tuskegee University Archives.

would like to send you to school in the hope that you may become a teacher. A bright girl like you could do so much good as a teacher among Negroes." Lacking adequate financial resources, Davis, if she was to be educated, had little choice but to follow their wishes. Her patrons defrayed her expenses while she attended Knoxville College. After graduation she taught history in one of the county schools, but she never relinquished her dream to nurse.[4]

Well beyond the age at which most black women entered nursing training, Davis, at age twenty-seven, took the first steps toward becoming a nurse. Afraid that she would be considered too old for admission, she changed her birth year from 1882 to 1889. Her decision to enter Freedmen's Hospital in Washington, D.C., and subsequent graduation in June 1913 signaled a growing confidence and independence. Like the vast majority of graduate nurses, Davis quickly entered private-duty work, earning twenty-five dollars per week. She never lacked work because, like many black nurses, she readily accepted those assignments avoided by white nurses, the care of chronically or terminally ill patients. After a year in private duty, however, she accepted a position as supervisor of nurses at all-black Provident Hospital in Baltimore. Again this was a typical career pattern of the more ambitious black nurses. She moved from private-duty to administrative and institutional nursing and eventually set her sights on a position in the public-health–nursing field. Racial discrimination and the reliance on student nurses meant that only a small fraction of black graduate nurses worked as visiting nurses or on hospital staffs.

While employed at Provident Hospital, Davis applied to the American Red Cross. Although her friends warned her that the Red Cross did not accept Negro nurses, Davis persevered. To her delight she was accepted into the program with the proviso that she take a special course in public-health or rural nursing in order to overcome a deficiency in her training and work background. Davis's good fortune continued when the Red Cross advanced her five hundred dollars to pay tuition for the one-year training course in rural nursing offered by Columbia University's Teachers College under the direction of M. Adelaide Nutting. Once in training, she acquired field experience working at Lillian Wald's Henry Street Settlement House in New York.[5] After much effort, Davis completed the training, and in July 1917 she received summons to Jackson, Tennessee.

After her first week on the job with the Red Cross visiting-nurse service, Davis received a package in the mail. It was her Red Cross nursing pin. As she examined the pin and admired the laurel wreath on the outer edge, she noticed the *1A* inscribed on the back. She later learned that "the letter A designated the wearer as a Negro." Thus Davis was designated "the first Negro Red Cross nurse." Only in 1949 did the organization discontinue the practice of inscribing the letter *A* on the pins of all black nurses. In 1919 Davis became director of nurses' training at John A. Andrew Hospital. She later pursued a long and distinguished career in the child welfare division of the Detroit Health Department, and from 1945 to 1951 she worked at Eloise Hospital in Detroit. She died May 2, 1965, in Mount Clemens, Michigan, shortly before she was to be honored at the American Red Cross national convention.[6]

Personal and familial influences were undoubtedly important motivations; still the lack of choices and opportunities played a more decisive role in channeling blacks into nursing. The majority of black women did not have ample employment or educational opportunities. Because of their sex and race, the larger society provided little for, and expected less of, them. For this reason young black women relied heavily, whenever it was available, upon the advice of caring guardians and patrons. But this does not mean that they always followed the counsel proffered.

Nurses Davis and Salaria Kee O'Reilly shared the experience of being raised by foster parents. At six months of age, Kee's recently widowed mother left her in the care of a friend in Akron, Ohio, and went to live and work in Georgia. While living in a succession of foster homes, Salaria eventually was graduated from high school. She secured employment in the office of the successful black Akron physician Dr. Bedford Neal Riddle (future husband of Elizabeth Massey Riddle). Eager and young, Salaria thirsted for a career. In 1930 she enrolled in evening classes at the local university, working for the doctor during the day. She informed Dr. Riddle of her desire to become a teacher of physical education, and he advised a more accessible course. Riddle was convinced that Kee "was better suited for nursing than teaching physical education." But it was not until Kee suffered rebuff at the university that she decided to pursue nursing. Still smarting years later from the rejection, she explained why she was forced to give up on becoming a teacher of physical education. "No Negro had been permitted to register for that course [swimming] as they were not allowed in the swimming pool." She resolutely declared, "Since I wasn't allowed to swim, I didn't mind becoming a nurse."[7]

Like many black women before her, Salaria Kee soon discovered that deciding to become a nurse was easier than gaining admission to a training school. But she was fortunate. Of the numerous institutions to which she applied, the Harlem Hospital nursing school in New York accepted her. She observed, "I had received letters from all schools of nursing in Akron, Cleveland, and Detroit." She mused ironically, "They must have had a conference with the agenda Salaria Kee, Colored. Each letter read: 'We have no provision for training colored nurses.' To this day I wonder if they have obtained black sheets and black bed pans."[8]

On February 1, 1931, Kee entered the Harlem Hospital school and encountered New York. The city initially shocked the young midwesterner: "There was much too much noise, the people were in too much of a hurry going nowhere and they spoke too many different languages to be in America."[9] Other surprising customs and practices within the training school added to her disquiet. The student nurses were all black, whereas the administrators and instructors were predominantly white. She simply could not accept the prevailing racial etiquette observed at Harlem Hospital. She found most distressing the segregated seating arrangements in the nurses' dining room. According to custom, Kee wrote, "white teachers and white nurses had special tables. White social workers had special tables while Negro teachers and Negro nurses in the same professional category had separate facilities."[10]

In late 1932, unmindful of the potential consequences, Kee seized the opportunity to make known her distaste for dining-room segregation at the school. When "by some shift in the program, staff and students went into the dining room at the same time," Kee and five members of her class claimed for themselves the one vacant table. The dining-room staff promptly refused to serve the students because the table they had chosen was "reserved for whites." Salaria, leading the angry students, "rose quickly, caught up the corners of the tablecloth and upset the whole dining room." The nursing students demanded that the superintendent arrange a meeting to discuss the matter. Meanwhile, they organized a student committee, elected Salaria the chairman, and circulated a petition, collecting signatures from 90 percent of the student body.

The student committee prepared well for the meeting with the white hospital administrators. After discussion of their grievances, they presented a list of three demands. They insisted that the school end racial segregation in the dining room; urged the addition of a black dietitian to the existing staff of five whites; and called for the granting of more authority to head nurses, who they charged functioned only as "straw bosses" and "petty foremen." Fortuitously the student protest occurred during a heated mayoralty contest, and to quell the disturbing rumors seeping out of the hospital, the incumbent mayor quickly, according to Kee, "sent up a committee to investigate segregation in the dining room." In what surely must be a record for speedy resolution of racial segregation, within a matter of hours of the committee's visit, "the entire system of 'reserved tables for whites' was abolished in one day!"[11] The administration met all of the student demands.

Once armed with the hard-earned diploma, most black and white nurses entered private-duty nursing; Salaria Kee's career, however, followed a different course. In 1934 Kee, now a graduate nurse, accepted a job at Sea View Hospital, one of only four institutions (Harlem, Lincoln, and Riverside were the other three) in New York City then employing black graduate nurses. Apparently memories of her outspokenness had faded, for in 1935 Harlem Hospital invited her to return as a regular staff member. A delighted Kee eagerly accepted the assignment to the obstetrical division. Her return to her alma mater signaled to others, or so she hoped, that protesting against unacceptable racist conditions and practices did not necessarily damage or destroy one's career chances.

Within a very short period, Kee found herself again embroiled in protest. She railed against the horrors she encountered in the obstetrical division at Harlem Hospital. Her subsequent written reports elaborated the dangers of overcrowding, inadequate staff, and poor-quality medical service. A public investigation ensued. Kee described in detail the situation:

> The ward was overcrowded and understaffed. One nurse in charge of a maternity ward and a nursery of fifty babies. Fifty babies to be fed and cleaned three times each night—one-hundred and fifty feedings and one-hundred and fifty changes, and one nurse to do it. In addition there was the ward for abnormals. This usually contained about twelve babies and as many infected or abnormal mothers, many infected with communicable

diseases. These, of course, should have been isolated and cared for by one nurse exclusively. Sometimes these diseased mothers wandered off into the ward of healthy babies.[12]

Not surprisingly, Kee's tenure at Harlem was destined to be brief. Admonished more than once to "mind her own business," the embattled Kee remained at Harlem Hospital only two years. In her mind she was simply being a good nurse. Of course, her definition of what constituted good nursing bore scant resemblance to the docile, obedient, and mindless stereotype.

Working as a staff nurse at Harlem Hospital provided both good and bad experiences. On the positive side, Kee thoroughly enjoyed working with the black nurses, who in spite of their own problems remained sensitive to and aware of world events. As she became more acculturated to the city, Kee discovered New York to be an exciting place, and of course, the Harlem area was still the cultural capital of black America. While the rest of the country suffered through the Great Depression, blacks in Harlem remained attuned to pressing political issues. Interest in international affairs reached an all-time high. Kee joined with a group of black nurses to organize an Ethiopian Club. They attended and sponsored lectures and discussions dealing with medical matters, local politics, and international events.[13]

Involvement in political activities increased Kee's understanding of the interconnection between the racism black Americans suffered and the oppression others abroad endured as German Nazism and Italian Fascism took hold in Europe. When Italy invaded Ethiopia in 1935, hundreds of Afro-Americans attempted unsuccessfully to join the Ethiopian forces to fight the aggressors. This concern motivated black New Yorkers to send a seventy-five-bed field hospital to Ethiopia. Kee worked closely with other black physicians and nurses to gather the first two tons of medical supplies and dressings sent there from this country. When Mussolini later advanced Italian troops into Spain, black Americans understood that this was the same fight. When the Spanish Civil War erupted, the hundreds of black men who had been prevented from going to Ethiopia volunteered to fight against Franco in Spain. To black Americans, Spain became a battlefield upon which Italian Fascism might be defeated. A victory there could perhaps force Italy completely out of Ethiopia.[14] Accordingly, hundreds of black and white men formed the Abraham Lincoln Battalion of the International Brigade of Volunteers, and went to do battle for freedom in Spain.[15]

Although Kee maintained a strong interest in the events unfolding in Spain, she did not initially plan to go there. A peculiarly American twist of fate propelled her on her Spanish journey. She asserted, "In 1936, the Ohio River flooded and they put up a notice asking for volunteer nurses to go to help relieve the suffering." Affixed to one side of the bulletin board was a similar plea for nurses for Spain. "When I went to volunteer for Ohio, they told me they had no place for me—that the color of my skin would make me more trouble than I'd be worth to them." With characteristic insight and appreciation of irony, she declared, "It seemed so funny, me being turned down in a democratic country and then being allowed to go to a fascist one."[16]

On March 27, 1937, Kee sailed from New York with the second American medical unit to republican Spain. The small party consisted of twelve physicians and nurses, Kee being the only Negro. In the course of the Spanish Civil War, approximately fifty American women went to Spain, under the official auspices of the American Medical Bureau to Aid Spanish Democracy. The six-day voyage proved an eventful one, as Salaria again encountered the ugly specter of racism. The physician in charge of the group refused to sit at the dining table as long as she sat there. He objected to eating with a Negro because that implied an acceptance of social equality. The ship's captain settled the dispute by arranging for Kee to take all of her meals at his table.[17]

Kee's party reached Port Bou, Spain, on April 3, and soon set up their hospital at Villa Paz near Madrid. The beds quickly filled with soldiers of every degree of injury and ailment, representing almost every race and tongue from all over the world. In such a setting where people were literally dying to make Spain the tomb of Fascism, divisions of race, creed, religion, and nationality lost significance.[18] For the first time in her life, Kee worked free of racial discrimination or limitation. She even married a wounded soldier from Ireland whom she nursed back to health, thus acquiring the surname O'Reilly. Eventually the health-care staff received orders to move the hospital to the front. During the remainder of her Spanish sojourn, the field hospital was moved several times, from Tervel, to Pueble De, to Barcelona. It was while in Barcelona that the hospital suffered a particularly heavy bombardment, leaving Kee wounded and furloughed home.

As she convalesced stateside, Kee served the Medical Bureau in New York by lecturing and cajoling Americans to contribute medical supplies, food, and clothing for the Spanish poor, especially the women and children. She declared before numerous audiences, "Negro men have given up their lives there [Spain] as courageously as any heroes of any age. Surely Negro people will just as willingly give of their means to relieve the suffering of a people attacked by the enemy of all racial minorities—fascism—and its most aggressive exponents—Italy and Germany." When, toward the end of World War II, the army and navy lifted the ban against recruiting black nurses into the U.S. Armed Forces Nurse Corps, Kee was one of the first to be summoned. She was assigned to basic training at Camp McCoy in Wisconsin.[19] In many ways Kee's nursing career was atypical. After all, no other black nurse served during the Spanish Civil War. Only her encounters with intractable racism and her unending struggle to practice in her profession with dignity and skill link her with every other black nurse in America.

Securing the requisite training posed a major hurdle to many a would-be nurse. The young black woman—and unlike Frances Elliott Davis, most entering students were in their late teens and early twenties—encountered a host of restrictions on admission to the limited number of accredited schools of nursing.[20] Competition to gain entrance into the better schools, such as Lincoln in New York, Provident in Chicago, Freedmen's in Washington, D.C., or John A. Andrew remained intense. Thus women sometimes went to great lengths to secure a place in the entering classes. Not infrequently a young woman would lie about her age, adding two or three years. If the exaggeration was discovered, she faced dismissal. As long as educational and occupational opportunities remained so circumscribed for black women, even the possibility of being expelled was traumatic. But as late as the 1930s, the threat of dismissal also helped to ensure unquestioning obedience and loyalty among the young student nurses.

Fear of being dismissed, therefore, yielded in the nursing student the required subservience to all authority within the rigidly hierarchical world of the nursing training school. Not all were daunted by the strict discipline. Many of the young women derived comfort in knowing their exact position and appropriate behavior relative to all others, including the doctors, upperclassmen, supervisors, and head nurses who constituted the hospital hierarchy. Certainly during the probationary period, which lasted anywhere from three to nine months, the young student quickly had to master the formal, and often unwritten, rules and customs governing interaction between her and fellow students. Lillian Harvey described her first year as a student at Lincoln Hospital: "It was in the 1930s and you really looked up to seniors because they were the ones on the units with you and you felt as if you had a friend and an ally—a comrade really."[21]

Although freshmen valued the support and friendship of seniors, they had to be ever mindful not to transgress rigid codes of behavior and deference. As Harvey observed, "Lincoln was one of those authoritarian schools where freshmen dared not walk in front of sophomores; sophomores dared not march in front of juniors; juniors respected seniors; and seniors were the last word and the first word as far as nursing was concerned, yet they were friends."[22] The nature of the friendship or bonding that developed among the student nurses had a lot to do with individual needs for protection, respect, pride, and information. Harvey recalled, "You would rather ask a senior a question than to ask a teacher. They didn't snitch on you either which was wonderful. Teachers had a way of teaching you something or correcting you and then mocking you on it or writing anecdotes about it." To Harvey, Lincoln's "very developed degree of military approach to nursing" flourished "because everyone got something"—"a senior got respect and a sense of dignity; freshmen got protection."[23]

Henrietta Smith Chisholm, a 1931 graduate of Freedmen's Hospital, described her training period as "three of my happiest years." Chisholm had decided to become a nurse at the age of twelve when she saw a cousin in a nurse's uniform. The image of a black woman dressed in a crisp, clean, white uniform left an indelible impression on the young girl. Chisholm confessed that she wanted to be like that and to have all that the white uniform represented. She thrived on the regimentation of nursing training. "I liked training. . . . Regimentation meant nothing to me. I like order and I like schedules. I'm that type of person so it was nothing. I enjoyed it."[24] Some of her fellow students, however, did not enjoy the military regime and authoritarian nature of the training. This, among other reasons, accounted for the high attrition of nursing students. Out of the thirty-three students who entered the Mercy Hospital training program in Philadelphia in 1930, only ten survived to receive their diplomas.[25]

Another survivor of nursing training at Mercy, Elizabeth Sharpe, confided that "peer pressure" to conform was central to the whole training experience. She observed, "At that time there was quite a bit of peer pressure. We didn't step on an elevator ahead of a senior. We didn't step out of a door ahead of any upperclassmen. As we got to those stages we had someone else to do the same things too." She recalled, "The senior student nurse was in charge. There was no such thing as graduate nurses who were head nurses. The senior nurse was in charge—she was the charge nurse."[26]

Actually, at Mercy Hospital, a formidable superintendent of nurses, Lula G. Warlick, called the shots. Warlick, a 1910 graduate of Lincoln Hospital, had assumed the reins of the floundering nursing program at Mercy in 1920. At that time the school had only sixteen students. Undaunted, Warlick helped to increase the number of students to forty within a decade. She commented in the 1923–24 annual report that "the minimum amount of education required by the State of Pennsylvania for entrance to accredited schools is one year's high school work but from the many applicants, we are selecting our students mostly from those having completed the four years course." Under her supervision the faculty grew from three to nine. Moreover, she was largely responsible for the Pennsylvania State Board of Examiners' according the school Class A status.[27]

Warlick, like her counterparts around the country, ruled Mercy with an iron hand. Sharpe spoke of her with a mixture of awe and reverence: "She made a nurse out of us. If there was anything to be gotten out of us, she got it. She was quite a disciplinarian. We all worked from 7:30

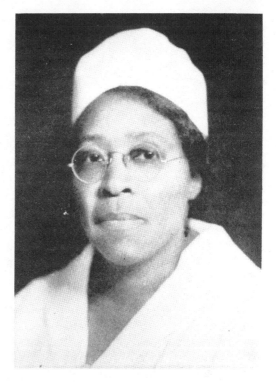

Lula G. Warlick, a 1910 graduate of Lincoln Hospital School for Nurses in New York, held supervisory positions at Provident Hospital in Chicago and Kansas City General Hospital No. 2 in Missouri before becoming, in 1920, the superintendent of nurses at Mercy Hospital in Philadelphia. She received the Mary Mahoney Medal of the NACGN in 1940. Mercy-Douglass Alumnae Association Collection. Courtesy of the Center for the Study of the History of Nursing, University of Pennsylvania.

A.M. to 7:30 P.M. and we had to be in by ten at night." All of the student nurses resided in the home adjacent to the hospital. Thus there existed scant opportunity to escape Warlick's watchful eye. Sharpe continued, "She watched to see that we got in by ten at night. If we had a boyfriend we would have to introduce them to her and she would pass on them." For the hapless student nurse caught disobeying one of Warlick's rules, two forms of punishment awaited: "Her favorite punishment was campus bounding us. We weren't allowed off the campus. The other favorite punishment was taking our caps away." According to Sharpe, the latter punishment constituted a painful public humiliation. "It was quite a disgrace to have your cap taken. Someone knew you had done something if your cap was taken."[28]

As the 1930s wore on, student nurses increasingly resented and resisted the rigid authoritarianism prevalent in all of the hospital nursing schools. Salaria Kee's initiative in the protest against segregated dining-room tables at Harlem Hospital was but one of the more graphic illustrations of student nurses' unwillingness to accommodate the racial status quo. Perhaps more occurrences of this sort happened than received media coverage. In any event, the general trend of resistance to the dictates of hospital and nursing-school supervisors prompted L. Bibb, a student nurse at General Hospital No. 2 in Kansas City, to write an essay on the problems of student adjustment to nursing-school life.

Bibb's critical essay on why contemporary students appeared less pliable and more angry appeared in the October-November 1937 issue of the NACGN's *National News Bulletin*. In it she speculated that the increasing difficulty of student adjustment "lies in the fact that the young woman of today has less home life than the one of twenty years ago. She has acquired more formal and less practical knowledge. She has more pre-conceived notions of the nursing profession; has more often selected it as a means of livelihood and less often as a means of service." Accordingly, Bibb insisted that the student nurse of the late 1930s was "keener in her judgements, less easily controlled, asks more questions, is quicker to detect supposed flaws in the system of education, in professional ethics, and in the professional demands for conformity rather than its reasons for conforming." Bibb concluded, "The spirit of independence which dominates her must necessarily come into abrupt conflict with the aged and conservative rules of hospital life."[29]

Whatever its origin, the new spirit challenged long-held views as to the proper professional conduct black student and graduate nurses should exhibit. This restlessness was reflected in the increased number of appeals black nurses made both to the headquarters of the National Association of Colored Graduate Nurses and to the officers of the NAACP. Throughout black America, militant voices expressed a similar reluctance to tolerate Jim Crow practices. Seemingly everyone was becoming more resentful of racial subordination, and the nursing students were no exception. Throughout the Great Depression and into the early 1940s, approximately half of the black nursing schools remained under the direction of white head nurses or white academic supervisors. Racial clashes over differences of opinion on critical matters were common. White administrators sometimes distrusted their allegedly aggressive and overly sensitive black subordinates. Blacks, on the other hand, believed the whites in charge to be hostile and indifferent to their needs and views.[30]

Black student nurses, especially those attending the two New York City–based training schools, Harlem and Lincoln, seemed least reluctant about appealing to the NAACP for assistance when confronted with overt discrimination at the hands of the white supervisors and administrators. Undoubtedly the student nurses were influenced by the growing militance of the black community in Harlem. This made it possible for them to ignore somber preachings of professional propriety. Furthermore, the proximity of the NAACP headquarters encouraged the solicitation of assistance, as did the fact that the NAACP officers responded quickly to the charges of racial discrimination brought to it by the black nurses. When investigations revealed that such discrimination or unfair treatment had occurred, the association sought redress and immediately publicized its involvement in its official organ, the *Crisis*. On occasion the NAACP would be called in to investigate a complaint of racial discrimination only to discover that the white supervisor was justified in the reprimand or dismissal of a black nursing student. Frequently, though, the investigators discovered that the treatment accorded black student and graduate nurses was flagrantly racist and the complaints were justified.

After 1935, Mabel K. Staupers, as the executive secretary of the NACGN, had to devote considerable attention to resolving the racial problems black student and graduate nurses brought to her. The NACGN, however, never had the reservoir of financial and legal resources that the NAACP had at its disposal. Apparently, the most urgent issue demanding the attention of the two associations was black women's limited access to nursing training and to postgraduate courses in special areas of nursing. Thus both organizations sought to open educational doors closed to black women, albeit using quite different strategies. While the NAACP officers believed that public exposure and scrutiny would lead to the discontinuation of discriminatory policies and practices, NACGN officers were somewhat reluctant to embarrass their white friends and fellow professionals. In the early years of its revitalization, the NACGN relied mostly on behind-the-scenes negotiation and maneuvering to bring about desired change and improvement in the status of black nurses.

When black graduate nurse Alyce Eugenia Greene received a rejection notice in response to her application to begin postgraduate study at the Division of Nursing in the Department of Hospitals in New York City, she contacted the NAACP. The rejection letter announced in part, "At present there are no post-graduate courses in New York City for Negro nurses."[31] Roy Wilkins went immediately to S. S. Goldwater, the commissioner of hospitals, warning him that "such a flagrant and brazen statement of race and color prejudice" would not be tolerated. Wilkins asserted that the letter Greene had received represented only the tip of the iceberg of "intolerant color prejudice which seems to run throughout the Department of Hospitals of the City of New York."[32] Moreover, the NAACP's Walter White put top city officials on notice when he declared that the organization would fight any efforts to institutionalize a Jim Crow strategy to silence black objections to being denied admission to city-operated postgraduate programs. Specifically, White warned that "the establishment of a segregated post-graduate course would not be satisfactory." He declared, "If a post-graduate course is established at Harlem Hospital, that is one matter; but if all colored applicants are sent exclusively to Harlem Hospital, this would be merely a form of segregation which we would be constrained to oppose vigorously."[33]

Thus, by appealing directly to prominent white political officials, the NAACP officers were, on a case-by-case basis, able to force an end to the more overt discriminatory policies and actions. Of course, an implied threat of legal action and damaging publicity went a long way toward motivating and sensitizing career-minded policy makers to the need for reforms. The NAACP's handling of the controversy surrounding the appointment of black nurses to the staff of the Glen Dale Sanitarium in Washington, D.C., is yet another example of the approach the organization employed in helping black nurses while simultaneously attracting favorable press coverage for its work.

In 1939 the District of Columbia commissioners of the Glen Dale Sanitarium, a facility for tuberculosis patients, over half of whom were black, decided to appoint sixteen new nurses selected from the lists of names provided by the civil service. When it became known that a few blacks would likely win appointment, Glen Dale's white nurses announced that they would resign rather than work with black nurses. The NAACP wasted little time entering into this fray. Walter White sent a telegram to West Virginia representative Jennings Randolph, chairman of the House District Committee, and Senator William H. King, chairman of the Senate District Committee, urging them to hold steadfast and not "bow to the demand of some white nurses at Glen Dale Sanitarium that qualified Negro nurses who had met civil service tests not be appointed."[34] Randolph subsequently ignored the white nurses' protests and threats of resignation and assured White and the NAACP that black nurses would be appointed "when they are certified by the Civil Service Commission and when vacancies occur for which they might qualify." In keeping with their threats, two white nurses resigned as soon as the first black nurse entered the sanitarium.[35]

The threat issued by the white nurses, to quit their jobs should black nurses receive appointments, was a common ploy used by white women workers throughout the thirties. More often than not it achieved the desired end, in industry, at least, if not always in nursing. Historians Susan M. Hartman and Karen Tucker Anderson have convincingly demonstrated that while white women enjoyed expanded employment opportunities, black women continued to be the last hired and the first fired throughout the Depression and World War II years. Employers seeking to avert threatened walkouts, slowdowns, and violence caved in to white women's objections to working beside or, most particularly, sharing restroom and toilet facilities with black women. To be sure, many employers harbored the same racist assumptions and beliefs in black inferiority, but camouflaged them behind white women's objections and threats.[36]

The black media were not easily fooled by such ploys and remained attuned to all excuses that rationalized the denial of job opportunities to black women. In their official organ, *Opportunity*, National Urban

League officers catalogued the thinly veiled rationalizations white employers offered for discriminating against black women:

> "There must be some mistake"; "No applications have heretofore been made by colored"; "You are smart for taking the courses, but we do not employ colored"; "We have not yet installed separate toilet facilities"; "A sufficient number of colored women have not been trained to start a separate shift"; "The training center from which you came does not satisfy plant requirements"; "Your qualifications are too high for the kind of job offered"; "We cannot put a Negro in our front office"; "We will write you . . . but my wife needs a maid"; "We have our percentage of Negroes."[37]

But the NACGN was more than a protest organization; it was first and foremost an organization of professional nurses. Its mission as defined by Staupers and her supporters was to win integration of black nurses into the mainstream of American nursing, establish open access to the best nursing schools, and increase job opportunities with equitable salaries for all. As one of many strategies, NACGN officers encouraged potential black nursing students to ignore previous histories of discrimination and to apply to the best schools. More and more black women heeded the advice, only to "feel the pain of rejection" when officials offered an array of creative excuses for why they could not be admitted. Gladys Lowe of Jacksonville, Florida, received the following note in 1935 in response to her application: "I am terribly sorry to say that it is not possible to admit colored nurses to our course in State College, Pennsylvania principally because the town is small and it is difficult to find living quarters."[38] When a concerned citizen and NAACP branch member, John R. Barreau of New Bedford, Massachusetts, inquired as to why black women were being denied admission to the city's St. Luke's Hospital Nurse Training School, a member of the institution's board of directors informed him that the exclusionary policy operated because "some patients would object to a colored nurse." A dejected Ruth Logan Roberts lamented to Barreau, "Unfortunately the situation which you describe at St. Luke's Hospital in New Bedford is fairly typical of conditions generally."[39]

Just how typical the discrimination against black student nurses was is readily documented. Indeed, by 1941 Roberts and Staupers had grown impatient with the continued rejection of good black applicants by some of the nation's best schools. They grew especially alarmed when Harriet M. Towns, a graduate of Spelman College in Atlanta, received letters of rejection from the nursing schools at Yale University and Case Western Reserve University in Cleveland, Ohio. The dean of the Yale University School of Nursing informed Towns, "I have read your autobiographical sketch with some interest, and regret to tell you that we have no Negro students in the School nor Negro nurses on the staff." She recommended that Towns contact Hulda Lyttle, head of nursing at the all-black

Meharry Medical College in Nashville, Tennessee.[40] The admissions officer at Case Western Reserve explained, "It is not possible for us to accept your application because at the present time our own clinical facilities do not make it possible for us to accept Negro applicants for the basic programs."

Cornelia Erf, chair of the Western Reserve Nursing School admissions committee, took pains to describe the problems involved in admitting a black into the program. She confessed that the school had "no difficulty in obtaining clinical facilities for Negro women who are already graduate nurses and who wish to specialize in some phase of nursing such as public health or hospital work where experience may be obtained in a community hospital." The problem, however, was that "the students in our basic program use the clinical facilities of the University Hospitals for their basic experience." Apparently, the University Hospitals did not allow black students to use its facilities. Erf therefore suggested that Towns pursue training at the black division of Grady Hospital in Atlanta.[41] Towns contacted neither Meharry nor Grady. Instead she wrote NACGN headquarters for help and advice.

Staupers registered confusion and alarm when she first learned of Towns's rejections. She had assumed, because of their previous record of integration, "that neither nursing school would deny admission to a qualified Negro applicant." Towns's rejection was of dual significance inasmuch as neither institution had indicated that she failed to meet university standards for admission. Staupers was determined to find out whether this was a case of racial exclusion or a change in admission policies. She and Roberts feared that if the matter were left unaddressed, it would "become a pattern for denying admission to other Negro students applying to these and other university schools of nursing." As it turned out, neither school had rejected Towns because of poor qualifications. They had rejected her because they could not provide guarantees of, or access to, clinical facilities for the black nursing student. The exclusionary policy, therefore, emanated from the university hospitals affiliated with the respective nursing schools.[42]

Upon receipt of Towns's request for assistance, Staupers and Roberts immediately contacted influential whites closely associated with both institutions—Anson Phelps Stokes, a former member of the Yale board of trustees, and Ohio congresswoman Frances Payne Bolton. Careful to avoid any publicity which would expose this instance of racial discrimination in two of the nation's highly regarded schools of nursing, Roberts and Staupers worked behind the scenes. Staupers confided to T. Arnold Hill, head of the Division of Negro Affairs of the National Youth Administration, "Our policy here has been not to embarrass our friends; that is why there has not been a great deal of publicity about much of our work in proportion to the publicity received by other organizations."[43] Hill in turn reassured Stokes that in light of his pledge to investigate and remedy the denial of admission of Negro students to the Yale School of Nursing, the leaders of the NACGN would put a lid on publicity. He wrote, "I know that with your interest and tactful approach, we will be able to make progress."[44]

While Staupers probed the Yale situation, Roberts communicated directly with Bolton, who was then serving on the NACGN's National Advisory Council and was a proven ally of black nurses. Roberts minced no words, declaring, "With Democracy so definitely on the defensive in the world today, it seems to me deplorably short sighted and stupid for educational institutions to foster and promote philosophies of racial exclusion."[45] Although she was determined to find a suitable remedy to the incident, Bolton cautioned calm, advising Roberts that "this whole matter of so-called racial discrimination is one which cannot be judged overnight." Bolton admitted sympathy with Towns's hurt. Nevertheless, she insisted that the NACGN shoulder some of the responsibility for precipitating the problem. She admonished that the NACGN should have advised the student about the policies of these schools and thus spared her "the pain of rejection." Bolton continued, "So far as Miss Towns, I am wondering if she will follow the suggestions made to her of getting her basic nursing experience and then getting an M.A. degree elsewhere. You will remember that Estelle Massey Riddle did this most successfully, and that she is now Superintendent of a very fine school in St. Louis. Possibly this might be just the place for Miss Towns to begin her nursing."[46]

Unchastened, Roberts rejoined that the NACGN should "advise a student to seek the educational experience for which she is fitted rather than one geared to a lower level of qualification."[47] Roberts discussed Bolton's remarks with Staupers, who, while refraining from commenting on Riddle's Homer G. Phillips experience, offered an unflattering evaluation of Grady Hospital. It "does not in any way develop leadership among Negroes," she declared. In fact, she pointed out, "leadership is discouraged even in the Negro Division of Grady Hospital. . . . I have visited the institution and I am sure that Miss Towns, who comes from one of our fine Negro families, would not be happy living under the conditions which Negroes are now forced to live at Grady Hospital." Staupers did not bother to conceal her annoyance with the suggestion that Towns attend Grady, where "she would be happier." She viewed it as "an old cliché, often used while denying opportunity to Negroes."[48]

Still, Bolton, while quietly investigating the admissions policies of the Case Western Reserve University School of Nursing, urged Roberts to try to understand the institution's position: "Is it not possible that they found a more difficult situation than suggests itself at first sight?" She pressed on: "The closest kind of intimate living conditions are part of a nursing school. . . . This surely you must appreciate, although your letter indicates that you may not have thought of that side of nursing training."[49]

Clearly the three women, Staupers and Roberts on one side and Bolton on the other, were talking at cross-purposes. Roberts's concerns went far beyond the racist policies and actions of specific institutions. She explained, "I have strong convictions on this point, not because of Harriet Towns and what happens immediately in her educational experience, but because of the larger implications of the racial and educational philosophies involved." She declared, "I feel that our real job is one of questioning the exclusion policies of the other schools." As the shadow of a world catastrophe loomed menacingly near, Roberts challenged, "Certainly in times like these we in America can ill afford the luxury of a racial superiority philosophy, and we should be able to look to our great institutions of learning to teach the fallacy of such arguments." In Roberts's opinion the NACGN had to continue to fight against exclusionary policies and racial discrimination. There was no other course to follow. She elaborated,

> This practice of exclusion remains so firmly entrenched in most such institutions, however, that it continues a real challenge not only in the area of educational opportunities for Negroes, but to the democratic principles which we in America are working so intensively to defend against other ideologies. The members of the Council feel impelled to protest against this policy of racial discrimination until it has been entirely eliminated.[50]

For her staunch, unwavering championing of the cause of the black nurse, the NACGN dispensed with tradition, and in 1942 awarded the Mary Mahoney Award to the only nonnurse ever to receive it, Ruth Logan Roberts.[51] The records do not indicate whether Towns ever became a nurse. Bolton, on the other hand, in keeping with her usual style of operation, continued to work behind the scenes to establish a clear policy of integration at the Case Western Reserve School of Nursing. It was mid-1945 when Bolton informed Staupers that "the dean of the school of nursing at Western Reserve had sought and received from the Medical Council of the university hospitals assurances that would make it possible for the school of nursing to process further applications from qualified Negro students."[52]

The urgency of Staupers's and Roberts's struggle to clarify the Towns episode is understandable, considering that fifty years after the founding in 1891 of Provident Hospital, black nursing schools had produced only 2 percent of the total nursing population of approximately 280,000 (see Appendix). Thus integration of white nursing schools represented the only viable way of increasing the number of black women in the profession. Estelle Massey Riddle reported that in 1941 "only 29 schools other than those exclusively for Negroes were open to Negro students."[53] Of the segregated schools for black students, twenty-three were controlled by hospitals, and the remaining four were programs operated at black colleges and universities. By 1944 the number of all-black schools had dwindled to twenty. Yet these schools enrolled 1,600 of the 2,000 students, while the remaining 400 black students were distributed among twenty-two integrated schools.[54]

Not until the passage of the Bolton Bill in 1943, establishing the United States Cadet Nurse Corps under the administration of the United States Public Health Service, did Riddle report significant improvement in the expansion of educational opportunities available to aspiring black women interested in nursing careers. The NACGN leaders quickly heralded the potential significance of the Bolton Bill and mobilized black nurses and others into pressure groups to ensure the inclusion of an antidiscrimination clause prior to its passage. Staupers, Riddle, and Roberts feared that in the absence of an antidiscrimination amendment, black nurses would not be in a position to take advantage of new opportunities. Never one to miss a chance to promote and protect the interests of black nurses, Staupers enlisted the aid of Thomasina W. Johnson, a lobbyist for the Alpha Kappa Alpha sorority, to direct and coordinate the fight for inclusion of the clause. As a direct consequence of Johnson's skillfully executed lobbying activities, New Jersey senator Warren W. Barbour introduced an antidiscrimination amendment to the Bolton Bill. Then Staupers urged black graduate nurses across the country to write their representatives and senators pressing them to support passage of the bill. Once it was law, Staupers publicized the legislation throughout the black nursing profession and described the specifications of the Cadet Nurse Corps program.[55]

The Cadet Nurse Corps, composed entirely of student trainees, proved a tremendous boost to black nursing in more ways than strictly educational. Nearly 125,000 nurses received training at 1,225 schools through grants awarded from the corps program. These grants enabled the schools to pay for the students' tuition, fees, and uniforms, and to give them stipends of from fifteen dollars to thirty dollars per month depending on their class status. The students accepted into the program were also provided special uniforms with special insignia. In return for this aid the prospective nurse pledged to serve in the armed forces or essential civilian posts until at least six months after the war ended.[56]

The black nurse educator Rita Miller, on leave from her position as chair of the Division of Nursing at Dillard University in New Orleans, was hired as a part-time consultant to acquaint black nursing-school administrators with the benefits to be derived from participation in the Cadet Nurse Corps programs.[57] Her efforts, combined with the generous grants awarded, allowed the stronger all-black schools dramatically to increase their student enrollment. The number of nursing students at Freedmen's Hospital grew from 77 in 1939 to 166 in 1944.[58] Among the

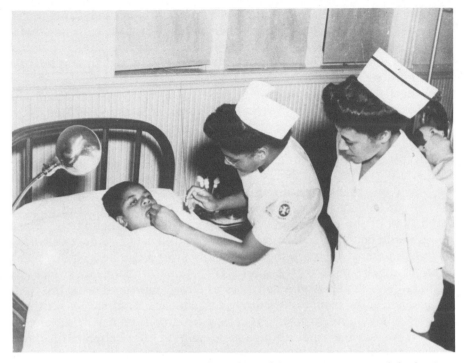

Mary Elizabeth Lancaster providing clinical instruction to one of the basic baccalaureate nursing students in the Cadet Nurse Corps, at Hampton Institute, 1943–1944. (Note insignia on left shoulder of student nurse's uniform.) Photo by Ruben Burrell. Courtesy of the M. Elizabeth Carnegie Nursing History Archives, Hampton University School of Nursing.

black schools fortunate enough to take advantage of the Cadet Nurse Corps program were John A. Andrew Memorial Hospital, Tuskegee, Alabama; University Hospital (Lamar School of Nursing), Augusta, Georgia; Provident Hospital, Chicago; Flint-Goodridge Hospital, Dillard University; Homer G. Phillips Hospital, St. Louis; Meharry Medical College, Nashville, Tennessee; Columbia Hospital, Columbia, South Carolina; and St. Phillip Hospital, Richmond, Virginia. Under the program, nursing schools were obliged to cut their training periods from the usual thirty-six months to twenty-four or thirty months. The remaining six to twelve months were to be devoted to supervised practice work.[59]

In order to qualify for a share of the Bolton Bill windfall, some white schools abandoned their discriminatory policies and extended equitable consideration to black applicants. By 1945 approximately 2,600 black students were enrolled in schools of nursing, a 135 percent increase over the 1939 figure. By the end of World War II, "49 schools of nursing with black and mixed enrollments had admitted black students, as compared with 29 in 1941."[60] Furthermore, in addition to the outbreak of World War II, as Riddle and others observed, one of the indirect benefits of the Bolton Bill to black nurses was an enhancement of their chances to secure employment in institutions previously closed to them. As Riddle indicated, "Pressure upon the over-all nursing supply helped to reduce racial barriers within the employment and educational areas of nursing. Hospitals and public health agencies which lost large numbers of their nurses to the Army and Navy Corps found it expedient to meet their needs with Negro nurses, although many of them had not previously employed this group."[61]

Writer Gerald A. Spencer likewise noted that "only the pressure of war with its shortages of nursing power brought about Negro nurses' admission to the staffs of Sydenham Hospital [in New York] and others."[62] Thus, during the 1940s, the intersection of a constellation of forces—pressure-group politics, behind-the-scenes negotiations, the crisis of a world war, the enactment of government legislation, the constant vigilance of NACGN officers, and the growing assertiveness of black student and graduate nurses—helped to improve, somewhat, the educational and employment opportunities for black nurses. While their professional status remained low, it was considerably higher than had been the case during the years following the First World War. Black nurses were inching toward parity within the profession.

Other developments begun in the 1930s led a larger number of black nurses than at any time previously to seek and secure employment in the field of public health. For the fortunate few, public-health nursing represented a significant step in the growth of employment opportunities. No longer were most black nurses limited to working in segregated black hospitals or in private duty. As the number working in the public-health arena increased, black nurses anticipated greater job security and even aspired to find more jobs as staff nurses in integrated hospitals. To be sure, full realization of the latter was still a long way off. In public-health nursing, as various oral histories attest, the black nurse became an even more effective mediator between the physicians and the patients. The black public-health nurse's practice usually was, in keeping with American racial customs, restricted to the care of black patients. By 1942, of the approximately 6,000 black nurses in America, 341 worked as public-health nurses in the South.[63]

Henrietta Smith Chisholm embarked upon a public-health–nursing career in 1931, after she was graduated from Freedmen's Hospital in Washington, D.C. "I liked public health very much. This was brand new. I never knew anything about it. . . . I was interested—that was the main thing." She elaborated, "Public health was the right field for me because I enjoyed it because it wasn't all morbidity—you felt like you were giving people help before they got into trouble. We hoped we were. I especially liked the infant and maternity program and worked mostly in infant, maternal and child welfare clinics." She lamented, however, that "at that time in Washington the child welfare clinics were separate, everything was separate." About her first job with a Washington, D.C., visiting nurses' association, Chisholm exulted, "I . . . was one of the lucky ones who got a permanent job making $1620 a year and this was good salary. $1620 a year and that was good salary during the Depression. Many heads of families were making $100 a month, $90 and $40. We were really on top." According to Chisholm, "visiting nurses were paying more than the hospitals. At that time in Washington, Freedmen's was the only hospital at which Negro nurses could work."[64] They worked either in municipal or state public-health agencies or in visiting nursing associations.

In many southern black communities, the black nurse, especially the public-health nurse, was the most prominent, if not the first, professional health-care giver to interact with the population. Thus it fell to her to establish the foundation and to define the nature of the professional-client relationship. As one writer put it, "The nurse, therefore, forms the hub around which much of a community's well-being revolves."[65] Black nurse Willa M. Maddux identified the requirements and characteristics black public-health nurses needed in order to work successfully with, as she phrased it, "the masses of untrained and indifferent people." Maddux contended, "It is imperative that the nurse be a person with broad sympathies, profound understanding and tact, and possess the requisite professional background." Writing in 1937, another black nurse from Florida observed similarly, "It is the job of the pioneer nurse to find an acceptable starting point to meet the approval of the people that she hopes to serve."

Commencing in the late 1920s, black nurses began securing positions as public-health nurses with state, local, and federal health departments and agencies. Few of them possessed more than a nursing diploma, but this was more education than the majority of their clientele had received. On January 1, 1923, Eunice Rivers, having recently completed her training at Tuskegee Institute, reported for work, joining the three-member team of Georgia's Macon County Movable School. The unit consisted of a teacher, carpenter, and nurse. Nurse Rivers had many wide-ranging responsibilities. She was expected to teach the rural tenant-farmer families the rudiments of home nursing, how to bathe a patient, how to take a temperature, how to give a massage. In summing up in an oral interview her decade of service with mothers and infants, she enumerated her accomplishments. In addition to teaching maternity care to new mothers, she trained "the midwives how to deliver, how to wash their hands, cut their nails and . . . how to make the pads, how to prepare the bed for the delivery, because at that time most of the women had the babies on the floor."

> We had an awful time trying to train the mothers to use the bed instead
> of the floor. We took paper—and there was no such thing as a draw sheet,
> a rubber sheet—so we carried old newspapers all the time, on the truck,
> and clean rags and this kind of thing, trying to teach the people how to
> do this. If we'd get in a home where we could find somebody who had an
> old ragged sheet, we'd show them how to make a pad, paper pad, to protect
> the bed. And also how to bathe the babies, feed them and prepare their
> meals, their bottles and this kind of thing.[66]

After nine years Rivers left the Movable School to become the nurse
for the black men involved with the now-infamous government-run study
of venereal disease, the Tuskegee Syphilis Experiment, in Macon County,
Alabama.

To achieve success as a public-health nurse required well-developed
interpersonal-relations skills. None were more adept or possessed of more
personality, tact, and determination than Eunice Rivers. Rivers over-
came the fears and suspicions of Macon County rural blacks both during
her years with the Movable School and as the nurse with the Tuskegee
Syphilis Experiment. Most of her clients evidenced a strong distrust of
physicians, refusing to heed their advice or even to seek their services
until it was often too late. Rivers lay part of the blame for this reluctance
on the heads of the physicians, who quite often simply did not know how
to talk to the people. She asserted that she won confidences by first ac-
knowledging that "they're people as far as I'm concerned. I don't go there
dogging them about keeping the house clean. I go there and visit a while
until I know when to make some suggestions. When I go to the house,
I accept the house as I find it. I bide my time." She continued, "Sometimes
I don't do a thing but go there, sit down there and talk." This tactic proved
especially effective and won for her the respect and admiration not only
of the black people whom she served but of the black and white physicians
with whom she worked.

The white doctors of the experiment marveled at Rivers's ability to get
patients to obey instructions. On occasion, however, she even had to step
out of the nurse's posture of professional subservience and deference to
physicians' authority. In at least one instance she took to task a young
white government doctor assigned to the syphilis study. She admonished
him, "If anything happens that you can't get along, that you can't get it
through their heads, just call me. We'll straighten it out. But don't holler
at them. These are grown men; some of them are old men. Don't holler
at them." The fact that she interceded and on occasion defended them
won their trust. This perhaps explains why many of the black patients
involved in the syphilis experiment continued to participate longer than
they should have. Rivers was, of course, convinced that the experiment
was a good and honorable effort.

Rivers admitted that as a nurse she was rewarded and sustained by

the devotion and respect her patients showered upon her. "They depended
on me . . . they would take whatever I said." Elaborating on her philosophy of the nurse-patient relationship, she added,

> After all, the doctor saw the patient and he was gone. And it was up to
> you to help that patient carry out his orders, do whatever the doctor sug-
> gested. The doctor said, you do so and so. . . . First thing, the patient doesn't
> know how to do it. He doesn't know what his reaction is going to be. He
> doesn't want to be stuck, this kind of thing. So the nurse plays an impor-
> tant part there. She's closer to the patient. Patients would get to the point
> where if they're not sure, they're going to ask you. They get you in the
> middle.[67]

Rivers was more than a good country nurse. Her more than forty-year
involvement in the Tuskegee Syphilis Experiment, in which treatment
was deliberately withheld from patients, raises questions concerning relationships between the black nurses and the black community and between black nurses and white health-care professionals. Indeed, it is fair
to say that without her the white "government doctors" would not have
been so successful in engaging so many black males in such a detrimental
and ethically bankrupt experiment. It was their unquestioning faith in
Rivers as someone selflessly looking out for and protecting them that led
the men to continue in the experiment for so many unrewarding years.
Though they remained fundamentally suspicious of the motives of the
"government doctors," they always tended to do what Rivers told them.
According to historian James H. Jones, "More than any other person,
[Rivers] made them believe that they were receiving medical care that
was helping them."[68] They were not.

Rivers's motives for collaborating in this experiment and deliberately
manipulating these black men are complex. It is possible that she viewed
the study as a way of ensuring for at least some blacks an unparalleled
amount of medical attention. Jones offers several compelling explanations for Rivers's complicity: As a nurse, she had been trained to follow
orders, and probably it simply did not occur to her to question a—or for
that matter, any—doctor's judgment. Moreover, she was incapable of
judging the scientific merits of the study. For Rivers, a female in a male-
dominated world, deference to male authority figures reinforced her ethi-
cal passivity. Finally, and perhaps most significant, Rivers was black,
and the physicians who controlled the experiment were white. Years of
conditioning and living in the South made it virtually impossible for Rivers to have rebelled against a white male government doctor, the ultimate authority figure in her world.[69] In this case the needs and interests
of the black community of Tuskegee were not addressed and protected
by the black nurse.

Black public-health nurses, regardless of region, had to fight to secure

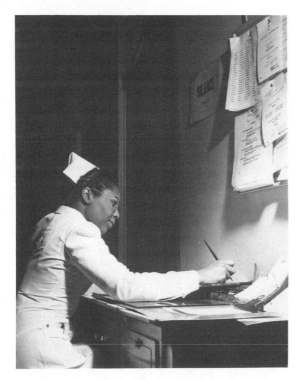

In the 1940s, as is the case today, nursing involved a lot of paperwork. This is Nurse Helen Butler at her desk in Provident Hospital in Chicago. Courtesy of the Library of Congress.

and maintain their positions. Chisholm's reflections on her public-health work in Washington, D.C., further illuminate the limitations placed on the career aspirations of these nurses. She remained with the visiting nurses' association for several years. In 1937 she transferred to the health department, later renamed the Department of Human Resources. She mused, "You wonder why you stay in one job, but there weren't any jobs. You had the best job. Except at Freedmen's there wasn't any place you could get a job and advance at all. No hospital until World War II in Washington accepted Negro nurses for anything. They did not let you come in to special your own friends. If you did, you didn't wear your cap or pin. This is demeaning, you know."[70]

Recurrent expressions of frustration over the lack of opportunities to advance to supervisory positions even after they had secured additional credentials bedeviled black public-health nurses. One nurse confided to Riddle, "Five of the Negro nurses on our staff have certificates in public health nursing and have been with the agency eight years or more, yet none of us has been advanced to a supervisory position." She continued, "We get good ratings on our work and some increases in salary. All of us have seen white nurses on the staff, with less experience and before

they received their public health certificate, advanced to supervisory positions." Another black nurse working toward an M.A. degree in public-
health nursing declared unhappily. "I do not feel, however, that my extra
study will gain for me any advancement. I may get a small salary increase, but I doubt there will be any change in the status of my duties."[71]

It was while working in the visiting nurses' association and in the District of Columbia Department of Health that Chisholm came to grips
with the reality of professional segregation. In recalling those early experiences, she reflected both personal and professional ambivalence. As
she explained, "Negro nurses took care of only Negro patients. In the
VNA they had what they called hourly service and this was if people
wanted special appointments but these were mostly white people. Negroes never did hourly service. Negroes never did home delivery service
because they might be white. There weren't enough to assign a white and
a Negro nurse so they had a white nurse because the patient might be
white."[72]

The years of discriminatory treatment had a telling effect on Chisholm.
When she could not alter the racist policy, she concentrated instead on
providing to poor black Washingtonians the best nursing service possible.
At one point, she defensively insisted, "I didn't want to go in those poor
white dirty homes, and they were dirty." Perhaps this was rationalizing
after the fact. Regardless, by the time the World War II crisis brought
its attendant destruction of certain segregationist practices, Chisholm
acknowledged that she was "as much of a segregationist as they were."
Still recoiling from a sudden policy change, she exclaimed, "Overnight
they said, 'You will visit any patient.'" She balked at this policy shift: "I
have as much feeling against visiting white people as they have. I am
not ready mentally. I am not ready, I have not prepared myself to visit
them any more than they have prepared themselves to accept me." Of
course, Chisholm soon got over her immobilizing distress, resolving, "I
had to have my job."[73]

Mary L. Steele Reives was graduated from Lincoln Hospital in 1929
and went to work for the Henry Street Visiting Nurse Service. She remarked, "I had applied for a job there and at that time they did not have
many black nurses."[74] Actually, the Henry Street Visiting Nurse Service
had a long history of having employed black nurses. The first one was
Elizabeth Tyler, a 1906 graduate of Freedmen's Hospital in Washington,
D.C. In addition to being an excellent nurse, she was described as being
"especially alive to social movements and organized preventive work."[75]

Whether in Macon County, Georgia, Washington, D.C., or New York,
public-health nursing involved the same duties, responsibilities, and
challenges. Reives elaborated: "You had a certain number of cases to do

each day. You went from one place to another. They would give you a work slip with the name and address of the patients. We had to report to work at 8:20 A.M. and obtain our assignment, and we were in the field from 9 A.M.-12 noon and 1 P.M.-5 P.M. each day." Reives confessed to enjoying the visiting nurse service: "Most of these people we saw were poor people and we were not allowed to accept anything from them," but there was a feeling of being appreciated.[76]

After passing the civil service examination, Reives secured a position in the New York City Department of Health. She recalled, "At that time it was not a generalized program. You either had to be a school nurse or a nurse in contagion. I had decided first to be a school nurse. . . . You had to learn how to give lectures to the students on health problems and childhood diseases." Two years of school nursing behind her, Steele moved into contagion nursing:

> We had to make home visits. We visited homes where there was a case of measles, scarlet fever, spinal meningitis, infantile paralysis, typhoid fever—any of the contagious diseases. You were given a list of cases you were to visit by your supervisor and you received a list every day in your district. If you didn't find anyone at home—sometimes they would feel bet-ter and would be out—you would go to the next person on the list and then double back before the work day was over.[77]

Later Reives was assigned to work at a tuberculosis clinic in the city, and after six years she moved on to become a school nurse at one of the city's trade schools.

Reives apparently spent the longest stretch of her career working at a new child-health station concerned primarily with newborn babies. She described a typical day in the life of a public-health nurse specializing in infant and maternal care:

> If a patient had delivered a baby at home, you had a certain length of time you had to give the mother full care. You had to give her a bed bath and bathe the baby. After the third day you would give her a partial bath and gradually let her get back into the routine of giving herself care so that when she was able to get out of bed she could do these things. You would give the baby his baths, watch his navel and keep it bandaged until the cord fell off, and give her instructions on how to care for the baby. This usually took about nine days. Then you would check in a certain number of days to see how she was getting along, and if anything abnormal had developed you would contact her doctor. Records and charts were kept each day, and if the doctor came he would know what you had done. You also had to give general care to people with diseases. For instance, adult fe-males, adult males, and children with pneumonia and contagious diseases. If they had a contagious disease, like scarlet fever or diphtheria, a quaran-tine sign would be put on the door and the family would be instructed as

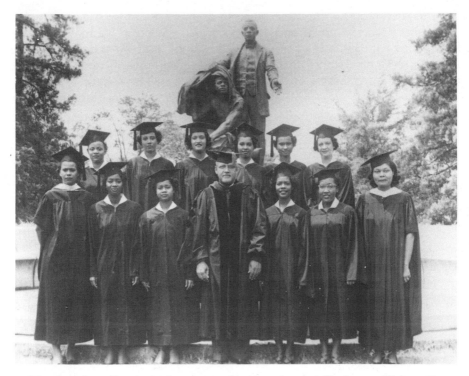

The first baccalaureate-degree graduating class at Tuskegee University, 1953. *First row, far right,* Lillian H. Harvey, dean of the School of Nursing; *first row, far right,* President Frederick D. Patterson; *first row, far left,* Queen E. Carter, assistant dean. Courtesy of Tuskegee University Archives.

to what to do. With diphtheria, cultures had to be taken when they began to improve—the cultures would be taken until two negative cultures were gotten in succession.[78]

While becoming a black nurse involved a two-tiered process of first deciding upon nursing as a career and then winning admission to a program, the actual development of a successful career involved coming to grips with the twin forces of racism and professionalism. These two realities intersected in such a way as to create a divergence between the experiences of black and white nurses. Throughout the first half of the twentieth century, racist policies and behaviors dictated that black nurses would, for the most part, serve only in the black communities or administer only to the black clientele of various public and private agencies. Nevertheless, because they considered themselves professionals, black nurses yearned to advance in their careers and tried to adhere to the highest ideals of the profession. With few exceptions, they fervently wished the freedom to provide service to all in need regardless of race, sex, or social and economic status. White nurses, as a group, never had to contend with racism or to suffer the "pain of rejection" in their quest for professional autonomy and advancement—though most did encounter the "pain of sexism," and many experienced putdowns from higher-ranking supervisors. Much, however, was expected of those black women in white whose paths were littered with so many obstacles and often insurmountable barriers. Yet as the country moved inexorably toward a global holocaust, black nurses had reason to anticipate improvement in their status. Black nurse leaders, at least, suspected that the days of Jim Crow were numbered.

"We Shall Not Be Left Out": World War II and the Integration of Nursing

8 It is a supreme irony that nursing's fortune is so often connected to war. Florence Nightingale's experiences in the Crimean War, the appalling casualties of the American Civil War, and the death and destruction of World War I all influenced the emergence and development of nursing training and practice. In the wake of these shocking episodes of massive carnage, nursing reaped increased status and greater public esteem.

As global war loomed ominously on the horizon in the late 1930s and early 1940s black nurse leaders were mindful of past opportunities lost to prove their value and to amass the rewards of a grateful public. They were determined, therefore, to take full advantage of the coming emergency. World War II was a watershed both in black nursing history and in black history in general. Nurses were not the only segment of the black population to resolve to take advantage of the situation to push for the full realization of their citizenship rights. Scholars have justifiably dubbed this period "the forgotten years of the Negro Revolution."

Stimulated by the limited reforms of the New Deal and the democratic ideology stressed by U.S. anti-Nazi propaganda, blacks became much more militant in attacking the racial status quo. Already situated on the bottom rung of the socioeconomic ladder, blacks, like private-duty nurses of both races, had suffered to a remarkable degree during the Great Depression. Much of the New Deal relief legislation designed to ameliorate the deprivation and suffering of impoverished Americans actually preserved Jim Crow practices. To be sure, blacks received significant amounts of work, housing, and federal relief, but this was certainly not sufficient to solve the basic problems arising from white prejudice and discrimination.[1]

The resurgence of economic activity at the outset of World War II effected only imperceptible changes in the overall condition of blacks, especially of black women, who remained the last hired and the first fired of all American workers.[2] Private industries, with and without government defense contracts, continued to discriminate against blacks in hiring, wages, and promotions. Many white unions excluded blacks, while the U.S. Employment Service, a federal agency, continued to fill "white only" requests from employers of defense labor. However, within the federal government, the army and navy displayed the strongest adherence to, and defense of, the ideology and practice of racial discrimination and segregation. Military leaders saw nothing amiss in sending a segregated army and navy to obliterate the forces of Fascism and Nazism to make the world safe for democracy. These contradictions were not lost upon black Americans. As Walter White observed at the time, "World War II has immeasurably magnified the Negro's awareness of the disparity between the American profession and practice of democracy."[3]

Black leaders such as A. Philip Randolph of the Brotherhood of Sleeping Car Porters, organizer of the 1941 March on Washington movement; Lester Granger of the National Urban League; Claude Barnett of the Associated Negro Press; James Farmer and Bayard Rustin of the Committee (later Congress) of Racial Equality; and Walter White of the National Association for the Advancement of Colored People employed a variety of tactics in the struggle to dismantle the entire edifice of white supremacy and racial proscription. They were not the only warriors seeking to slay Jim Crow. Black women, too, adopted variations of tried and true strategies to battle for black rights during the war years. Black nurses were no exception.

With any movement of consequence, a high caliber of leadership imbued with a clear vision of what is desired is essential to success. Mabel Keaton Staupers, as the leader of the successful campaign to integrate black women into the segregated Army and Navy Nurse Corps during World War II, surely belongs among the ranks of the better-known female leaders of this era of the black-rights quest. Without her leadership it is doubtful that the overall struggle for recognition, status, and acceptance of black nurses into the institutional structures of American nursing— the American Red Cross Nursing Service, the Army and Navy Nurse Corps, and the American Nurses' Association—would have advanced. In this hard-fought, often frustrating struggle, Staupers had to seek assistance from First Lady Eleanor Roosevelt; form coalitions with black professional and civil-rights organizations such as the National Medical Association and the National Association for the Advancement of Colored People; gain the support of the black press; cement ties with leading white philanthropists; negotiate alliances with sympathetic white nurse leaders; and win the hearts and minds of the general black public. Fortunately she proved capable of meeting these challenges.

As the 1940s commenced, two developments seemingly boded well for the future of the black nurses' struggle for integration. The first was the establishment of the National Nursing Council for War Service, and the

second was the creation of the previously discussed United States Cadet
Nurse Corps. On July 29, 1940, five leaders of the nursing profession—
Julia C. Stimson, president of the American Nurses' Association and for-
mer superintendent of the Army Nurse Corps; nurses Stella Goostray and
Grace Ross; Mary Beard, director of the American Red Cross Nursing
Service; and Mary Roberts, former editor of the ANA's *Journal of
Nursing*—met in the conference room of the ANA's New York headquar-
ters to discuss the issue of nursing preparedness for the inevitable war.
Isabel Stewart, president of the NLNE, had first suggested the need to
establish an official nursing committee representing the profession as a
whole. Joining the nurse leaders at this meeting were representatives of
several federal agencies: the Army Nurse Corps; Navy Nurse Corps;
Children's Bureau; United States Public Health Service, Division of
State Relations and Hospitals, Nursing Service; Veterans' Administration Nursing Service; Department of Indian Affairs; and American Red
Cross.

The meeting resulted in the founding of the National Nursing Council
for War Service (later National Defense). Each state subsequently formed
a Council for War Service, with essential subcommittees functioning in
cooperation with the main body.[4] In spite of the substantial number of
federal agencies represented at the initial meeting, the Nursing Council,
as one War Department memorandum described it, had "no official function." The council, however, was not without power and influence. It existed primarily "to estimate war and civilian needs for nurses, to assist
in recruiting nurses, and to advise with public officials."[5]

Black nurses were heartened and delighted to be included among the
membership of the National Nursing Council. Mabel Staupers and
Frances Foulkes Gaines, a twenty-one-year employee of the Chicago Department of Health, represented the National Association of Colored
Graduate Nurses on the council. Later, Estelle Massey Riddle, with the
aid of a grant from the General Education Board, would become a full-
time staff member of the National Nursing Council for War Service. Riddle's special assignment was to hold institutes and to visit schools of nursing and colleges to improve the preparation and utilization of black
nurses in the event of war. Staupers confidently opined, "I have every
belief that since we were voluntarily requested to become a part of the
Nursing Council on National Defense and since the national survey of
nurses is being sent to Negro nurses, we will not be left out."[6] Riddle,
too, was delighted to be a part of the National Nursing Council. She saw
it as occupying a strategic position from which to provide leadership for
the improvement of race relations within the profession and in the country at large. Riddle later recalled, "Through the relationships established, in this connection, information relative to the progress and the

problems of Negro nurses was more widely disseminated than ever before."[7]

At the same time that nurses organized the Nursing Council, President Franklin Delano Roosevelt set up in the Federal Security Agency the Office of Defense, Health, and Welfare with a subcommittee on Negro health. Mabel K. Staupers, as executive secretary of the NACGN, was invited to join her black male colleagues on this subcommittee chaired by her good friend Dr. Midian O. Bousfield, director of Negro health for the Julius Rosenwald Fund. Also serving on the committee were Albert W. Dent, superintendent of Flint-Goodridge Hospital in New Orleans; A. M. Vaughn, president of the NMA; and Russell A. Dixon, dean of the Howard University School of Dentistry.[8] Thus as far as the official and semiofficial committees of importance to black nurses were concerned, they were well represented.

Yet black nurses did not feel completely sanguine about membership on nursing councils and health subcommittees. They remained uneasy that these groups alone guaranteed their inclusion in national defense plans developed by the War Department and the federal government. No one would fight their battles or advance their interests as well as they. Therefore, to ensure that their unique problems and interests would have a special hearing, Staupers, ever determined that black nurses would not again experience the pain of rejection and exclusion that had been theirs during World War I, created an NACGN National Defense Committee. She appointed as chair of the committee a Washington, D.C.–based nurse, Marian Seymour of Freedmen's Hospital. Each of the other carefully selected members represented black nurses from every region of the country: Estelle M. Riddle of St. Louis and Carrie E. Bullock of Chicago, both former NACGN presidents; Janice Jones of Tulsa, Oklahoma, president of the Southern Region; Sylvia Daily Hines of Richmond, Virginia, president of the St. Philip Hospital Alumnae Association; and Ferrol G. Bobo, chair of the Los Angeles NACGN.[9] It was an inspired stroke of her political acumen.

The timing of the formation of the NACGN Defense Committee was propitious, as two subsequent meetings with government military officials demonstrated. In October 1940, Staupers journeyed to Washington to attend a hastily arranged meeting with Major Julia O. Flikke, during which she discussed her concern about the possible rejection of black applicants for appointment to the Army Nurse Corps. Then a month later Staupers quickly summoned the leaders of the NACGN Defense Committee to Washington, this time to meet with Surgeon General of the United States Army James C. Magee and his top aides.

The meeting with Magee was arranged in response to his announcement on October 25 of the War Department's "plan for the use of colored personnel." According to the plan, no "colored personnel" would be called to service until separate black wards could be designated in station hospitals, and this only where the number of black troops was sufficient to warrant separate facilities. The War Department established a quota of 56 nurses, 120 doctors, and 44 dentists to man the wards designated for the black troops. Magee, in declaring that this official policy was "segregation without discrimination," reflected the prevailing views of his colleagues at the War Department. In areas, particularly in the South, where the overwhelming majority of black troops were to be located, two separate wards in existing station hospitals were to be established: Fort Bragg in North Carolina and Camp Livingstone in Louisiana. In a subsequent clarification, Magee stated, "Where only a few of that race are to be hospitalized in any given hospital . . . it would . . . be poor economy to set aside separate wards for the segregation of such cases."[10]

In the face of criticism of this policy, Undersecretary of War Robert P. Patterson argued that establishment of separate units was entirely consistent with racial policies and customs operating in the larger society. Actually, Patterson believed that the War Department was acting in a rather progressive fashion. He wrote at one point:

> The Medical Department has not discriminated in any sense against the Negro medical profession, nurses, or enlisted men. It has assigned Negro personnel in keeping with War Department policy and provided field and service units in support of Negro troops with Negro personnel. For the first time in the history of the Army opportunity has been furnished the Negro medical profession and ancillary services to exercise full professional talent through the establishment of separate departments at two of our large cantonment hospitals for the care of Negro soldiers. These departments are completely manned by Negro doctors, nurses, and enlisted men.[11]

Thus, as far as War Department officials were concerned, segregation, implying only separation, was nondiscriminatory if equal facilities were provided. Blacks, on the other hand, considered the concept of enforced segregation discriminatory. From their perspective, separation prevented freedom of movement, as well as fostered unequal facilities and restricted professional opportunities. Traditionally, minority groups possessed few means of enforcing equality guarantees. Staupers, for one, argued, "My position is that, as long as either one of the Services reject Negro nurses, they are discriminated against and as long as either Service continues to assign them to duty as separated units, they are segregated."[12]

The meeting between the black nurses and War Department bureaucrats proved disappointing. Joining Magee were General Albert G. Love, Colonel Larry B. McAfee, and Captain Florence A. Blanchard of the

Army Nurse Corps. During the meeting and afterwards, Magee elaborated the official government policy, stating, "Negro nurses [will be] assigned to negro hospitals provided separate mess and housing facilities are available." In a letter to Mary Beard he declared, "It is not intended that colored nurses or colored physicians be engaged in the care and treatment of military personnel other than colored."[13] There could be no mistake. Magee and the others had made their positions clear.

During this meeting with Magee and his associates, Staupers found herself in a dilemma frequently experienced by black leaders. She had fervently envisioned a broader use of black women in the Armed Forces Nurse Corps, and what Magee announced fell far short of her desires. Yet she knew that the establishment of quotas was an advance over the total exclusion black nurses had suffered in World War I, when only eighteen of them had been called to service, after the cessation of hostilities. Now Staupers reasoned that once a handful of black nurses won a place in the Armed Forces Nurse Corps, the NACGN could intensify agitation against the quotas and fight for total integration. It was a gamble she was willing to take for the moment. Staupers refused to give in without a struggle, and on one point she held firm. She adamantly rejected Love's proposal that the NACGN assume responsibility for the recruitment of a few black nurses for the Army Nurse Corps as the need arose. She reminded the colonel that such tasks were the responsibility of the American Red Cross Nursing Service, and while the NACGN would assist the Red Cross, it would not assume total responsibility for this activity.[14]

The War Department's discriminatory policy for the use of "colored personnel" did not catch any one of the Afro-American leaders entirely off guard and therefore unprepared quickly to protest. Throughout the early fall of 1940, various groups, anticipating the continuation of Jim Crow policies and practices, had formed committees and written numerous letters to, and attended meetings with, the president, Mrs. Roosevelt, and other federal government officials, urging a fair consideration and equitable treatment of blacks in the war mobilization. On September 27, 1940, a group of prominent black medical and civil-rights leaders had even received assurances from President Roosevelt that forthcoming war-policy announcements would "insure that Negroes are given fair treatment on a non-discriminatory basis."[15]

Three weeks before the War Department announced the policy, the special Liaison Committee of the National Medical Association, composed of black physicians Roscoe C. Giles, Clarence H. Payne, and Carl G. Roberts, had appealed to the president to "give full and equitable representation in those services, in proportion to our population, among the enlisted and officer personnel with respect to the medical and combat troops." The doctors noted with dismay that no or inadequate provisions had been made for the inclusion of black professionals in the organization of base hospitals or in the expansion of the medical corps. As the official representative of "the 5,000 Negro physicians of the National Medical Association of America," the letter ended, "we have been singularly slighted."[16]

Skepticism and cynicism abounded among many blacks, who expected that blacks would be unfairly treated inasmuch as previous War Department policy decisions had rarely, if ever, accorded them an even chance. Mary McLeod Bethune, president of the National Council of Negro Women and a member of Roosevelt's Black Cabinet, wrote to Eleanor Roosevelt after discussing the matter with black leaders Robert C. Weaver, Channing Tobias, and T. Arnold Hill. Anticipating the worst, she informed the First Lady, "We feel there should be attached to the War Office, some strong person who will implement the statement of policy we understand the War Department will soon make to the effect that Negroes will be used throughout all branches of the Services."[17] Staupers, along with other black leaders, pleaded to President Roosevelt after Magee's announcement: "We have prepared ourselves and many of us are holding responsible executive positions, and can see no reason why we should be denied service in the Army Corps."[18]

Perhaps it was the concatenation of appeals which informed, in part, Secretary of War Henry Stimson's decision to invite William H. Hastie to become a member of his staff. In any event, on the same day that Magee announced the plan for the use of black health-care personnel, Stimson announced the appointment of Hastie, then dean of the Howard University Law School in Washington, D.C., as his civilian aide on Negro affairs. In light of the War Department's plan for the rather limited use of black health-care personnel, it is ironic that within less than a year, one official memorandum described Hastie's chief function as liaison between the War Department and the President's Committee on Fair Employment Practices. He was to oversee "all matters wherein the War Department as contracting agency is vested with or shares responsibility for carrying out the provisions of Executive Order No. 8802," which Roosevelt issued on June 25, 1941.[19] The executive order was intended to reaffirm the policy of full participation in the defense program by all persons regardless of race, creed, color, or national origin. Inasmuch as Magee announced his plan in October 1940, not June 1941, he perhaps felt immune from having to comply with Executive Order No. 8802.

The indomitable Staupers was not one to walk away without a struggle and silently tend to the pain of rejection and discrimination. She resolved to fight back, even if it meant challenging the whole War Department, insisting to Mary Beard, "We fail to understand how America can say to the world that in this country we are ready to defend democracy when its Army and Navy are committed to a policy of discrimination."[20] As a first move she sent Barnett and black newspapers a steady stream of

Plans to effect the complete integration of black women into the Armed Forces Nurse Corps unfolded as the war progressed. During the first year of peacetime mobilization, 1940–41, Staupers, in concert with the NACGN Defense Committee, struggled both to prevent the exclusion of black nurses and simultaneously to encourage them to apply for service through the American Red Cross.[26] Once the war began, she and her colleagues fought to abolish the quotas established by the army. They continued to protest even when, in July 1942, the Army Nurse Corps accepted sixty new black nurses, assigning them to the recently opened large black station hospital at Fort Huachuca in Arizona. Throughout 1943 and 1944, Staupers and the NAACP challenged the army's practice of assigning black nurses only to care for German prisoners of war.[27] In addition, she maintained a constant vigil over all impending congressional legislation, insisting that antidiscrimination clauses be included whenever possible. However, in spite of continuous NACGN pressure, the Navy Nurse Corps proved unalterably opposed to the induction of black women nurses.

As had been the case in World War I, the American Red Cross Nursing Service was (this time under Mary Beard's leadership) again designated the official agency for the procurement of nursing personnel for the armed services. As early as the summer of 1939, assistant director Virginia Dunbar had solicited Staupers's aid in formulating requirements for black nurses who desired to serve in the Armed Forces Nurse Corps. Inasmuch as most black nurses residing in southern states were prohibited from membership in state nurses' associations, Staupers and Dunbar agreed to consider membership in the NACGN an accepted substitute.[28] With some justification, perhaps, Dunbar feared that large numbers of black women would decline to enroll, given the hostility many blacks harbored toward the American Red Cross. Indeed, many black leaders questioned the propriety of designating the Red Cross the chief procurement agency for nursing personnel in the armed forces. They pointed out that the organization continued to maintain blood banks in which blood donated by blacks was separated from that of whites. Accordingly, the National Urban League adopted a resolution declaring:

> Although the National Urban League commends the American Red Cross for certain steps that have been taken to serve more effectively the needs of Negro men and women in the armed forces, the League feels nevertheless that these steps do not go far enough and are in some respects not wisely planned. . . . The policy of racial blood segregation must be discontinued as it affronts the respect of 13,000,000 Negroes and undermines their morale in a period of national peril.[29]

Pushing aside all misgivings, Staupers decided to cooperate fully with the Red Cross and urged Dunbar to send letters and application blanks to black training schools, nurse superintendents, and hospitals. She alerted Marian Seymour, chair of the NACGN Defense Committee, to get "this information to the nurses through the newspapers" in order to encourage black enrollment, and suggested that she contact the Washington, D.C., representative of the Associated Negro Press. Pausing to commend Seymour for the "grand job" she was doing, Staupers added that increased involvement of the black nursing-school alumnae associations and local health organizations as well as community NACGN defense committees would result in securing a large enrollment of black nurses.[30]

In spite of massive publicity, superb local organizing, and untiring effort, black nurses proved reluctant to enroll in the Red Cross Nursing Service. Perplexed, Mary Beard and Virginia Dunbar wondered if there was something else they could do. Staupers patiently explained that at the heart of their reluctance to register was an understandable inability to forget past discrimination. She pointed out, "It is not easy for a group of people who have been restricted as long as we have to put our entire heart and soul into something, however noble the cause may be, when we find at every turn of the road the hand of discrimination being placed upon us." Staupers declared, "When I talked with you, I understood that the Army would need about five hundred Negro nurses. We set machinery in motion for enrollment, and every day blacks were coming to our office to be signed." She lamented, "I am sure that the slowing down is due to the fact that the nurses do not approve of the Surgeon General's [Magee's] attitude." Nevertheless, Staupers reassured Beard that though she too was personally "discouraged over the attitude of the War Department," she would work even harder to encourage black nurses to enroll.[31] Still smarting from her own encounter with Magee the previous fall, Staupers elaborated to Dunbar, "It is not so much what he [Magee] states . . . but it was his implication that we were inferior to other nurses."[32]

Although it was a slow, tedious process to overcome black nurses' hesitancy, eventually Staupers's hard work bore fruit, and the first fifty-six black women nurses won induction into the Army Nurse Corps in April 1941. Staupers, ever mindful of the value of good press, arranged for the New York *Amsterdam-Star News* to publish pictures of the two black women nurses from Lincoln Hospital as they left the city to join their twenty-four colleagues at Fort Bragg. Another twenty-six were stationed at Camp Livingstone. Staupers advised black nurse Della Raney similarly to seek press coverage of their activities whenever possible. "One of the things our nurses fail to do is get constructive publicity," she declared. "I hope that all of you from time to time will try to get as much valuable publicity as possible."[33]

In seeking good publicity, and as much as she could, Staupers anticipated the advice that Claude Barnett would give to her as her ongoing struggle to lift the Nurse Corps quotas unfolded. Barnett said, "There is a fine possibility at this time for you to do your association a lot of good through publicity and the cause of the nurses also—not through complaint alone but by effective, clear description of what is going on." He added, "Just protest is not enough. Folks want to know what they can do for the profession and how to do it."[34] Barnett did not have to repeat his counsel, for Staupers, a quick learner, used every opportunity available to tell the black nurses' story and to win community support.

To be sure, few black as compared to white nurses were called to serve during the early part of 1941, yet like their white counterparts, they endured the same arbitrary and discriminatory treatment meted out to women in the Army Nurse Corps. In addition to the requirement of membership in a professional nurses' association, all armed-forces nurses had to be no younger than eighteen or older than thirty-five. The Surgeon General's Office preferred younger women, deeming them "more flexible" and allegedly able to adjust better to the hardships encountered in foreign service, including "sleeping in tents, meager laundry facilities and adverse working conditions." There was, in addition, a strong bias against married women. Armed-forces nurses had to be single, divorced, or widowed, for according to male military officials, only single women would willingly transfer to all parts of the world on short notice. The officials defended their positions on the grounds that they had to "preserve at all cost the sanctity of the family." These men asserted that it would be very difficult for a woman to break up her home and leave her husband and children.[35] Presumably this was not true for a man.

Not surprisingly, some nurses chafed under these restrictions and stereotypes, and as quietly and unobtrusively as possible they pressed for modification or loosening of the more objectionable regulations. They succeeded in having the age limit raised and forced a revision of the proscription against marriage. Some white nurses especially objected to the ban on marriage, informing the secretary of war, "If you were to revise the law that Army nurses must be single, perhaps there would not be so much mumbling in our heads. The point is, there are several of us who wish to be married. All Army personnel except nurses are given this privilege."[36] In September 1942, the adjutant general received a memo from Colonel John A. Rogers of the Medical Corps to the effect that a change had been made in army policy regarding the discharging of nurses who married. The new ruling stated, "Hereafter a member of the Army Nurse Corps who marries will, at the discretion of the Surgeon General, be continued in active service for the duration and for six (6) months thereafter or until such time as she is found physically disqualified for further active military service." The ruling ended by declaring, "An Army nurse so continued in service will be assigned to duty as the needs of the service require."[37]

Another set of stipulations required that the potential nurse corps recruit provide references of her good moral character. Unwed pregnancies, of which there were apparently many, were punished by dishonorable discharges and loss of pension benefits. A galling inequity was the practice of paying armed-forces nurses lower wages for their services than those paid to other comparable workers. Indeed, nurses in the Army and Navy Nurse Corps received a lower initial salary than any other nurse in government employ. Corps nurses collected a mere $70 per month, while dietitians and nurses on civilian status earned a monthly income of $125. To add insult to injury, the waiters who served the nurses' meals were paid at least $100 per month. Even the nurse ensign, for example, received a base salary of $90 a month, compared to the $150 for a male ensign.[38]

Added to the list of grievances pertaining to military nursing was the practice of the "relative rank" granted army nurses by Congress on June 4, 1920, and continued until the advent of World War II. "Relative rank" conferred an officer's title and uniform but accorded less power and pay than their male counterparts received. Some nurse leaders strongly believed that they should have the same privileges and perquisites as commissioned officers. Not until June 22, 1944, did Congress enact a law providing members of the Army and Navy Nurse Corps with officer's rank. The struggle for rank was actually a quest for the power and right to manage the nursing care they themselves delivered and the nursing functions performed by the enlisted men. In the final six months of the war, military nurses won equal initial pay allowances, rights benefits, and privileges as prescribed by law for commissioned officers.[39]

The second confrontation between black nurses, black medical men, and U.S. government officials over the issue of health-care personnel quotas occurred on March 7, 1941. While the grievances of armed-forces nurses were many and not easily addressed, uppermost among Staupers's concerns was that the black nurse be allowed an equal opportunity to protest along with her white colleagues. Staupers and the members of the Negro Health and Advisory Committee of the Council of National Defense had requested the meeting with Surgeon General James C. Magee in order to try to persuade him to lift the quotas on the procurement and assignment of black medical personnel. Adamant, Magee still refused to reconsider the original quotas. Those were his terms, and black nurses could either accept or reject them. Never one to mince words, Staupers warned the surgeon general that "since Negro nurses recognize that service to their country [is] a responsibility of citizenship, they [will] fight with every resource at their command against any limitations on their services, whether a quota, segregation, or discrimination."[40]

Behind the scenes, Hastie labored untiringly to convince his coworkers and superiors to do away with all quotas. As civilian aide on Negro affairs, he suffered, none too quietly, the intransigent racism of his bosses.

He endeavored to persuade the War Department of the inherent unfairness of quotas and the adverse consequences of continued segregation. Hastie urged that the quotas be abolished before they became an institutionalized manner of treating black Americans. His entreaties and meticulously drafted recommendations calling for the desegregation of the army fell upon deaf ears and eyes blinded by adherence to racial separation. Specifically, when Hastie inquired as to the possibility of using more black nurses, he received a curt memorandum declaring, "No additional negro nurses will be procured until additional negro wards are activated."[41] Ultimately the War Department administrators treated Hastie with no more respect than that accorded to Staupers and her fellow committee members.

The general staff at the War Department objected that if Hastie had his way, he would have the army "carry out a complete social revolution against the will of the nation." Conflict raged through 1941 until days before the Japanese bombed Pearl Harbor, when Hastie and the army's high command reached an impasse. General George C. Marshall remarked in response to one of Hastie's desegregation memorandums that "the War Department cannot ignore the social relationships between Negroes and whites which have been established by the American people through custom and habit." Marshall added, reflecting the racist tenor of the times, "Either through lack of opportunity or other causes, the level of intelligence and occupational skill of the negro population is considerably below that of the white." He predicted that were the army to engage in social experiments, only "danger to efficiency, discipline, and morale" would result. Finally, he observed that the army had attained maximum strength by properly placing its personnel in accordance with the individuals' capabilities.[42]

Eventually Hastie's impatience and exasperation reached the limit. Too many of his recommendations were ignored. Thus left with no alternative, he resigned as civilian aide to the secretary of war on January 31, 1943.[43] With his resignation, however, black nurses and other black healing professionals lost a valued, highly placed ally in their quest for integration.

Compared to the navy and the position it adopted, the army was a model of racial enlightenment. The navy found the establishment of quotas unnecessary, for it held black women simply ineligible and undesirable for service in its nurse corps. According to Lt. Commander Sue S. Dauser, superintendent of the Navy Nurse Corps, navy nurses were special nurses. They combined the responsibilities and roles of teacher, counselor, dietitian, laboratory technician, x-ray operator, bookkeeper, and confidante of the sick. The navy nurse was required to instruct hospital corpsmen in modern nursing methods. In turn, the men so taught would be responsible for the welfare of the patients in the sickbays of battleships, cruisers, destroyers, and other combat vessels to which members of the Nurse Corps were not assigned. While the army nurse engaged in some teaching activity, this was considered incidental when compared to ward or bedside duties. In sum, a navy nurse had to be a "tactful, clearminded administrator and teacher."[44] Presumably black women were devoid of such qualities. Furthermore, there were very few black sailors in the navy.

After months of protesting the exclusionary policy, Staupers received notice, midway through the war in 1943, that the navy had at last decided to take the matter of inducting black nurses "under consideration." The army, on the other hand, raised its quota of black nurses to 160; 30 of them were assigned to foreign duty, and another 31 were deployed to form a new separate unit at Fort Clark, Texas.[45] While welcome news, these cosmetic changes failed to appease Staupers. Still troubled by her inability to persuade the army, navy, and War Department to abolish quotas and immediately institute plans for the full integration of black nurses, she resolved to present her case to America's First Lady. In her mind, little had changed since the time she had first admitted to Beard, "I am discouraged over the attitude of the War Department."[46]

To prepare Eleanor Roosevelt for their meeting, Staupers sent the First Lady copies of letters she had received from black nurses serving at the various segregated posts. While too lengthy to quote in their entirety, the letters offer a poignant glimpse into these nurses' wartime experience. An unidentified black nurse at the 168th Station Hospital in England called her own disappointment "a bitter pill." She lamented having traveled such a great distance only to take care of German prisoners. Staupers tactfully observed that "the nurses in India seem to be getting along all right so far. At least they are not taking care of prisoners."

Closer to home, at Fort Huachuca, black nurses were justifiably dissatisfied. One nurse complained, "There is some kind of recreation on the post for everyone but us.—Thus every night week after week, and month after month we sit and stare at each other. It is not a normal life for anyone, after spending eight and a half hours with the Germans every day." Reproachingly she went on, "Apparently we are not considered officers by those in command, for we are never included in the command affairs and meetings called for all officers of the post to attend." More specifically, the nurse conveyed the latest insult: "Last night there was a large reception given at the officers' club to welcome the new post commander. It is a command affair and every officer, besides being urged to attend, was given an invitation. That is, all the officers on the post but the five Negro nurses."[47]

Shortly after Staupers's contact, Eleanor Roosevelt sent discreet inquiries to Secretary of War Stimson and Beard. In her classic understatement, she wrote, "I have several protests lately that due to the shortage

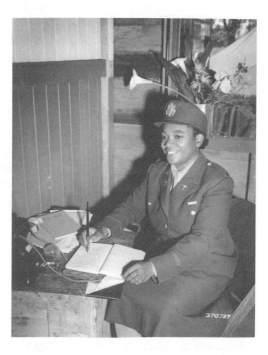

Second Lieutenant Inez E. Holmes from Norfolk, Virginia, was one of the first fifteen black nurses to arrive in Australia. She is seated at her desk in the 268th Station Hospital, Camp Columbia. 29 November 1943. Courtesy of the National Archives, photo no. 111–SC–370739.

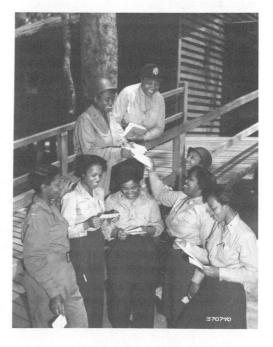

The first contingent of black nurses to arrive in the Southwest Pacific area in 1943 receives a batch of mail from home at their station at the 268th Station Hospital. Second Lieutenant Inez Holmes is handing a letter to Lieutenant Prudence L. Burns, Mounds, Illinois. Observing is Chief Nurse First Lieutenant Birdie E. Brown, New York City. Courtesy of the National Archives, photo no. 111–SC–370740.

of nurses, the colored nurses be allowed to serve where there is no serious objection to it."⁴⁸ While Stimson's response was essentially defensive and noncommittal, Beard confessed that the American Red Cross Nursing Service had been "greatly concerned with the unequal treatment of qualified Negro nurses as compared with the white nurses" serving in the armed forces. She reassured the First Lady that the National Nursing Council for War Service was attempting quietly to influence the assignment policy of the Army and Navy Nurse Corps. Beard also informed the First Lady that the Nursing Service of the Red Cross was then "looking for a qualified negro nurse to add to our staff here at Headquarters in order that she may advise and aid us with this problem." She made it clear that the Nursing Service functioned only as a recruiting agency for the army and navy and did not have any power to stipulate the assignment of nurses after referral. Elmira B. Wickenden, executive secretary of the National Council, offered similar reassurances. Indeed, the National Nursing Council had sent, in late 1943, a resolution to the surgeon generals of the Army and Navy Medical Corps: "Be it resolved that Negro graduate registered nurses be appointed to the Army (or Navy) Nurse Corps on the same basis as any other American nurses who meet the professional requirements, as was done in the last war."⁴⁹

Staupers's patience had grown very thin; she wanted results, not reassurances, promises, or resolutions. Propitiously, 1944 was a presidential election year. Staupers discreetly let it be known in the appropriate political circles that she was an avowed Roosevelt supporter and did not wish to make a fuss or "give any publicity to the present situation during this preelection period." The implied hint of a willingness to go public with black nurses' disaffection reached responsive ears. A mutual friend, Anna Arnold Hedgeman, the national executive secretary of the National Council for a Permanent Fair Employment Practices Committee, interceded and suggested to Eleanor Roosevelt that the time had come for her to invite Staupers to a meeting with her.⁵⁰

Staupers and Roosevelt met in November 1944, whereupon the NACGN executive secretary described in detail the black nurses' relationship with the armed forces. She informed the First Lady that eighty-two black nurses were serving 150 patients at the station hospital at Fort Huachuca at a time when the army was complaining of a dire nursing shortage. Staupers expounded at length on the practice of using black women to take care of German prisoners of war. She asked, rhetorically, if this was to be the special role of the black nurse in the war. Staupers elaborated, "When our women hear of the great need for nurses in the Army and when they enter the service it is with the high hopes that they will be used to nurse sick and wounded soldiers who are fighting our country's enemies and not primarily to care for these enemies."⁵¹

Roosevelt, apparently moved by the discussion, applied her own subtle pressure to Norman T. Kirk, surgeon general of the United States Army (who had replaced James C. Magee in June 1943), Secretary Stimson, and the Navy's rear admiral, W. J. C. Agnew. Kirk insisted that the Army Nurse Corps' personnel difficulties emanated not so much from the use of black nurses on the wards, "but in the many social complications related to quartering them and providing their off-duty subsistence allowances."⁵² Meanwhile the Army Nurse Corps continued to induct an occasional black nurse.

As 1944 faded into 1945, events on the black nursing front took a sudden upswing. In early January, Kirk announced to a crowd of three-hundred nurses, politicians, and private citizens assembled at the Hotel Pierre in New York City that in order for the army to be adequately supplied with nurses, it might be advisable to institute a draft. Staupers immediately rose to her feet and pointedly asked the surgeon general, "If nurses are needed so desperately, why isn't the Army using colored nurses?" She challenged, "Of 9,000 registered Negro nurses the Army has taken 247, the Navy takes none." Kirk, visibly uncomfortable according to press reports, corrected her numbers and then made an error himself: "There are 7,000 Negro nurses in comparison to 200,000 in the United States. I believe that the average share of colored nurses in the Army is equal to the total number of Negro troops."⁵³

Of course Kirk was being less than candid. According to nursing historians Kalisch and Kalisch, "If as many black nurses, in proportion to their numbers, had been accepted by the Army and the Navy as were white nurses, there would have been 1520 in the Army and Navy instead of only 330 in the Army at that date." A more reasonable and perhaps acceptable rationale would have been to point out that the black population could not have afforded the loss of 10 percent of its health-care providers without seriously jeopardizing black health.⁵⁴ News of the Staupers-Kirk exchange received nationwide coverage and made the headlines of virtually every black newspaper in the country.

The *Boston Guardian* declared, "It is difficult to find calm words to describe the folly which color prejudice assumes in the desperate shortage of nurses." The editor anticipated the kind of future action that occurred when he predicted that "the Commander-in-Chief will be backed up in this instance by the great majority of the people if he orders a cessation of the outrageous ban on nurses because of skin color and thus helps to modernize the armed forces by ridding them of the foggyism which is the greatest barrier to national growth."⁵⁵

Compounding the tension surrounding the Kirk-Staupers incident, on January 6, 1945, in a radio address to the U.S. Congress, President Roosevelt announced his strong support for the enactment of legislation amending the Selective Service Act of 1940 to provide for the induction of nurses into the army. He justified the need for such legislation on the grounds that volunteering had not produced the number of nurses required. Roosevelt adopted this position over the objections of Chief of Staff Marshall and Major General Stephen G. Henry, both of whom advised that the proposed legislation would be "most discriminatory in that it singles out a small group of especially trained women for induction under the Selective Service Act." One memorandum asserted that it was doubtful whether the War Department could defend this action, and continued, "nor can we present convincing factual data to support the need." As arranged, Representative Andrew J. May (Democrat, Kentucky) introduced the Draft Nurse Bill, H.R. 1284 79th Congress, on January 9, 1945, and it was immediately referred to the Committee on Military Affairs.[56]

The ensuing public outcry, quickly forthcoming and totally unexpected, jarred the military brass. Roosevelt apparently had not the slightest appreciation for the depth of the public's dissatisfaction with the armed services' restrictive quotas for black nurses. Staupers quickly sought to harness, direct, and channel the wave of public anger and sympathy. She urged black nurses, women's groups, and sympathetic white allies across the country to send telegrams directly to President Roosevelt and Congressman May protesting the exclusion, discrimination, and segregation of black nurses. In a joint statement by the National Nursing Council for War Service and the NACGN, Elmira Wickenden and Mabel Staupers, the executive secretaries of the two organizations, argued that the admission of black nurses into the navy would have positive, broadranging effects. They insisted that "it would demonstrate to young Negro women who are considering nursing as a career the fact that opportunities to serve will not be denied them, thus paving the way for a greater contribution by Negroes after the war to the health not only of Negroes but of the whole population." Staupers in numerous press releases pleaded, "We stress again for the Negro nurses all over the country that they rally now as never before to the support of the NACGN."[57]

And rally they did. The sheer hypocrisy of calling for a draft of nurses while excluding large numbers of black nurses willing to serve was too much for most Americans to swallow. Telegrams poured into the White House from the NAACP, the Catholic Interracial Council, the National Nursing Council for War Service, the Congress of Industrial Organizations, the American Federation of Labor, the National YWCA Board, the Alpha Kappa Alpha sorority, the Philadelphia Fellowship Commission, the New York Citizens' Committee of the Upper West Side, the National Council of Negro Women, the United Council of Church Women, and the American Civil Liberties Union. Acting secretary Thelma M. Dale of the National Negro Congress wrote to President Roosevelt, "The nation-wide support which the National Association of Colored Graduate Nurses in cooperation with the National Council for War Service has received on this specific issue, we believe, indicates that our nation and the armed forces generally are ready to accept Negro nurses on a basis of full integration."[58]

Buried beneath the avalanche of telegrams and seared by the heat of an inflamed public, Kirk, Agnew, and the War Department declared an end to quotas and exclusion. On January 20, 1945, Kirk stated that nurses would be accepted into the Army Nurse Corps without regard to race. Five days later Admiral Agnew announced that the Navy Nurse Corps was now open to black women, and within a few weeks Phyllis Daley became the first black woman to break the color barrier and receive induction into the corps. There was no outcry over the acceptance of black women nurses into the Armed Forces Nurse Corps.[59] Staupers's carefully orchestrated telegram campaign and tedious years of continuous effort had culminated in the breaking of at least this one link in the chain which oppressed, excluded, and prohibited black women from the full realization of their civil rights. This was by no means the end of their war. It was, however, a welcome victory in what had been a long struggle overwhelmingly characterized by defeat, rejection, humiliation, and frustration.

The proposed nurse draft legislation and ensuing congressional debate had been the catalyst in the struggle, bringing support and sympathy from both white and black Americans. Presidential and congressional speeches bemoaning the shortage of nurses had only fed the fire that Staupers's public protests had ignited. While Staupers and black nurses may have supported in principle the nurse draft legislation, they nevertheless used it to draw attention to the fact that they had been excluded, segregated, and discriminated against. Staupers again displayed a flawless sense of timing and political maneuvering.

White nurses' opinions on the proposed legislation varied. Some maintained that the prestige of the profession had been dealt a serious blow, while others expressed pride in the acknowledged essentiality of its service. Shortly after the bill was introduced, the board of directors of the American Nurses' Association endorsed the principle of a draft of nurses as the first step toward selective service for all women. The National League of Nursing Education, the National Nursing Council, and the National Organization for Public Health Nursing all approved the principle of selective service. Congresswoman Bolton on January 11, 1945 delivered a strongly worded speech before Congress urging passage of the legislation. In an unprecedented action, the House of Representatives passed by a large majority the bill to conscript nurses. In the meantime, more than twenty-five thousand nurses volunteered for service as a direct response to President Roosevelt's earlier appeal.

By May 2, 1945, the War Department and Surgeon General Kirk had reconsidered the advisability of draft legislation for nurses. Kirk subse-

First Lieutenant Nancy C. Leftenant, a graduate of Lincoln Hospital School for Nurses in New York, joined the Reserve Corps of the Army Nurse Corps in February 1945. In March 1948 she became the first black member of the Regular Army Nurse Corps. Mabel K. Staupers Collection. Courtesy of the Moorland-Spingarn Research Center, Howard University.

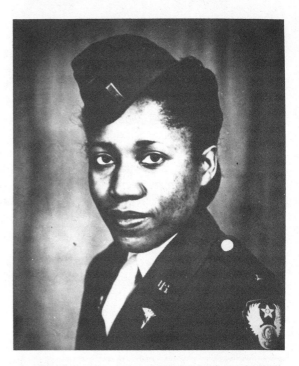

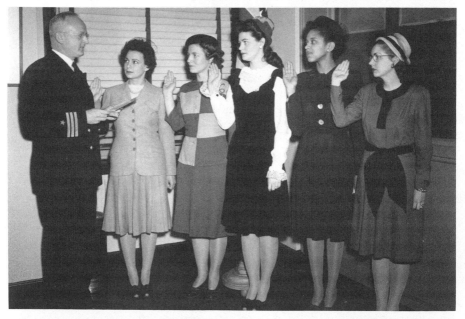

Commander Thomas A. Gaylord of the United States Navy administers oath to five new navy nurses commissioned in New York. A graduate of Lincoln School for Nurses, Miss Phyllis Mae Daley (*second from right*) became the first of four black nurses sworn into the Navy Nurse Corps as an ensign. 8 March 1945. Courtesy of the National Archives, photo no. 80–G–48365.

quently informed Katherine J. Densford, president of the American Nurses' Association, that "no further action was to be undertaken" in this regard. By abandoning the legislation, the War Department avoided and left unanswered the serious questions concerning the constitutionality of such a draft. In any event, by the time the war ended, approximately seventy-six thousand nurses had actually served in the Army and Navy Nurse Corps.[60]

The battle to integrate blacks into the Army and Navy Nurse Corps had been an exhaustive and draining one. In 1946 Staupers relinquished her position as executive secretary to take a much-needed and well-earned rest. It was to be of short duration, however, for Staupers considered her work incomplete. She had not accomplished her major objective, the integration of black women into the American Nurses' Association. Beginning in 1934, Staupers and Riddle had appeared before the House of Delegates at the biennial meeting of the ANA. After the 1944 meeting Staupers confided to Bolton her hope that "integration may be an accomplished fact before 1945." Indeed, so convinced was she of this possibility that she advised the black nurses attending the four NACGN regional conferences in 1944 to recommend to the board of directors that it be "ready and willing to vote for complete integration, if and when the American Nurses' Association House of Delegates accept us to full membership."[61]

General integration into the ANA did not come until three years after 1945. In 1948 the association's House of Delegates opened the gates to black membership, appointed a black nurse as assistant executive secretary in its national headquarters, and witnessed the election of Estelle Massey Riddle Osborne to the board of directors. Elizabeth Ann Edwards, the new assistant executive secretary, was a native of Portsmouth, Virginia, and a graduate of Harlem Hospital. She had earned an M.A. degree in personnel administration and guidance from Teachers College, Columbia University. Edwards was assigned the task of clearing the credentials of individual black nurses from the intransigent southern states of Georgia, Louisiana, South Carolina, Texas, Virginia, Arkansas, Alabama, and the District of Columbia. The decision to grant individual membership to black nurses barred from these state associations was followed by the adoption of a resolution to establish biracial committees in districts and state associations to implement educational programs and promote development of intergroup relations.[62]

The American Nurses' Association's individual membership program helped to bridge the way from exclusion to complete membership. The action elicited widespread commentary. Black nurse Alida C. Dailey observed, "Those of us who know the ugly sting of prejudice will gather courage from this hopeful step by the ANA."[63] Dr. Montague Cobb, editor of the *Journal of the National Medical Association*, applauded the move and asserted that it had a threefold significance: It represented the recognition of the injustice of black exclusion; it constituted a rebuke to local groups who refused to grow beyond obsolescent traditions; and it proved a sharp contrast to the "do-nothing" policy of the American Medical Association, which steadfastly refused to grant individual membership to black doctors in the South.[64]

For Staupers, the breakdown of the exclusion barriers was a triumphant vindication of her leadership acumen. Although she had ceased being the executive secretary in 1946, she remained a powerful force within the organization. She deftly managed to have the NACGN and its 1949 annual convention authorize the board of directors to inquire into the legal process necessary for dissolution. According to Staupers, the convention "unanimously accepted the ANA's suggestion that the functions of the NACGN be taken over by the ANA and its program be expanded for the complete integration of Negro nurses." The American Nurses' Association agreed to continue to award the Mary Mahoney Medal to the individual, regardless of race, or group contributing the most to intergroup relations within a given period.[65]

The move to integrate black nurses into the ANA occurred shortly before the publication of Esther L. Brown's much-heralded report *Nursing for the Future*. Brown's critically acclaimed study discussed the exclusion of "minority groups" from professional nursing organizations and the profession's "shameful attitude" toward and treatment of black graduate nurses. She wrote:

> That nursing has reflected the mores of America generally is true. By so doing, it has robbed the public of a larger amount of nursing care. It has also perpetuated injustice to members of "minorities," and, if the psychiatrists be right, the profession has damaged its own collective personality and that of its individual members by acts of discrimination against others.[66]

The significance of the Brown study cannot be overestimated. It precipitated the reorganization of the entire nursing profession, giving it "a dynamic sense of direction and an exciting new program."[67]

On January 26, 1951, NACGN executive secretary Alma Vessels John and president Mabel K. Staupers issued a press release announcing the dissolution of the association. The board of directors and members had returned symbolically to St. Marks Methodist Church in New York and voted the forty-year-old organization out of existence. The release claimed that, as far as was known, the NACGN was the first major black national organization to terminate its work "because it feels that its program of activities is no longer necessary." Staupers declared, "The doors have been opened and the black nurse has been given a seat in the top councils." She later exulted, "We are now a part of the great organization

of nurses, the American Nurses' Association." The press release pains-
takingly enumerated the successes realized by the NACGN and thus attempted to justify its demise. The number of state associations prohibiting black nurses from membership had been reduced from a high of
seventeen to five. The number of schools admitting all qualified students
had risen from approximately 28 prior to World War II to 330 by 1950.
It also emphasized that an unprecedented number of black nurses had
been integrated into the staffs of hospitals, public-health agencies, and
military and veterans' services.[68]

In a ceremony befitting the occasion, the NACGN officers invited one
thousand well-known black and white guests to a testimonial dinner to
celebrate the death of their organization. Ralph Bunche, the first black
U.S. ambassador to the United Nations, welcomed the jubilant crowd and
toasted, "This is a case for rejoicing, for this is evidence of American
democracy reaching its maturity."[69] The NAACP's executive secretary,
Walter White, exclaimed, "For the first time in my life I have enjoyed
a funeral. Instead of being lugubrious the obituaries were gay and
congratulatory."[70]

Judge Hastie delivered the keynote address, an insightful speech filled
with somber reflections on the meaning of "integration" and the significance of the dissolution of the NACGN. Hastie cautioned that "integration" would create problems of adjustment and reorientation for both
blacks and whites. He advised blacks that as oppressed people it would
be difficult to throw off the ways of thinking and acting which had grown
out of their oppression. He pointedly criticized "all pseudo-benevolent
apologists for segregation in American life." "They are anxious that the
Negro remain 'happy' and hence, that he not be disturbed by distressing
problems of reorientation in a larger and not always friendly environment." Hastie characterized whites who ascribed to these notions as
being "the spiritual grandchildren of the apologists for slavery."

Hastie commended the NACGN leaders for the dissolution of their organization. He described the event as symbolizing "the dynamics of constructive social evolution at its best." He concluded praising the officers
of the NACGN for "cheerfully giving up the preeminence of organization
leadership." He added, "People love rank and status; and that is not a
racial characteristic. There is a measure of self-satisfaction in being a big
fish which is not lessened by the area, however small the pool. I am not
sure how many of us here would gracefully, even eagerly, surrender such
honored organizational leadership as is being given up tonight."[71]

Staupers received many accolades for her leadership in the dissolution
of the NACGN. Alma C. Haupt of the NOPHN exulted, "Hail to the tri-
umvirate! You have led the NACGN through successful stages of development to its glorious conclusion."[72] One writer referred to the entire process as "the symphony of the nursing world," of which Staupers was

apparently composer and conductor.[73] Months later, the executive secretary of the Washington State Nurses' Association informed Staupers that it had nominated her for membership on the board of directors of the American Nurses' Association.[74]

By far the crowning acknowledgment of Staupers's role in and contribution to the quest of black nurses for civil rights and human dignity came from an unexpected source. The Spingarn Committee of the NAACP chose her to receive the Spingarn Medal for 1951. Channing H. Tobias, director of the Phelps-Stokes Fund, confided to Staupers, "I know the committee was especially appreciative of the fact that you were willing to sacrifice organization to ideals when you advocated and succeeded in realizing the full integration of Negro nurses into the organized ranks of the nursing profession of this country."[75]

Staupers well deserved the praise, awards, and recognition heaped upon her in the aftermath of the dissolution of the NACGN. For over fifteen years she and Riddle had labored to develop cooperative relations with leading white women and black male heads of organizations. More significant, they had cultivated and sustained mutually beneficial ties with the leaders of the NAACP, the National Medical Association, the National Urban League, and the National Council of Negro Women. Staupers, furthermore, manipulated the press extremely well by releasing statements at the most strategic moments. Her public remarks unfailingly emphasized the cause for which she was fighting. In so doing, she constantly reminded the country of the plight of black nurses, of the racism and sexism that robbed them of the opportunities to develop their full human potential. Small of frame, energetic, and fast-talking, Staupers knew when to accept a half-loaf of advancement and when to press on for total victory. It is unlikely that the eventually complete integration of black women into American nursing on all levels could have been accomplished without Staupers at the helm of the NACGN.

Conclusion

As formidable a task as overcoming racism proved, black nurses by the middle of the twentieth century had garnered sufficient resources to make them more than equal to the challenge. Several factors contributed to their empowerment, not the least of which was the substance of the training students received and the connections graduate nurses forged with the diverse communities they served. The constructive relations black nurses enjoyed with their communities had a significant impact on their professional identities and on their self-esteem. Regardless of how they were perceived or portrayed by whites, black nurses found confirmation of their worth from their people. Thus they could never imagine themselves as so many victims, powerless to combat racism. Most of the black hospitals and training schools had been launched in the 1890s. By the 1950s their days were numbered, and their closing in the late sixties and early seventies signaled the end of a unique social, political, and professional environment which had both nurtured and exploited black women.

From the outset the nursing training provided black women in the black hospitals emphasized collaborative teamwork. As students they learned that healing was not simply a matter of attending an isolated patient's disease. The patient was part of a multilayered system of social and interpersonal relations. Thus the student and the trained nurse had to concern themselves with issues pertaining to family, kin, and the health environment of the broader community, for all of these forces affected patient recovery.

The black nurse was a vital component of a complex system of healthcare delivery. Although the quality of her skill and training may have been judged deficient by her white colleagues, the black community held its nurses in high esteem. Likewise, those whites who argued that the preservation of the white race depended upon improving black health and eradicating infectious disease in that segment of the population clearly recognized the strategic importance of black nurses. Black physicians and the founders and administrators of hospitals similarly admitted that without the presence of nurses, their efforts to induce blacks to seek hospitalization and to abandon excessive reliance on folk remedies would have failed miserably.

One of the most distinguishing characteristics of black nursing was the extent to which individual practitioners were expected to become intimately involved in the life of the communities in which they worked. They joined and participated in the women's clubs, lectured in the community's schools, attended local churches, and visited the homes of the poor and the middle class with equal grace. Out of this bonding emerged a social contract of reciprocal obligations and expectations. The community trusted its nurses to be patient and race advocates, constantly seeking improved health care.

Conversely, the nurses expected and received support and cooperation from the community whenever they needed it, whether to save an institution threatened with collapse, to equip newly created hospitals, to pay for a new nurses' home, or to send thousands of telegrams to the president of the United States and to the generals and admirals in the War Department to protest quotas and discrimination in the Armed Forces Nurse Corps. Leaders of black protest groups, sororities, and religious bodies joined with newspaper editors, journalists, physicians, and educators to assist the nurses when called upon.

There were essentially three kinds of nursing work. Black nurses concentrated, however, in only two of the three areas of practice, private duty and public health. They did not enter hospital staff nursing in any appreciable numbers until the 1960s. Black hospitals relied heavily on student labor and were slow to make the transition to a graduate nursing staff. Largely in response to the civil rights movement and the accompanying federal-rights legislation, white hospital personnel departments began to drop racial bars. By the 1970s black nurses had become, along with other minority nurses, the mainstay of many inner-city, municipally operated hospitals.

Black private-duty nurses, from the 1890s through the 1950s, attended patients of both races, especially in the South. It is ironic, but well in keeping with the contours of southern race relations, that whites who denied black women admission to the major white training schools in the region had few reservations about employing them in their homes. This contradiction suggests two things, that whites perceived all black women to be essentially servants, regardless of their training, or that black nurses performed nonnursing tasks, as their white colleagues charged, while on private assignments and accepted lower wages for their work. Undoubtedly white private-duty nurses chafed at the economic competition black nurses posed and became even more hostile to them as the general demand for private work declined during the 1920s and 1930s. Whatever the reasons, the deep-seated identification of black women with domestic servitude exacerbated the difficulties black nurses encountered trying to win acceptance and integration into a status-starved and prestige-hungry profession.

Elite white nurse leaders had their own battles to fight. Their quest for authority, autonomy, and power over nursing practice and education met strong, often vituperative, objections from male physicians and hospital administrators determined to keep nurses subordinate to the medical profession. The problems growing out of the intersection of gender, class, and race that black women's presence brought to the profession were too much for most elite white nurses to handle.

As public-health work among white nurses declined, its significance to black nurses increased. The Rosenwald Fund and other philanthropic foundations played a critical role in the opening up of opportunities in public health to black nurses. Philanthropists provided the scholarship monies to facilitate black nurses' advanced education. They contributed to the establishment of public-health–nursing programs, most notably at St. Philip Hospital in Richmond, Virginia, and at North Carolina Central College in Durham. Finally, the foundations paid the salaries of the first group of black public-health nurses hired by southern state departments.

Black public-health nurses tended to work exclusively with black clientele in segregated and isolated black communities and neighborhoods. For the most part, when they were in the field they enjoyed considerable professional autonomy. Within the evolving black nursing hierarchy, those working in public health ranked higher than those in private duty. More credentials were required; in addition, the income in public health was steady, and the distance from domestic servitude more pronounced.

On the down side, however, public-health work was fraught with frustration. The needs of the black communities were such that the public-health nurses could address only a fraction of the problems they encountered. Moreover, virtually all of the supervisors and administrators of public-health agencies and visiting nurses' associations were white. Thus the black public-health nurse met with tensions at both ends of the employment spectrum. Again, before the 1960s ambitious black public-health nurses encountered a very low ceiling blocking advancement to upper-level administrative positions.

Black nurses, like many of their white colleagues, desired to advance as nurses, to contribute toward the growth and development of their chosen profession. The majority aspired to excellence and wanted to earn and receive recognition for their skill and service. They too wanted the indices of success, appointment to managerial and responsible positions within the hospital, school, or organization hierarchy, and to reap the financial rewards and increased public esteem and social status accorded other social-service–oriented professionals. Confronted with entrenched racism, however, black nurses duplicated white nurses' professionalization efforts. Exclusion from membership in the American Nurses' Association, denial of opportunities to attend conventions or to publish in key journals, and the compulsion to take separate and ostensibly less demanding licensure examinations left them no alternative but to pursue a parallel process of professionalization. However, their activities had a double mission: they pursued professionalization in order to make a stronger case for their eventual integration into the mainstream of American nursing.

The essential difference between white nurses' professionalization and that of black nurses was the powerful impact of racism and the concomitant necessity to struggle. Each step taken on the road toward higher status, greater recognition, and more control and responsibility was achieved only after the black nurses had removed some major stumbling block born of racism. It is fair to conclude that the white nursing establishment simply did not want black women to be nurses and could not treat them as equal professionals. It is equally fair to suggest that the 1940s was a propitious decade. Massive federal funding and the successful antisegregation campaigns of black nurses made it both possible and worthwhile for the nursing profession to change the policies and practices proven detrimental to the advance of all minorities within nursing.

Today, there exists an acute shortage of nurses in the country. By the turn of the century the demand will double the supply. This more than anything else points up the urgency of the need for the larger society to dispense with outmoded views and attitudes toward the profession of nursing. Nurses must be treated with the respect generally accorded male medical professionals. They have earned the right to be considered as complementary, not subordinate, health-care professionals. If the country is to meet the challenge of producing more nurses, then certain steps must be taken at once. Future recruits must be assured of salaries commensurate with the skill required and the work that they perform. Efforts need to be launched to help nurses deal with the high incidence of burnout and to provide them with the necessary hospital support staff instead of requiring them to do extra duties that have little to do with caring for patients.

Black nurses have long played a critical role in extending care to poor black people imprisoned in inner-city ghettos. Now more than ever, it is imperative that the black community have access to quality care and that the larger society devote the necessary resources and attention to the ills which plague that most vulnerable segment of the polity. The health and future of large segments of the black community remain inextricably connected to the fortunes of black professional nurses.

The year 1950 was a high point in black nursing history. The dissolution of the NACGN and the integration of black nurses into the ANA was both a symbolic and real victory for the struggle-weary leaders. They had earned the right to enjoy the momentary euphoria. But that, alas, was all it was to be, a momentary high.

The last four decades have witnessed improvement in racial relations within the profession. Indeed, a black nurse, Barbara Nichols, secretary of the Wisconsin Department of Regulation and Licensing—the first black to hold a cabinet-level post in the state—was elected president of the ANA in the early eighties. By 1984, 26 black nurses were numbered among the 492 fellows of the prestigious American Academy of Nursing (founded in 1973). Numerous black nurses have achieved high visibility and occupy positions of influence within the profession: Rhetaugh Dumas, dean of the University of Michigan School of Nursing; Juanita Fleming, associate vice-chancellor for academic affairs at the Medical Center, University of Kentucky; Geraldine Felton, professor and dean of the College of Nursing of the University of Iowa; Gloria Smith, appointed director of the Michigan Department of Public Health in 1983 by Governor James Blanchard—the first nurse ever to be appointed to head a state agency in Michigan; Verdelle B. Bellamy, associate chief, nursing service for geriatrics, Veterans' Administration Medical Center, Atlanta; and Vernice Ferguson, deputy assistant chief medical director for nursing programs and director of nursing services, Veterans' Administration, Washington, D.C. In 1981 Ferguson was elected president of the American Academy of Nursing.[1]

The end of overt discrimination and segregation, however, did not mean the eradication of more subtle and sophisticated forms of institutionalized racism. Few of Mabel Staupers's generation could have foreseen the evolving racial stratification within nursing that portended future marginalization and greater subordination for black nurses. Today, for example, as M. Elizabeth Carnegie points out, more black students are enrolled in associate nursing degree programs than in any other type. The first such programs, based primarily in community colleges, came into existence in 1952. Carnegie observed, "Were it not for the associate degree programs in community colleges, with low cost to the students and flexible standards in terms of age, marital status, sex, and race, many qualified Black students would be lost to the field of nursing."[2]

What this means, of course, is that fewer black nurses will be available to assume future leadership roles or occupy the influential positions in the profession, institutions of higher education, or government as long as so many have access only to associate degree programs in community colleges. To be sure, this is not so much a fault of the nursing profession as it is a reflection of the persistent effects of racism and economic impoverishment of blacks in the larger society. Indeed, the ANA launched, and received funding for in 1974 from the National Institute of Mental Health, a program designed to increase the number of black and minority doctorates in nursing research. According to project director Hattie Bessent, a total of 122 minority nurses enrolled in fifty-one universities throughout the country have received funding since the first fellowships were awarded in 1975.[3]

But there were other problems that black nurses continued to encounter which related more directly to their perceptions of lingering white insensitivity within the profession. In the twenty years following the dissolution of the NACGN and the ostensible integration of black nurses into the ANA, only imperceptible improvements had been registered in the actual status of black women within the profession. Some black nurses were beginning to feel that dissolution of the NACGN had been, at best, premature.

In 1970 approximately 150 black nurses attending the annual convention of the ANA met to discuss ways in which to better articulate the health needs of the black community and to share frustrations with their lack of mobility within the health-care system. In subsequent meetings the nurses delineated a host of grievances, chief among which was the absence of blacks in leadership positions within the ANA. At that time there had never been a black president or vice-president of the ANA. Furthermore, few black nurses won appointment to committees and commissions or were invited to present papers at the annual conventions. They were rightly alarmed that there had been no significant increase in the number of black registered nurses, and that the ANA failed to acknowledge significantly the black nurses' contribution to nursing. In a fashion reminiscent of the actions of Martha Franklin and Adah Thoms in 1908, a group of black nurses under the leadership of Lauranne Sams of Cleveland, Ohio, soon organized a new independent association of black nurses. In December 1971, the National Black Nurses' Association was formed, with Sams as its first president.[4]

Of the ten published objectives of the NBNA, four concerned the obligation of black nurses to act as advocates for improving the health care of black people. The remaining six focused on efforts to promote the professional development of black nurses. Specifically the NBNA endeavored to "serve as the national body to influence legislation and policies that affect Black people and work cooperatively and collaboratively with other health workers to this end." The leaders were equally as determined to "set standards and guidelines for quality education of Black nurses on all levels by providing consultation to nursing faculties and by monitoring for proper utilization and placement of Black nurses." The members of the NBNA pledged to recruit more black nurses into the field, to compile and maintain a national directory of black nurses, and, importantly, to "be the vehicle for unification of Black nurses of varied age groups, educational levels, and geographic locations to insure continuity and flow of our common heritage." According to Carnegie, today the organization has several thousand members in more than forty chapters.[5]

These modern-day organizing activities of black nurses are fascinating for what they reflect about the process of professionalization when race is a factor. Again it is ironic that a group of black nurses, a generation removed from the one which dissolved the NACGN, perceived so little substantive improvement in the group's status that they had to form a new separate association in order to force the mainstream organization to accord blacks the same consideration and access to resources available to white professionals. The inequity in their situation is readily evident. These nurses are now required to support two organizations, to pay double membership dues, to develop and hone a dual consciousness of themselves as *black* professionals.

If ever a group wanted integration to work, it was black nurses. They still do. Maybe someday there will be a truly warranted occasion for jubilation. Meanwhile they are wise to hold fast to the new organization. Inarguably, black nurses and the masses of black people have little to gain and everything to lose under a separate and unequal health-care system. But segregation was not their choice or their creation. Separate institutions and organizations founded by and under the control of black people remain, however, important weapons against racism.

The actions of turn-of-the-century black leaders who founded and sustained hospitals and nursing training schools, clinics, and other health-related facilities are justly commended, and the passing of these institutions in the past few decades has left a tremendous void in poor rural and inner-city black communities. The specter of death still haunts millions of black people because of neglect and inaccessible health care. This is not to say that all of those race-created hospitals and training schools were first-rate; clearly they were not. But the majority of the schools, in producing the first three generations of black nurses, performed a service no other sector of the society was willing to assume. The difference these women made to the survival and well-being of black people cannot be measured.

APPENDIX

Data on Black Hospitals and Nurse Training Schools

TABLE 1

PROFESSIONAL NURSING SCHOOLS IN THE UNITED STATES: 1880–1950

Year	Number of Schools	Number of Students	Number of Graduates
1880	15	323	157
1893	35	1,552	471
1900	432	11,164	3,456
1905	862	19,824	5,795
1910	1,129	32,636	8,140
1915	1,509	46,141	11,118
1920	1,755	54,953	14,980
1927	1,797	77,768	18,623
1929	1,885	78,771	23,810
1931	1,844	100,419	25,971
1932	1,781	84,290	25,312
1935	1,472	67,533	19,600
1936	1,417	69,589	18,600
1937	1,389	73,286	20,400
1938	1,349	74,305	20,655
1939	1,328	82,095	22,485
1940	1,311	85,156	23,600
1941	1,303	87,588	24,899
1942	1,299	91,457	25,613
1943	1,297	100,486	26,816
1944	1,307	112,249	28,276
1945	1,295	126,576	31,721
1946	1,271	128,828	36,195
1947	1,253	106,900	40,744
1948	1,245	91,643	34,268
1949	1,215	88,817	21,379
1950	1,203	98,712	25,790

SOURCE: *Historical Statistics of the United States: Colonial Times to 1970,* Bicentennial Ed., 2 vols., United States Department of Commerce, Bureau of the Census (Washington, D.C.: Government Printing Office, 1975), pt. 1, p. 76.

TABLE 2

BLACK HOSPITALS AND NURSE TRAINING SCHOOLS, 1912

State	Name of Hospital	Location
Alabama	Burwell's Infirmary	Selma
	Cottage Home Infirmary and Nurse Training School	Decatur
	Hale's Infirmary	Montgomery
	Northcross Sanitarium	Montgomery, 6 Shepherd St.
	Tuskegee Institute Hospital	Tuskegee Institute
	Virginia McCormick Hospital	Normal, A and M College
District of Columbia	Freedmen's Hospital	Washington, D.C.
Florida	Brewster Hospital	Jacksonville
	Mercy Hospital and Nurse Training School	Ocala
Georgia	Burrus Sanitarium	Augusta
	Charity Hospital	Savannah
	Fairhaven Infirmary	Atlanta
	Lamar Hospital and Nurse Training School	Augusta
	MacVicar Hospital	Atlanta, Spelman Seminary
Illinois	Provident Hospital	Chicago
	Kenniebrew's Infirmary	Jacksonville
Indiana	Charity Hospital	Indianapolis
	Colored Hospital	Evansville
	Lincoln Hospital	Indianapolis
Kansas	Douglass Hospital and Training School	Kansas City
	Mitchell Hospital	Leavenworth
Kentucky	Citizens National Hospital	Louisville
	Red Cross Sanitarium	Louisville
Louisiana	Providence Sanitarium	New Orleans
	Sarah Goodridge Hospital and Nurse Training School	New Orleans
Maryland	Provident Hospital	Baltimore
Massachusetts	Plymouth Hospital and Training School	Boston
Missouri	Provident Hospital	St. Louis
	Perry Sanitarium	Kansas City, 1214 Vine St.

Continued

TABLE 2—*Continued*

State	Name of Hospital	Location
North Carolina	Good Samaritan Hospital	Charlotte
	Lincoln Hospital	Durham
	Slater Hospital	Winston-Salem
	St. Agnes Hospital	Raleigh, St. Augustine School
	Leonard Hospital	Raleigh, Shaw University
Ohio	Colley's Hospital	Cincinnati
Oklahoma	Morrison Hospital	Muskogee, 805 N. Main St.
Pennsylvania	Frederick Douglass Memorial Hospital and Training School	Philadelphia
	Mercy Hospital and School for Nurses	Philadelphia
	The Booker T. Washington Hospital and Nurse Training School	Pittsburgh
South Carolina	Colored Hospital and Nurse Training School	Charleston
	Taylor Lane Hospital	Columbia
	Mrs. Dr. Rhodes' Private Hospital	Columbia
Tennessee	Dr. J. T. Wilson's Infirmary	Nashville
	Hadley's Private Infirmary for Women Only	Nashville
	Hariston Infirmary	Memphis
	George W. Hubbard Hospital	Nashville
	Hospital Training School	Knoxville, Knoxville College
	Negro Baptist Hospital	Memphis
	Rock City Sanitarium	Nashville, 316 Foster St.
	Mercy Hospital	Nashville
Texas	Hubbard Sanitarium	Galveston
	Dr. Bluitt's Sanitarium	Dallas, 2034 Commerce St.
	Feagin's Hospital	Houston
	Tent Colony for Colored People	San Antonio, 324 W. Commerce St.
	Wright Cuney Memorial Nurse Training School	Dallas
	Dr. Sheppard's Santarium	Marshall, 214 N. Wellington St.
Virginia	Dixie Hospital	Hampton
	Epps Memorial Hospital	Petersburg
	Richmond Hospital	Richmond
	Woman's Central League Hospital	Richmond
West Virginia	North Mountain Sanitarium	North Mountain
	Mercer Hospital	Bluefield
	Harrison Hospital	Kimball

SOURCE: Monroe N. Work, *Negro Year Book and Annual Encyclopedia of the Negro, 1912* (In Charge of Research and Records, the Tuskegee Normal and Industrial Institute), pp. 155–157.

TABLE 3

SCHOOLS OF NURSING ADMITTING BLACK STUDENTS, 1924

State & City	Name of Hospital	Beds	Remarks
Alabama			
Anniston	St. Luke's Hospital*	25	
Birmingham	Norwood Hospital*	100	
Birmingham	St. Vincent's Hospital*	100	
Birmingham	South Highland Infirmary*	140	
Fairfield	Employees Hospital, Tennessee Coal, Iron & Railway Co.*	300	
California			
Loma Linda	Loma Linda Hospital*	208	
Los Angeles	Los Angeles County Hospital*	1,150	
Los Angeles	White Memorial Hospital*	87	
San Francisco	University Hospital*	237	Would be admitted if they qualified educationally.
District of Columbia			
Washington	Freedmen's Hospital (Colored)*	225	
Florida			
Jacksonville	Brewster Hospital (Colored)*	28	
Georgia			
Athens	St. Mary's Hospital* (In Colored Ward)	50	
Atlanta	Municipal Training School (Colored), Grady Hospital*	400	
Atlanta	MacVicar Training School (Colored), Spelman Seminary*	35	Colored students only.
Augusta	Lamar Win Colored Nurses, University Hospital*	138	
Columbus	Columbus City Hospital*	60	Practice training in colored hospital.
Griffin	Griffin Hospital*	50	
LaGrange	Dunson Hospital (Colored)	70	Combined capacity of white and colored hospitals.
Macon	Macon Hospital*	113	

*Listed in 1924 List of Schools of Nursing Accredited by the State Boards of Nurse Examiners.

Continued on next page

TABLE 3—*Continued*

State & City	Name of Hospital	Beds	Remarks
Illinois			
Chicago	Chicago Lying-in Hospital	225	Three at one time, affiliates from Provident Hospital.
Chicago	Provident Hospital (Colored)*	50	Colored students only.
Hinsdale	Hinsdale Sanitarium and Hospital*	150	
Indiana			
Indianapolis	Indianapolis City Hospital*	400	
Kokomo	Good Samaritan Hospital*	36	
Kansas			
Kansas City	Douglass Hospital and Training School (Colored)*	20	
Kentucky			
Louisville	Red Cross Sanitarium (Colored)*	30	
Louisiana			
New Orleans	Flint-Goodridge Hospital (Colored)*	41	
Massachusetts			
Boston (Roxbury)	New England Hospital for Women and Children*	150	Two at a time.
Lawrence	Lawrence General Hospital*	111	
Mississippi			
D'Lo	Pineview Hospital	20	
Jackson	State Charity Hospital*	100	
Meridian	East Mississippi Charity Hospital*	256	
Missouri			
Kansas City	Kansas City Colored Hospital*	200	
Kansas City	Wheatley-Provident Hospital (Colored)*	25	
St. Louis	St. Louis Hospital No. 2 (Colored)*	175	
New York			
New York City	Harlem Hospital (Municipal Colored)	390	
New York City	Lincoln Hospital (Private Colored Training School)*	314	

*Listed in 1924 List of Schools of Nursing Accredited by the State Boards of Nurse Examiners.

Continued on next page

TABLE 3—*Continued*

State & City	Name of Hospital	Beds	Remarks
North Carolina			
Durham	Lincoln Hospital (Colored)*	38	
Goldsboro	Spicer Sanatorium	35	Have not admitted heretofore. Expect to admit colored students at some future time.
Raleigh	St. Agnes Hospital (Colored)*	75	Colored students only.
Sanatorium	North Carolina Sanatorium	197	
Pennsylvania			
Philadelphia	Mercy Hospital (Colored)*	70	
Philadelphia	University of Pennsylvania Hospital	546	No ruling against. Applications very rare.
South Carolina			
Chester	Pryor Hospital*	50	
Columbia	Good Samaritan Hospital & Nurse Training School*	60	
Rock Hill	Fennell Infirmary*	35	
Spartanburg	Spartanburg County Hospital for Colored People*	92	
Tennessee			
Memphis	Jane Terrell Baptist Hospital*	80	
Nashville	George W. Hubbard Hospital (Colored)*	97	
Virginia			
Hampton	Dixie Hospital (Colored)	75	All colored pupils.
Newport News	Whittaker Memorial Hospital (Colored)*	25	Other directory gives bed capacity as 100.
Richmond	Richmond Hospital (Colored)	10	
Richmond	St. Phillip Hospital (Colored, Medical College of Virginia)*	146	
West Virginia			
Huntington	Barnette Hospital (Colored)*	30	

*Listed in 1924 List of Schools of Nursing Accredited by the State Boards of Nurse Examiners.

TABLE 4

SCHOOLS IN HOSPITALS FOR BLACKS
WHICH ADMITTED BLACK STUDENTS, 1924

None of these schools were on the accredited list used.

State & City	Name of Hospital	Beds	Remarks
Alabama			
Montgomery	Hale Infirmary*	35	
Selma	Good Samaritan	30	
Arizona			
Phoenix	B. T. Washington Hospital	25	Will be when they work up to it.
Arkansas			
Little Rock	Royal Circle Hospital	45	
Georgia			
Statesboro	Statesboro Sanitarium		In colored hospital.
Kansas			
Topeka	Topeka Industrial Institute Hospital		
Maryland			
Baltimore	Provident Hospital	24	
Michigan			
Detroit	Mercy Hospital		
North Carolina			
Asheville	Blue Ridge Hospital		
Charlotte	Good Samaritan Hospital*	20	
South Carolina			
Charleston	Hospital & Training School for Nurses	18	
Columbia	Benedict College Hospital		
Tennessee			
Knoxville	Eliza B. Wallace Memorial Hospital		
Memphis	Negro Baptist Hospital	100	
Nashville	McMillan Infirmary*		
Nashville	Millie Hale Hospital*	100	
Texas			
Fort Worth	Booker T. Washington Sanitarium	25	
Virginia			
Richmond	Piedmont Sanitarium		
Roanoke	Burrell Memorial Hospital Association	45	
West Virginia			
Bluefield	Lomax Sanitarium		
Bluefield	Mercer Hospital		

*Has since been reported as accredited.

TABLE 5

HOSPITALS AND NURSING SCHOOLS VISITED BY
ETHEL JOHNS IN 1925

Name of Hospital	City & State	No. of Pupils	No. of Beds
Lincoln Hospital	New York	97	450
Harlem Hospital	New York	66	348
Grady Hospital	Atlanta	60	230
Freedmen's Hospital	Washington	50	278
John A. Andrew Hospital	Tuskegee	48	75
Provident Hospital	Chicago	34	65
Kansas City No. 2	Kansas City	32	200
Hubbard Hospital	Nashville	32	140
Mercy Hospital	Philadelphia	31	100
St. Agnes Hospital	Raleigh	31	100
City Hospital No. 2	St. Louis	31	275
T.C.I. Employees Hospital	Birmingham	30	300
St. Philip Hospital	Richmond	30	176
Dixie Hospital	Hampton	30	65
Willie T. Hale Hospital	Nashville	26	60
MacVicar Hospital (Spelman)	Atlanta	19	45
Douglass Hospital	Philadelphia	16	100
Wheatley Hospital	Kansas City	16	25
Red Cross Hospital	Louisville	12	38
Fraternal Hospital	Montgomery	10	20
Tuggle Institute Hospital	Birmingham	6	40
St. Vincent's Hospital	Birmingham	3	25
Veterans Bureau Hospital	Tuskegee	Graduate Nurses Only	621
		710	3,776

SOURCE: Ethel Johns, "A Study of the Present Status of the Negro Woman in Nursing," unpublished report (New York: Rockefeller Foundation, 1925).

TABLE 6

BLACK NURSING SCHOOLS AND THEIR GRADUATES, 1927

Name	Location	Year Established	Total No. of Graduates	Minimum Age At Entrance	Minimum Entrance Requirement (Years of High School)	Superintendent of Nurses
Lincoln	New York	1898 (Proprietary)	493	(18)	4	Sarah Jones Ford, R.N.
Freedmen's	Washington, D.C.	1894 (Academic)	439	(18)	4	Charlotte K. May, R.N.
Dixie-Hampton	Hampton	1891 (Academic)	281	(21)	4	Martha L. Studley, R.N.
Provident	Chicago	1891 (Proprietary)	226	(18)	4	Belva L. Overton, R.N.
St. Agnes	Raleigh	1896 (Proprietary)	172	(18)	4	Frances A. Worrall, R.N.
Hubbard	Nashville	1900 (Academic)	138	(18)	4	Hulda Little, R.N.
Flint-Goodridge	New Orleans	1896 (Academic)	137	(18)	2	Eola V. Lyons, R.N.
Mercy	Philadelphia	1907 (Proprietary)	136	(18)	4	Margaret M. Jackson, R.N.
Hospital & Training School	Charleston	1897 (Proprietary)	127	(18)	8th-grade graduate	Anna D. Banks
Tuskegee Institute	Tuskegee	1892 (Academic)	125	(18)	3	Mary S. Booth, R.N.
Kansas City General	Kansas City	1911 (Municipal)	86	(18)	4	Lorinda S. Harris, R.N.
Grady	Atlanta	1917 (Municipal)	80	(18)	2	Annie B. Feeback, R.N.
Harlem	New York	1923 (Municipal)	72	(18)	4	Sadie J. O'Brien, R.N.
Brewster	Jacksonville	1902 (Municipal)	63	(18)	2	Bertha E. Dean, R.N.

Total number of black graduate nurses to January 1, 1925: 2,784.
List of Schools of Nursing Accredited by the State Boards of Examiners as of January 1, 1928 mentions 36 schools for black nurses.

Source: Adah Thoms, *Pathfinders*, chap. 4.

TABLE 7

NEGRO HOSPITALS APPROVED BY THE
AMERICAN COLLEGE OF SURGEONS AND THE
AMERICAN MEDICAL ASSOCIATION, 1930

Name of Hospital	*Location*
John A. Andrew Memorial (1) (2)	Tuskegee
United States Veterans No. 91 (1)	Tuskegee
Freedmen's (1) (2)	Washington, D.C.
Grady Memorial (Emory Division) (1) (2) (3)	Atlanta
Provident (1) (2)	Chicago
Flint-Goodridge (1) (2)	New Orleans
Provident (1) (2)	Baltimore
Wheatley Provident (1)	Kansas City
General No. 2 (1) (2)	Kansas City
St. Agnes (1) (2)	Raleigh
Frederick Douglass Memorial (1) (2)	Philadelphia
Mercy (1) (2)	Philadelphia
George W. Hubbard (1) (2)	Nashville
Millie E. Hale (1)	Nashville
Dixie (1)	Hampton
St. Philip (1) (2) (3)	Richmond
Burrell Memorial (1)	Roanoke
St. Louis No. 2 (2)	St. Louis
Lincoln (2)	Durham

(1) Approved by the American College of Surgeons.
(2) Approved for internship by the American Medical Association.
(3) Approved for residency in specialties by the American Medical Association.

SOURCE: *Negro Hospitals: A Compilation of Available Statistics,* published by the Julius Rosenwald Fund (Chicago: February 1931), p.17.

TABLE 8

PRESIDENTS OF THE NATIONAL ASSOCIATION OF COLORED GRADUATE NURSES, 1908–1951

1908–1910 Miss Martha Franklin New Haven, Connecticut	1926–1929 Miss Carrie E. Bullock Chicago, Illinois
1910–1912 Mrs. Mary Tucker Philadelphia, Pennsylvania	1929–1930 Mrs. Hallie Avery West Memphis, Tennessee
1912–1913 Mrs. Mary Clark Lemus Richmond, Virginia	1930–1934 Miss Mabel C. Northcross St. Louis, Missouri
1913–1914 Mrs. Rosa Williams Brown Palm Beach, Florida	1934–1939 Mrs. Estelle M. R. Osborne New York, New York
1914–1916 Miss Carrie Sharpe Petersburg, Virginia	1939–1947 Mrs. F. Foulkes Gaines Chicago, Illinois
1916–1923 Mrs. Adah B. Thoms New York, New York	1947–1949 Mrs. Alida C. Dailey Montclair, New Jersey
1923–1926 Miss Petra A. Pinn Wilberforce, Ohio	1949–1951 Mrs. Mabel Keaton Staupers New York, New York

SOURCE: Herbert M. Morais, *The History of the Negro in Medicine* (1970), p. 282.

Notes

Introduction

1. Barbara Melosh, "Every Woman Is a Nurse: Work and Gender in the Emergence of Nursing," in *"Send Us a Lady Physician": Women Doctors in America 1835–1930*, ed. Ruth J. Abrams (New York: W. W. Norton, 1985), pp. 121–123.

2. Interview with Estelle Massey Riddle Osborne, 21 June 1976, conducted by Patricia Sloan. The author is grateful to Professor Sloan for sharing this and a series of other interviews that she conducted with black nurses who practiced during the 1930s and 1940s. Transcripts of these interviews are located at the M. Elizabeth Carnegie Nursing History Archive, Hampton University School of Nursing, Hampton, Va. Also see Patricia Sloan, "Geneva Estelle Massey Riddle Osborne, 1901–1981," in *American Nursing: A Biographical Dictionary*, ed. Vern L. Bullough, Olga Maranjian Church, and Alice P. Stein (New York: Garland Publishing, 1988), pp. 250–252). Osborne was a 1923 graduate of the segregated St. Louis Hospital No. 2 in St. Louis, Missouri.

3. Interview with Mary L. Steele Reives, 17 July 1976, conducted by Sloan.

4. Interview with Elizabeth Sharpe, 17 July 1976, conducted by Sloan.

5. Interview with Lillian Kemp, 14 June 1976, conducted by Sloan.

6. Darlene Clark Hine, "'They Shall Mount Up with Wings as Eagles': Historical Images of Black Nurses, 1890–1950," in *Images of Nurses: Perspectives from History, Art, and Literature*, ed. Anne Hudson Jones (Philadelphia: University of Pennsylvania Press, 1988), pp. 177–196.

7. Sheila Rothman, "Women's Special Sphere," in *Women and the Politics of Culture: Studies in the Sexual Economy*, ed. Michele Wender Zak and Patricia P. Moots (New York: Longman, 1983), pp. 213–223; Mary Beth Norton, "The Paradox of 'Women's Sphere,'" in *Women of America: A History*, ed. Carol Ruth Berkin and Mary Beth Norton (Boston: Houghton Mifflin, 1979), pp. 139–149; Linda K. Kerber, "Separate Spheres, Female Worlds, Woman's Place: The Rhetoric of Women's History," *Journal of American History* 75 (June 1988): 9–39; Dorothy Sterling, ed., *We Are Your Sisters: Black Women in the Nineteenth Century* (New

York: W. W. Norton, 1984), pp. 322–328. Sterling includes among an array of revealing documents the words of Mattie Curtis: "I got married before de war to Joshua Curtis. I always had craved a home an' plenty to eat, but freedom ain't give us notin' but pickled hoss meat an' dirty crackers an' not half enough of dat. Josh ain't really care 'bout no home but through dis land corporation I buyed dese fifteen acres on time. I cut down de big trees dat wus all over dese fields an' I hauled out de wood an sold hit, den I plowed up de fields an' planted dem. Josh did help to build de house an' he worked out some. All of dis time I had nineteen chilluns an' Josh died, but I kep' on" (p. 323).

8. Althea T. Davis, "Adah Belle Samuels Thoms, 1870–1943," in *American Nursing*, p. 314; John A. Kenney, "Some Facts concerning Negro Nurse Training Schools and Their Graduates," *Journal of the National Medical Association* 11 (April–June 1919):53–68. Reprinted in *Black Women in the Nursing Profession: A Documentary History*, ed. Darlene Clark Hine (New York: Garland Publishing, 1985), pp. 11–19.

9. Janet Wilson James, "Isabel Hampton and the Professionalization of Nursing in the 1890s," in *The Therapeutic Revolution: Essays in the Social History of American Medicine*, ed. Morris J. Vogel and Charles E. Rosenberg (Philadelphia: University of Pennsylvania Press, 1979), pp. 201–244; Martha Vicinus, *Independent Women: Work and Community for Single Women, 1850–1920* (Chicago: University of Chicago Press, 1985), pp. 28–29, 85–120.

10. Celia Davies, "Professionalizing Strategies as Time- and Culture-Bound: American and British Nursing circa 1893," in *Nursing History: New Perspectives, New Possibilities*, ed. Ellen Condliffe Lagemann (New York: Teachers College, Columbia University, 1983), pp. 47–63; Susan M. Reverby, *Ordered to Care: The Dilemma of American Nursing, 1850–1945* (Cambridge: Cambridge University Press, 1987), pp. 121–128; Barbara Melosh, *"The Physician's Hand": Work Culture and Conflict in American Nursing* (Philadelphia: Temple University Press, 1982), pp. 39–47; Penina Migdal Glazer and Miriam Slater, *Unequal Colleagues: The Entrance of Women into the Professions, 1890–1940* (New Brunswick, N.J.: Rutgers University Press, 1987), pp. 3–23.

11. Darlene Clark Hine, "The Ethel Johns Report: Black Women in the Nursing Profession, 1925," *Journal of Negro History* 67 (Fall 1982): 212–228; Mary Elizabeth Carnegie, *The Path We Tread: Blacks in Nursing, 1854–1984* (Philadelphia: J. B. Lippincott Co., 1986), pp. 69–70.

12. Carnegie, *The Path We Tread*, p. 106.

13. Helen Sullivan Miller, *The History of Chi Eta Phi Sorority, Inc., 1932–1967* (Washington, D.C.: Association for the Study of Afro-American Life and History, 1968), p. 34.

14. Ludie Andrews to Mrs. Kemper Harrold, 24 February 1926; J. T. Singleton to Whom It May Concern, Spelman, 23 May 1901; Peter Cline to Whom It May Concern, Spelman, 4 June 1901; Ludie Andrews's Application Blank, 28 May 1901. Copies of this correspondence are included in *History of Grady Memorial Hospital School of Nursing, 1917–1964*, ed. Verdelle B. Bellamy (Atlanta, Ga.: Chi Eta Phi Sorority, circa 1985), typescript without pagination.

15. Ibid.

16. Charles E. Rosenberg, *The Care of Strangers: The Rise of America's Hospital System* (New York: Basic Books, 1987), pp. 212–236, 238–258; David Rosner, *A Once Charitable Enterprise: Hospitals and Health Care in Brooklyn and New York, 1885–1915* (Princeton, N.J.: Princeton University Press, 1982), pp. 62–93.

17. Rosenberg, *The Care of Strangers*, p. 220. See: Vanessa Gamble, *Black Community Hospitals: A Historical Perspective* (New York: Garland Publishing, 1987).

1. Origins of the Black Hospital and Nurse Training School Movement

1. Todd L. Savitt, *Medicine and Slavery: The Disease and Health Care of Blacks in Antebellum Virginia* (Urbana: University of Illinois Press, 1978), p. 180; Susie King Taylor, *Reminiscences of My Life in Camp with the 33rd United States Colored Troops Late 1st South Carolina Volunteers* (Boston: privately printed, 1902), pp. 17, 21. Also see Philip A. Kalisch and Beatrice J. Kalisch, "Untrained but Undaunted: The Women Nurses of the Blue and the Gray," *Nursing Forum* 15, no. 1 (1976): 26.

2. Ann Douglas Wood, "The War within a War: Women Nurses in the Union Army," *Civil War History* 18 (September 1979):197–222.

3. "Report of the Committee for the Training of Nurses," *Transactions of the American Medical Association* 20 (1869):161–173.

4. Richard H. Shryock, *The History of Nursing: An Interpretation of the Social and Medical Factors Involved* (Philadelphia: Saunders, 1959), p. 300; John Duffy, *The Healers: A History of American Medicine* (Urbana: University of Illinois Press, [1976], 1979 ed.), pp. 280–281; Richard H. Shryock, "Nursing Emerges as a Profession: The American Experience," *Clio Medica* 3 (1968):131–147; Mary Elizabeth Carnegie, *The Path We Tread: Blacks in Nursing, 1854–1984* (Philadelphia: J. B. Lippincott Co. 1986), pp. 2–4.

5. Duffy, *The Healers*, pp. 280–281.

6. Charles E. Rosenberg, "Inward Vision and Outward Glance: The Shaping of the American Hospital, 1880–1914," *Bulletin of the History of Medicine* 53 (1979):347; also see Charles E. Rosenberg, *The Care of Strangers: The Rise of America's Hospital System* (New York: Basic Books, 1987); David Rosner, *A Once Charitable Enterprise: Hospitals and Health Care in Brooklyn and New York, 1885–1915* (Princeton, N.J.: Princeton University Press, 1982).

7. Alfred Worcester, *Small Hospitals: Establishment and Maintenance* (New York: John Wiley and Sons, 1909), p. 3. Also see Susan Reverby, "The Search for the Hospital Yardstick: Nursing and the Rationalization of Hospital Work," in *Health Care in America: Essays in Social History*, ed. David Rosner and Susan Reverby (Philadelphia: Temple University Press, 1979), pp. 206–208; Morris J. Vogel, *The Invention of the Modern Hospital: Boston, 1870–1930* (Chicago: University of Chicago Press, 1980), pp. 1–4.

8. Helen S. Miller, *Mary Eliza Mahoney, 1845–1926: America's First Black Professional Nurse* (Atlanta: Wright Publishing Co., 1986), pp. 19–21; "Mary Eliza Mahoney, First Negro Nurse," *Journal of the National Medical Association* 46 (July 1954):299; Mabel Keaton Staupers, *No Time for Prejudice: The Story of the Integration of Negroes in Nursing in the United States* (New York: Macmillan Co., 1961), p. 2.

9. J. Morgan Kousser, "Separate but *Not* Equal: The Supreme Court's First Decision on Racial Discrimination in Schools," *Journal of Southern History* 46 (February 1980):17–44.

10. Report of Acting Surgeon-in-Chief, Louisiana, January 1867, submitted to General O. O. Howard. Records of the Bureau of Refugees, Freedmen and Abandoned Lands, Record Group 105, National Archive, Washington, D.C.; John W. Blassingame, *Black New Orleans, 1860–1880* (Chicago: University of Chicago Press, 1973), pp. 50–51. Also see Thomas Holt, Cassandra Smith-Parker, and

Rosalyn Terborg-Penn, *A Special Mission: The Story of Freedmen's Hospital, 1862–1962* (Washington, D.C.: Howard University Press, 1975).

11. William Ivy Hair, *Carnival of Fury: Robert Charles and the New Orleans Race Riot of 1900* (Baton Rouge: Louisiana State University Press, 1976), pp. 72, 87, 89; Edward H. Beardsley, *A History of Neglect: Health Care for Blacks and Mill Workers in the Twentieth-Century South* (Knoxville: University of Tennessee Press, 1987), pp. 16, 28–30; James H. Jones, *Bad Blood: The Tuskegee Syphilis Experiment* (New York: Free Press, 1981), pp. 23–25, 36–33; Allan M. Brandt, *No Magic Bullet: A Social History of Venereal Disease in the United States since 1880* (New York: Oxford University Press, 1985), pp. 157–158; Antonio A. René, "Racial Difference in Mortality: Blacks and Whites," in *Health Care Issues in Black America: Policies, Problems, and Prospects*, ed. Woodrow Jones, Jr., and Mitchell F. Rice (Westport, Conn.: Greenwood Press, 1987), pp. 21–41; J. Lynn Smith and Homer L. Hitt, *People of Louisiana* (Baton Rouge: Louisiana State University Press, 1952), pp. 24, 34, 174–178; John S. Haller, Jr., "Race, Mortality, and Life Insurance: Negro Vital Statistics in the Late Nineteenth Century," *Journal of the History of Medicine* 25 (1970):247–261.

For the morbidity and mortality statistics in Jacksonville, Florida, see C. E. Terry, "The Negro: His Relation to Public Health in the South," *American Journal of Public Health* 9 (April 1913):300–310. Dr. Terry reported "their [Negroes'] average mortality for the four years 1908–1911 [as] being 23.2 per thousand against 15.2 for the whites, an excess of 8. per thousand. . . . While the white birth rate exceeds the death rate by 2.62 per thousand, the negro death rate exceeds the birth rate by 6.61 per thousand. . . . During 1910 and 1911 the stillbirths constituted 17.52 per cent. of all negro births against 7.49 per cent. of white births" (p. 301).

Similar disparities in black and white well-being were also reported by the health commissioner of Cincinnati, Ohio. See William H. Peters, "Negro Health and Race Relations," *Cincinnati Journal of Medicine*, May 1925, pp. 149–152. Peters wrote, "Our colored people, who constitute about nine per cent of the population, contribute twenty-eight per cent of the deaths from tuberculosis in Cincinnati. . . . Of the colored children born alive almost three times as many of them per 1,000 births recorded, perish during the first year of life. The Negroes contributed over 70 per cent of the cases reported last year [1924] in Cincinnati" (p. 149). Peters went on to offer an environmental explanation for the excess of black deaths: "Over one-half of Cincinnati's Negro population live in four down-town congested wards under conditions which make the Negro the victim of causes which lower resistance to disease. Among the most important may be mentioned bad housing, ignorance, race prejudice, lack of opportunity and dissipation" (p. 150).

12. Edwin R. Embree, *Investment in People: The Story of the Julius Rosenwald Fund* (New York: Harper and Brothers, 1949), pp. 11, 18, 29, 31; Carnegie, *The Path We Tread*, pp. 20–21.

13. Edwin R. Embree, Memorandum to Ethel Johns, 13 August 1924, Rockefeller Foundation Papers, Box 122, Folder 1509, Rockefeller Archive Center, Pocantico Hills, North Tarrytown, N.Y.

14. Florence Matilda Read, *The Story of Spelman College* (Princeton, N.J.: Princeton University Press, 1961), pp. 153, 214. Also see Patricia E. Sloan, "Black Hospitals and Nurse Training Schools: The Formative Years, 1880–1905," Paper presented at the fifth Berkshire Conference of Women Historians, Vassar College, Poughkeepsie, N.Y., 17 June 1981; Sloan, "Black Hospitals and Nurse Training

Schools: Spelman, Provident, Hampton, and Tuskegee" (Ed.D. dissertation, Teachers College, Columbia University, 1978). For a penetrating analysis of the emergence of the new charitable trusts, see Barry D. Karl and Stanley N. Katz, "The American Private Philanthropic Foundation and the Public Sphere, 1890–1930," *Minerva* 19, no. 2 (Summer 1981):236–270. Karl and Katz assert that "these new charitable trusts were mainly founded in response to the dilemmas concerning the status of Negroes in the 'New South'" (p. 245). Among the charitable trusts was John D. Rockefeller's General Education Board, created in 1902, which, as Karl and Katz insist, represented "the fusion of traditional charitable organisation, ancient methods for the perpetuation of family wealth and novel social, legal and intellectual ideas" (p. 245).

15. Perhaps the most authoritative discussion of the number and condition of black hospitals in the 1920s is contained in William H. Walsh's "Report of the Committee on Hospitalization of Colored People—1930," *Transactions of the American Hospital Association* 32 (1930):53–61. Under the direction of the Council on Medical Education and Hospitals, the American Medical Association appropriated $5,000 for a survey of black hospitals. The report was submitted to the AMA in 1928. In assessing conditions in the black hospitals, the committee declared, "Hospitalization for the negro is generally poor throughout the South, except for the indigent in public hospitals in larger centers. The negro race must therefore accept this situation, or assume the responsibility of new pay hospital development" (p. 54). The committee concluded:

> Of the 120 hospitals . . . twenty-nine were new or previously unreported institutions and ten others were reported as closed for various reasons. Previous to the investigation the American Medical Association had knowledge of 154 colored hospitals, and the newly discovered institutions raised the number to 183. This number, minus the ten reported closed, leaves a total of 173. There are sixty-three . . . most of which are located in Northern states, which need to be reinspected before the totals regarding all colored hospitals, nurses, and the like will be complete. (pp. 56–57)

Concerning the leadership of black hospitals, the committee distinguished between those institutions established by blacks and those founded by whites for the care of blacks. On the one hand they cautioned that "negro hospitals should not necessarily have negro executives and a negro hospital staff. Public hospitals, with beds for negro patients, should still have white executives and a white hospital staff, at least in the South." Yet on the other hand the committee held that "negro hospitals in general should be controlled by negroes, but at present in the South the assistance of the white people is often needed." The remaining two recommendations called for new, ongoing surveys of "hospital beds available, from all sources, for negroes; the standard of service rendered; and the proportion of pay and indigent patients." Finally the members asserted that "a survey of some of the most likely institutions, with the purpose of instructing them in methods of administration and routine procedure, would be a valuable philanthropy" (p. 55). Adah Thoms, *Pathfinders: A History of the Progress of Colored Graduate Nurses* (New York: McKay Co., 1929), pp. 12–13; *Crisis* 32 (June 1926):84; Darlene Clark Hine, "From Hospital to College: Black Nurse Leaders and the Rise of Collegiate Nursing Schools," *Journal of Negro Education* 51 (Summer 1982):223–237.

16. Philip A. Kalisch and Beatrice J. Kalisch, *The Advance of American Nursing* (Boston: Little, Brown and Co. 1978), pp. 558–559.

17. Embree, *Investment in People*, pp. 108–109; Julius Rosenwald to J. M. T. Finney, Jr., 25 September 1928, Julius Rosenwald Papers, Box 31, Folder 6, University of Chicago, Chicago, Ill.

18. Raymond Fosdick, W. Rose, James Hardy Dillard, Interoffice Memo on Negro Education, 6 October 1922, General Education Board Papers (GEB), Box 331, Folder 3490, Rockefeller Archive Center, Pocantico Hills, North Tarrytown, N.Y.

19. William Kenneth Boyd, *The Story of Durham: City of the New South* (Durham: Duke University Press, 1925), p. 221.

20. "Report of Committee on Medical Education on Colored Hospitals," *Journal of the National Medical Association* 2 (1910):283, 287, 290. For a discussion of the role played by black women physicians in the establishment of hospitals and nursing training schools, see Darlene Clark Hine, "Co-Laborers in the Work of the Lord: Nineteenth-Century Black Women Physicians," in *"Send Us a Lady Physician": Women Doctors in America, 1835–1920*, ed. Ruth J. Abrams (New York: W. W. Norton, 1985), pp. 107–120.

21. Daniel Hale Williams, "The Need of Hospitals and Training Schools for the Colored People of the South," *AME Church Review* 17 (July 1900):9–18.

22. Ibid.

23. Ibid.

24. Booker T. Washington, "Training Colored Nurses at Tuskegee," *American Journal of Nursing* 10 (December 1910):167–171.

25. Eugene H. Dibble, Jr., Louis A. Rabb, and Ruth B. Ballard, "John A. Andrew Memorial Hospital," *Journal of the National Medical Association* 53 (March 1961):103–105; John A. Kenney, *The Negro in Medicine* (Tuskegee, Ala.: Tuskegee Institute, 1912), pp. 12, 46.

26. Washington, "Training Colored Nurses at Tuskegee," pp. 167–171; *Tuskegee Normal and Industrial Institute Catalogue, 1896–1897*, p. 86. The more formal Tuskegee Institute training school for nurses, designed to produce women who would in fact become professional nurses, did not begin operation until September 1898. One catalogue explained, "The increasing demand for trained nurses in the South has necessitated the establishment of a regular Training School of Nurses in connection with the School Hospital," *Tuskegee Normal and Industrial Institute Catalogue, 1897–1898*, pp. 61–62.

27. Daniel Hale Williams, "Afro-Americans as Surgeons and Nurses," *AME Church Review* 10 (January 1894):425–431.

28. John A. Kenney, "Some Facts concerning Negro Nurse Training Schools and Their Graduates," *Journal of the National Medical Association* 11 (April–June 1919):53. For a provocative discussion of the cultural ideology of woman's place and the division of labor in health care, see Barbara Melosh, "Every Woman Is a Nurse: Work and Gender in the Emergence of Nursing," in *"Send Us a Lady Physician": Women Doctors in America, 1835–1920*, ed. Ruth J. Abram (New York: Norton, 1985), pp. 121–127.

29. Alonzo Clifton McClennan, "Editorial," *Hospital Herald: A Journal Devoted to Hospital Work, Nurse Training, and Domestic and Public Hygiene* 1 (December 1898):5. Also see issues of 25 January 1899; July 1899; and November 1899. All issues except December 1898 can be found in the Waring Library in Charleston, S.C. The December 1898 issue was found in the Caroliniana Library, University of South Carolina, Columbia. Additional information on McClennan was provided by his granddaughter Maude T. Jenkins to Darlene Clark Hine, 26 March 1987. She has turned over some additional letters and newspaper clippings to the Amistad Research Center, Tulane University, New Orleans, La.

30. Ibid.

31. John Edward Perry, *Forty Cords of Wood: Memoirs of a Medical Doctor* (Jefferson City, Mo.: Lincoln University Press, 1947), pp. 376, 382.

32. Alice Bacon, "The Hampton Training School for Nurses," *Fourth Annual Report of the Training School for Nurses and Dixie Hospital* (Hampton, Va.: 1895–1896), p. 16; *Sixth Annual Report* (1896–1897); *Thirteenth Annual Report* (1903–1904), p. 21.

33. Quotes from Alice M. Bacon, "The Dixie and Its Work," *Southern Workman* 20 (November 1891):244; Cora M. Folsom, "The Dixie Hospital: In the Beginning," *Southern Workman* 55 (March 1926):121–126.

34. Ibid.

35. Emery L. Rann, "The Good Samaritan Hospital of Charlotte, North Carolina," *Journal of the National Medical Association* 56 (May 1916):223–225.

36. W. Montague Cobb, "Saint Agnes Hospital, Raleigh, North Carolina, 1896–1961," *Journal of the National Medical Association* 53 (September 1961): 439–442. Quotes are taken from Mary V. Glenton, *The Story of a Hospital* (Hartford, Conn.: Church Missions Publishing Co., 1923), 13 pages.

37. Ibid.

38. "The History of Flint-Goodridge Hospital of Dillard University," *Journal of the National Medical Association* 61 (November 1969):553; *The Fifth Annual Report of the Flint-Goodridge Hospital* (31 December 1921). Annual Reports found in the Amistad Research Center, New Orleans, La.

39. Minutes of the eleventh Annual Convention of the South Carolina Federation of Colored Women's Clubs (14–16 June 1921), Florence, S.C., pp. 32–33. Found in the Papers of Mary Church Terrell, Container 23, Library of Congress, Washington, D.C.

40. Gerda Lerner, "Early Community Work of Black Club Women," *Journal of Negro History* 59 (1974):158–167. See especially her discussion of the Neighborhood Union in Atlanta, p. 164. Also see: Cynthyia Neverdon-Morton, *Afro-American Women of the South and the Advancement of the Race 1895–1925* (Knoxville: University of Tennessee Press, 1989).

41. Samuel U. Rodgers, "Kansas City General Hospital No. 2: A Historical Perspective," *Journal of the National Medical Association* 54 (September 1962):527. For a sound discussion of conditions on separate black wards in nonsegregated hospitals, see Rosenberg, *The Care of Strangers*, pp. 301–330.

42. *Crisis* 23 (April 1922):270; Clement Richardson, ed., "William J. Tompkins, M.D. and Old City Hospital," in *The National Cyclopedia of the Colored Race*, vol. 1 (Montgomery, Ala.: National Publishing Co., 1919), p. 305. For a detailed account of racial politics and conflict over the staffing of a hospital for blacks, see Pete Daniel, "Black Power in the 1920s: The Case of Tuskegee Veterans Hospital," *Journal of Southern History* 36 (1970):368–388.

43. Peter Marshall Murray, "Hospital Provision for the Negro Race," *Journal of the American Medical Association* 94 (May 1930):1414.

44. Rann, "The Good Samaritan Hospital of Charlotte, North Carolina," pp. 223, 225. The hospital opened a school of nursing in 1903 and held its first commencement in 1905. The white women from the St. Peters Church made up the board of management and continued to administer and raise funds for the hospital until 1947. The nursing school was closed on October 31, 1959.

45. Anna De Costa Banks, "The Work of a Small Hospital and Training School in the South," *Eighth Annual Report of the Hampton Training School for Nurses and Dixie Hospital* (1898–99), pp. 23–28.

46. Ibid.

47. Kenney, "Some Facts concerning Negro Nurse Training Schools and Their Graduates," pp. 53–58. Also see *Southern Letter* (March 1917), letter written by Euphemia A. Davis, Class of 1908, from Colosada, Ala., on February 22, 1917. Davis wrote, "Being a Tuskegee trained nurse has helped me more than any other thing. On a number of instances I have been chosen for work simply because the persons knew that I graduated from Tuskegee."

48. Thoms, *Pathfinders*, pp. 192–194. For a detailed description of the National Health Circle for Colored People, Incorporated, and the Blue Circle Nurses, see Darlene Clark Hine, "The Call That Never Came: Black Women Nurses and World War I—An Historical Note," *Indiana Military History Journal* 8, no. 1 (January 1983):23–27.

2. Northern Black Hospitals and Nurse Training Schools

1. Elliott M. Rudwick, "A Brief History of Mercy-Douglass Hospital in Philadelphia," *Journal of Negro Education* 20 (January 1951):50–66; W. Montague Cobb, "Nathan Francis Mossell, M.D., 1856–1946," *Journal of the National Medical Association* 46 (March 1954):118–129; idem, "Henry McKee Minton, 1870–1946," *Journal of the National Medical Association* 47 (July 1955):285–286; Aubre de L. Maynard, *Surgeons to the Poor: The Harlem Hospital Story* (New York: Appleton-Century-Crofts, 1978); Helen Buckler, *Daniel Hale Williams, Negro Surgeon* (New York: Putnam, 1968). Buckler's research papers, including scores of letters written by black physicians who knew and worked with Daniel Hale Williams, are located in the Moorland-Spingarn Library, Manuscript Section, Howard University, Washington, D.C. Also see Delora Mitchell, "Provident Hospital: A Black Institution Survives" (M.A. thesis, Northeastern Illinois University, 1962).

2. R. A. Lambert, Negro Hospitals in Chicago, 21–22 February 1939. General Education Board Papers, Box 699, Folder 7000, Rockefeller Archive Center, North Tarrytown, N.Y.

3. S. G. L. Dannett, "Nanahyoke Sockum Curtis," in *Profiles of Negro Womanhood*, vol. 2, *Twentieth Century* (New York: Negro Heritage Library, Educational Heritage, 1966), p. 104; Joyce Ann Elmore, "Black Nurses: Their Service and Their Struggles," *American Journal of Nursing* 76 (March 1976):435. For an excellent description of the important work of black women in the rise and development of Provident Hospital, see Susan Lynn Smith, "The Black Women's Club Movement: Self-improvement and Sisterhood, 1890–1915" (M.A. thesis, University of Wisconsin, 1986), chap. 5, pp. 79–100.

4. *Crisis*, September 1915, pp. 238–249; Henry B. Matthews, "Provident Hospital—Then and Now," *Journal of the National Medical Association* 53 (May 1961):209. For a lengthy discussion of the Williams and Hall controversy, see Buckler, *Daniel Hale Williams*, pp. 251–258; Allan H. Spear, *Black Chicago: The Making of a Negro Ghetto, 1890–1920* (Chicago: University of Chicago Press, 1967), pp. 99–100.

5. Robert McMurdy to William C. Graves, 24 May 1913, Julius Rosenwald Papers, Box 31, Folder 7, University of Chicago Library.

6. Ibid.

7. Embree to Johns, 13 August 1924, Rockefeller Papers, Box 122, Folder 1509; W. C. Graves to Abraham Flexner, 26 May 1925, Julius Rosenwald Papers, Box 31, Folder 7, University of Chicago Library. Also see in the same box and folder Albert B. George to Graves, 21 April 1927; George to Rosenwald, 24 September 1928; Alfred K. Stern to Henry P. Chandler, 31 December 1927.

8. Embree to Rosenwald, 24 January 1929, Julius Rosenwald Papers, Box 31, Folder 7, University of Chicago Library.

9. Embree to Richard M. Pearce, 5 July 1929, General Education Board Papers, Box 699, Folder 7000.

10. Allan H. Spear, *Black Chicago*, pp. 12, 141–146.

11. Embree to Rosenwald, 27 January 1919, Julius Rosenwald Papers, Box 31, Folder 7.

12. Rosenwald to Frank Billings, 19 December 1929, Julius Rosenwald Papers, Box 31, Folder 7.

13. Basil C. H. Harvey, "Provision for Training Colored Medical Students," *Journal of the American Medical Association* 94 (May 1930):1415.

14. Embree to Billings, 22 January 1930, Julius Rosenwald Papers, Box 31, Folder 7; and see 22 April 1930, Journal Voucher no. 91. I thank Dr. Vanessa Lee Gamble, M.D., for sharing a copy of her University of Pennsylvania graduate seminar paper, "The Provident Hospital Project: An Experiment in Black Medical Education," Gamble to Hine, 7 September 1980.

15. Joseph A. Berry and E. Milton Johnson to George R. Arthur and other Provident Hospital trustees, 29 December 1934, Julius Rosenwald Fund Papers, Box 243, Folder 1, Fisk University Library, Nashville, Tenn.

16. *Richmond Planet*, 11 February 1931. For a good discussion of the tensions existing between southern and northern black physicians, see Edward H. Beardsley, *A History of Neglect: Health Care for Blacks and Mill Workers in the Twentieth-Century South* (Knoxville: University of Tennessee Press, 1987), pp. 77–100.

17. *Richmond Planet*, 11 February 1931.

18. Ibid., 21 February 1923.

19. R. A. Lambert, "Negro Education: Provident Hospital," 29 November 1938, memo, GEB Papers, Box 699, Folder 7202, Rockefeller Archive Center.

20. Raymond B. Fosdick, *Adventure in Giving: The Story of the General Education Board* (New York: Harper and Row, 1962), p. 186.

21. Rudwick, "A Brief History"; Cobb, "Nathan Francis Mossell"; Edward S. Cooper, "The Mercy-Douglass Hospital," *Journal of the National Medical Association* 53 (January 1961):3. For an excellent study of the impact of racial discrimination, see Vincent P. Franklin, *The Education of Black Philadelphia* (Philadelphia: University of Pennsylvania Press, 1979).

22. Cobb, "Nathan Francis Mossell," p. 124; *Frederick Douglass Memorial Hospital Report for 1905–06* (Philadelphia, Penn.), p. 13, quoted in Rudwick, "Brief History," pp. 51 and 57; "Report of Committee on Medical Education on Colored Hospitals," *Journal of the National Medical Association* 2 (1910):284, last Mossell quote, p. 285.

23. Cobb, "Nathan Francis Mossell," p. 127; Rudwick, "Brief History," p. 51.

24. Cobb, "Nathan Francis Mossell," p. 124; Rudwick, "Brief History," p. 52; Cobb, "Nathan Francis Mossell," p. 123. See especially, for a detailed description of the general philanthropic work of black community women, Mrs. N. F. Mossell, *The Work of the Afro-American Woman* (Freeport, N.Y.: Books for Libraries Press, 1971, first published in 1894).

25. Quoted in Rudwick, "Brief History," p. 52; Cobb, "Nathan Francis Mossell," p. 124; Edward S. Cooper, "The Mercy-Douglass Hospital."

26. Rudwick, "Brief History," p. 52.

27. Cooper, "The Mercy-Douglass Hospital," p. 4.

28. Ibid.

29. "A Philadelphia Hospital," *Crisis* 35 (December 1928):425–426.
30. Rudwick, "Brief History," p. 53.
31. Cobb, "Nathan Francis Mossell," p. 126.
32. Cobb, "Henry McKee Minton."
33. Edwin R. Embree to Ethel Johns, 13 August 1924, Rockefeller Foundation Papers, Box 122, Folder 1509.
34. *Richmond Planet*, 11 February 1931.
35. Rudwick, "Brief History," p. 56.
36. Ibid.
37. Rudwick, "Brief History," pp. 56–57; Cobb, "Henry McKee Minton," p. 286; Russell F. Minton, "The History of Mercy-Douglass Hospital," *Journal of the National Medical Association* 43 (1951):153–159; Cooper, "The Mercy-Douglass Hospital," pp. 5–6.
38. Embree to Johns, 13 August 1924; Paul Starr, *The Social Transformation of American Medicine* (New York: Basic Books, 1982), p. 158. The early history of Lincoln is recounted in Fitzhugh Mullan, *White Coats, Clenched Fists: The Political Education of an American Physician* (New York: Macmillan, 1976), pp. 117–121. For a history of blacks in early twentieth-century Harlem, see Gilbert Osofsky, *Harlem: The Making of a Ghetto* (New York: Harper and Row, 1966).
39. Thoms, *Pathfinders: A History of the Progress of Colored Graduate Nurses* (New York: McKay Co., 1929), p. 74.
40. Ibid.
41. *Progress Reports*, 1920–27, Rockefeller Foundation Papers (1924), p. 3, Box 138.
42. Embree to Johns, 13 August 1924.
43. *Progress Reports* (1925), Rockefeller Foundation Papers, pp. 4–7, Box 138; *Progress Reports* (1924), p. 5.
44. For detailed coverage of racial tensions at Harlem Hospital, see "The Case of Harlem Hospital," *Crisis* 23 (January 1927):24–25; *Crisis* 41 (March 1934):83–84; *Crisis* 41 (April 1934):101–102; *Crisis* 40 (April 1933):44–45; Gerald A. Spencer, *Medical Symphony: A Study of the Contributions of the Negro to Medical Progress in New York* (New York: Arlain Printing Co., 1947), pp. 98–100; Aubre de L. Maynard, *Surgeons to the Poor*, pp. 15–25.
45. Alisan M. Bennett, "A History of the Harlem Hospital School of Nursing: Its Emergence and Development in a Changing Urban Community, 1923–1973" (Ed.D. dissertation, Teachers College, Columbia University, 1984), pp. 35–52, 173; Birdie E. Brown, *Face It with a Smile* (New York: Vantage Press, 1976), p. 13.
46. Maynard, *Surgeons to the Poor*, p. 23.
47. *Progress Reports* (1925), Rockefeller Foundation Papers, p. 7.
48. Ibid., p. 11.
49. Spencer, *Medical Symphony*, pp. 98–100; Maynard, *Surgeons to the Poor*, p. 25.; Bennett, "A History of the Harlem Hospital," pp. 157–160, 233.

3. Training Nurses in Southern Black Hospitals

1. Daniel Hale Williams, "Afro-Americans as Surgeons and Nurses," *AME Church Review* 10 (January 1894):425–431.
2. For the most complete listing of black hospitals and nursing training schools and the dates of founding and closing, see Mary Elizabeth Carnegie, *The Path We Tread: Blacks in Nursing, 1854–1984* (Philadelphia: J. B. Lippincott Co., 1986), pp. 23–25. For a good general treatment of four of the earliest institutions, see Patricia Sloan, "Black Hospitals and Nurse Training Schools: Spelman, Provi-

dent, Hampton, and Tuskegee" (Ed.D. dissertation, Teachers College, Columbia University, 1978).

3. Ethel Johns, "A Study of the Present Status of the Negro Woman in Nursing, 1925." Copy found in Rockefeller Foundation Papers, Box 122, Rockefeller Archive Center, Pocantico Hills, North Tarrytown, N.Y. The report consisted of a forty-page narrative and summary of findings followed by twenty-one exhibits (A to P), each describing a specific institution. Two appendixes provided general information on the National Association of Colored Graduate Nurses and the National Hospital Association and an array of miscellaneous statistical tables: Darlene Clark Hine, "The Ethel Johns Report: Black Women in the Nursing Profession, 1925," *Journal of Negro History* 67 (Fall 1982):213; Alice Bacon, "The Hampton Training School for Nurses," *Fourth Annual Report of the Hampton Training School for Nurses and Dixie Hospital, 1895–1896*, p. 16; *Thirteenth Annual Report, 1903–1904*, p. 21; *The Hospital Herald; A Monthly Journal Devoted to Hospital Work, Nurse Training, and Domestic and Public Hygiene* 1, no. 12 (November 1899):12; Joyce Ann Elmore, "A History of Freedmen's Hospital Training School for Nurses in Washington, D.C., 1894–1909" (M.A. thesis, Catholic University, Washington, D.C., 1965), pp. 54–55. Permelia Doty of the New York State Board of Nurse Examiners inspected the John A. Andrew Memorial Hospital nursing school at Tuskegee Institute on March 4, 1924. Doty noted that even at this late date many of the forty-two student nurses had not finished even the first year of high school and that during their first year they were "carrying this [high school] work in addition to their nursing training." Copy of the Report of Inspection of John A. Andrew Memorial Hospital by the National Organization for Public Health Nursing found in Rockefeller Foundation Papers, Box 122, Folder 1505–1509. Rockefeller Archive Center, Pocantico Hills, North Tarrytown, N.Y. For an excellent study of the training experiences of white nurses, see Nancy Tomes, "'Little World of Our Own': The Pennsylvania Hospital Training School for Nurses, 1895–1907," *Journal of the History of Medicine and Allied Sciences* 33 (October 1978):507–530.

4. *Hospital Herald*, November 1899, p. 7. According to the *Herald*, "Applicants for admission to the school should be between the ages of twenty and forty. They must possess a good common school education and be thoroughly sound, mentally, morally and physically. A certificate as to the moral character from some responsible person will be required, also the certificate of some regular physician as to physical condition." All issues except one found in the Waring Historical Library of the Medical University of South Carolina, Charleston. The 1898 issue of *Hospital Herald* was found in the Caroliniana Library, Columbia, S.C. See Johns, "Negro Woman in Nursing," pp. 19–20, Exhibit C—Kansas City General Hospital No. 2, Kansas City, Mo.; Exhibit G—St. Agnes Hospital and School for Nurses, Raleigh, N.C.; Hine, "The Ethel Johns Report," p. 214; *First Annual Report of the Flint-Goodridge Hospital*, 31 December 1916, copy found in the Amistad Research Center (now located at Tulane University), New Orleans, La.

5. Billings's quote, Johns Hopkins Hospital, *Reports and Papers*, no. 3, p. 11, taken from Janet Wilson James, "Isabel Hampton and the Professionalization of Nursing in the 1890's," in *The Therapeutic Revolution: Essays in the Social History of American Medicine*, ed. Morris J. Vogel and Charles E. Rosenberg (Philadelphia: University of Pennsylvania Press, 1979), p. 208.

6. Josephine St. Pierre Ruffin's remarks on this incident are included in *Lifting As They Climb*, by Elizabeth Lindsay Davis (Washington, D.C.: NACW, circa 1933), pp. 13–15; Darlene Clark Hine, "Lifting the Veil, Shattering the Silence: Black Women's History in Slavery and Freedom," in *The State of Afro-American*

History: Past, Present, and Future, ed. Darlene Clark Hine (Baton Rouge: Louisiana State University Press, 1986), p. 235.

7. *Hospital Herald* 1, no. 11 (November 1899):7.

8. W. T. B. Williams, "Hospital and Training School for Nurses," Charleston, S.C., A. C. McClennan, M.D., Surgeon-in-Charge, 28 November 1905, 13 pages. General Education Board Collection, Series 1, Box 200, Folder 1899, Rockefeller Archive Center, North Tarrytown, N.Y. I wish to thank especially Professor James D. Anderson for bringing this document to my attention.

9. *First Annual Report of the Flint-Goodridge Hospital, December 31, 1916.*

10. *Tuskegee Normal and Industrial Institute Catalogue, 1894–1895*, p. 55; ibid., *1896–1897*, p. 86; *1906–1907*, p. 27.

11. *First Annual Report of the Flint-Goodridge Hospital, December 31, 1916.*

12. Ibid.

13. *Fourth Annual Report of the Hampton Training School for Nurses and Dixie Hospital, Hampton, Virginia, 1895–1896*, pp. 9–12.

14. *1906–1907 Annual Catalogue of Tuskegee Normal and Industrial Institute*, p. 27; *First Annual Report of the Flint-Goodridge Hospital, December 31, 1916.*

15. Elmore, "A History of Freedmen's Hospital," pp. 47–48; Hine, "The Ethel Johns Report," pp. 215, 216; Johns, "Negro Woman in Nursing," pp. 20–21, Exhibit K—Grady Hospital, Atlanta, Ga.; Exhibit I—St. Philip Hospital, Richmond, Va.; Elmore, "A History of Freedmen's Hospital," p. 55.

16. *Eleventh Annual Report of the Hampton Training School for Nurses and Dixie Hospital, Hampton, Virginia, 1901–1902*, pp. 19–20.

17. *Hospital Herald* 1, no. 9 (October 1899).

18. *Fourth Annual Report of the Hampton Training School for Nurses and Dixie Hospital, 1895–1896*, p. 12.

19. *Eleventh Annual Report of the Hampton Training School for Nurses, 1901–1902*, p. 20.

20. Lucy Brown, "The Nursing Department," *Hospital Herald*, October 1899.

21. W. T. B. Williams, "Hospital and Training School for Nurses," pp. 8–9.

22. *Twenty-second Annual Catalogue of Tuskegee Institute, 1902–1903.*

23. Adah B. Thoms, *Pathfinders: A History of the Progress of Colored Graduate Nurses* (New York: McKay Co., 1929), p. 38.

24. Austin Curtis, quoted in Elmore, "A History of Freedmen's Hospital," pp. 43–44. For a description of the early years, see *Annual Report of Freedmen's Hospital to the Secretary of the Interior* (Washington, D.C.: Government Printing Office, 1900), pp. 440–441.

25. Nina Gage to Arthur Howe, 17 January 1938, Dixie Hospital Manuscript Collection, Hampton University Archives, Hampton, Va. (Papers are unprocessed, thus making it impossible to provide box and folder numbers.) For more background information, see Lilli Sentz, "Nina Diadamia Gage," *American Nursing: A Biographical Dictionary*, ed. Vern L. Bullough et al. (New York: Garland 1988), pp. 128–130.

26. Emily Green Allen, "Nursing Portraits," *National News Bulletin* 8, no. 12 (August 1936). Allen was a member of the graduating class of 1911.

27. John Kenney to Executive Council, Tuskegee Institute, 18 May 1905, Box 560; 4 February 1909, Box 591; 24 May 1910, Box 601. Booker T. Washington (BTW) Papers, Library of Congress, Washington, D.C.

28. Kenney to Executive Council, 4 February 1909, BTW Papers, Box 591; Kenney to Executive Council, Tuskegee Institute, 24 May 1910, BTW Papers, Box 601.

29. W. T. B. Williams, "Hospital and Training School for Nurses."

30. Ibid. Quotes of McClennan taken from *Hospital Herald*, December 1898, p. 4.

31. *Hospital Herald* 1, no. 5 (April 1899) and no. 6 (May 1899).

32. Brown, "The Nursing Department," *Hospital Herald*, October 1899.

33. Charles S. Johnson, *The Negro in American Civilization: A Study of Negro Life and Race Relations in the Light of Social Research* (New York: Henry Holt and Co., 1936), p. 188.

34. Herbert M. Morais, *The History of the Negro in Medicine* (Washington, D.C.: Association for the Study of Afro-American Life and History, 1967), pp. 151–153.

35. H. M. Green, "Hospitals and Public Health Facilities for Negroes," in *Proceedings of the National Conference of Social Work* (Chicago: University of Chicago Press, 1928), pp. 178–180; "Investigation of Negro Hospitals," *Journal of the American Medical Association* 80 (April 1923):1244; 92 (1929):1375–1376; John A. Kenney, "The Negro Hospital Renaissance," *Journal of the National Medical Association* 23 (July-September 1930):109. Also see H. M. Green, "Some Facts about the National Hospital Association That Should Interest You," undated typescript included in the Ethel Johns correspondence, Rockefeller Foundation Papers, Box 122.

36. *Negro Hospitals: A Compilation of Available Statistics* (Chicago: Julius Rosenwald Fund, 1931), pp. 6–7; Green, "Hospitals and Public Health Facilities for Negroes," p. 180.

37. Green, "A Plea for the Small Hospital for Negroes," *Trained Nurse and Hospital Review*, August 1926, p. 172.

38. "The Hale Infirmary, Montgomery, Alabama," in *National Cyclopedia of the Colored Race* (1919), p. 129.

39. Green, "A Plea for the Small Hospital for Negroes," p. 172.

40. W. T. B. Williams, "Hospital and Training School for Nurses."

41. Ibid.

42. Thoms, *Pathfinders*, pp. 34–35.

4. Black Collegiate Nursing Education

1. Esther Lucille Brown, *Nursing for the Future: A Report Prepared for the National Nursing Council* (New York: Russell Sage Foundation, [1948]), p. 177; Fred Davis, Virginia L. Olesen, and Elni Waik Whittaker, "Problems and Issues in Collegiate Nursing Education," in *The Nursing Profession: Five Sociological Essays*, ed. Fred Davis (New York: John Wiley and Sons, 1966), pp. 138–175; Margaret Bridgeman, *Collegiate Education for Nursing* (New York: Russell Sage Foundation, [1953]).

2. Isabel M. Stewart, "Next Step in the Education of Nurses," *National News Bulletin* 13 (December 1939). Copies of the National Association of Colored Graduate Nurses official organ found in the Schomburg Public Library, New York City; Stewart, *The Education of Nurses* (New York: Macmillan, 1943), p. 302.

3. Rheva A. Speaks, quoted in *National News Bulletin* 13 (April 1940); Darlene Clark Hine, "From Hospital to College: Black Nurse Leaders and the Rise of Collegiate Nursing Schools," *Journal of Negro Education* 51 (September 1982):222–237; Davis et al., "Problems and Issues," p. 149.

4. Estelle Massey Riddle, "The Training and Placement of Negro Nurses," *Journal of Negro Education* 4 (1935):48.

5. Riddle, "Negro Nurses: The Supply and Demand," *Opportunity* 15 (November 1937):329.

6. Riddle, "Sources of Supply of Negro Health Personnel, Section C: Nurses," *Journal of Negro Education* 6 (1937):492.

7. Riddle, "Negro Nurses: The Supply and Demand," p. 328; Also see Julianne Malveaux and Susan Englander, "Race and Class in Nursing Occupations," *SAGE* 3 (Spring 1986):41–45.

8. Mary Elizabeth Carnegie, *The Path We Tread: Blacks in Nursing, 1854–1984*, (Philadelphia: J. B. Lippincott Co., 1986), pp. 27–32.

9. Ibid., p. 32. Carnegie discussed the development of associate degree programs in community colleges since the 1950s. She maintained that "were it not for the associate degree programs in community colleges, with low cost to the student and flexible standards in terms of age, marital status, sex, and race, many qualified Black students would be lost to the field of nursing" (p. 33). For a discussion of the impact of federally funded health-care and nursing-education programs, see Riddle and Josephine Nelson, "The Negro Nurse Looks toward Tomorrow," *American Journal of Nursing* 45 (August 1945): 627–630.

10. "The History of Flint-Goodridge Hospital of Dillard University," *Journal of the National Medical Association* 61 (November 1969):553; *Fifth Annual Report of the Flint-Goodridge Hospital*, 31 December 1921. Annual reports of the hospital found in the Amistad Research Collection, Tulane University, New Orleans.

11. Memorandum on Flint-Goodridge Hospital, New Orleans, and Its Relation to the New Dillard University, 12 November 1929, General Education Board Collection, Box 89, Folder 788, Rockefeller Archive Center, North Tarrytown, N.Y.

12. Ibid.; Raymond Fosdick, *Adventure in Giving: The Story of the General Education Board* (New York: Harper and Row, 1962), p. 205.

13. Fosdick, *Adventure in Giving*, p. 205.

14. Ibid., p. 206; Jackson Davis to Raymond B. Fosdick, 11 April 1930, GEB Papers, Box 89, Folder 789.

15. Davis to Fosdick, 11 April 1930, GEB Papers, Box 89, Folder 789; "Report of the Joint Committee to the Board of Education of the Methodist Episcopal Church and the American Missionary Association," 14 October 1929, GEB Papers, Louisiana 66, Series I, Box 89.

16. Fosdick, *Adventure in Giving*, p. 206; Captain H. W. Knight, "Flint-Goodrich [*sic*] Hospital," *Journal of the National Medical Association* 22 (July–September 1930):130–131.

17. Fosdick, *Adventure in Giving*, pp. 206–207.

18. Press clippings, *Christian Educator* (1929), p. 5, copies in GEB Collection, Box 90, Folder 796.

19. Leo Favrot, Press Release (1929), GEB Collection, Box 90, Folder 796.

20. Mordecai W. Johnson, Remarks delivered at the laying of the cornerstone of Dillard University, 27 May 1938, Press Stories, GEB Collection, Box 90, Folder 796.

21. R. B. Eleazer, "Flint-Goodridge Hospital," *Crisis* 40 (July 1933):151–153; New Orleans *Times Picayune*, 8 May 1938; Claire and George Sessions Perry, "Penny-a-Day Hospital," *Saturday Evening Post*, September 1939, pp. 30ff.; "The History of Flint-Goodridge Hospital of Dillard University"; Moise H. Goldstein and B. C. MacLean, "A Hospital That Serves as a Center of Negro Medical Education," *Modern Hospital* 39 (November 1932, reprint):1–8; Horace Mann Bond, quoted in Charles S. Johnson, *Into the Main-stream: A Survey of Best Practices in Race Relations in the South* (Chapel Hill: University of North Carolina Press, 1947), pp. 246–248; "Albert W. Dent Elected President," *Dillard Bulletin* 5 (June

1941):1; Interview with Albert Dent, New Orleans, La., 15 October 1980; see Hine, "From Hospital to College," pp. 222–237, for a discussion of the transformation of the Florida A & M School of Nursing.

22. *Saturday Evening Post*, September 1939.

23. Leo M. Favrot to Trevor Arnett, 26 May 1936, Box 89, Folder 790; Diary of Mary Elizabeth Tennant, 5, 6 August 1940, Box 548, Folder 5864; Robert Lambert, Interoffice Memorandum, 5 December 1939, Box 90, Folder 795. Lambert wrote, "I am again most favorably impressed with Dent. I have no doubt about his being the ablest Negro hospital administrator in the country." GEB Papers, Rockefeller Archive Center, Pocantico Hills, N.Y.

24. Albert W. Dent to Jackson Davis, 6 March 1943, GEB Papers, Box 548, Folder 5864; Edgar B. Stern to Trevor Arnett, 7 November 1932, ibid., Box 89, Folder 790; Dent, "Annual Report of the Flint-Goodridge Hospital," 31 December 1935 (copies of all annual reports found in GEB Papers, Box 90). See *National News Bulletin* 7 (December 1934) for comments on nursing education by Eola V. Lyons. Throughout the 1930s, a hotly debated issue in nursing circles was whether it was cheaper to operate a hospital with a staff of graduate nurses or with all student nurses.

25. Albert W. Dent, "Hospital Services and Facilities Available to Negroes in the United States," *Journal of Negro Education* 18, no. 3 (1949 Yearbook): 326–332.

26. Carter G. Woodson, *The Negro Professional Man and the Community* (New York: Association for Study of Negro Life and History, 1934; reprinted by Negro Universities Press, 1969), pp. 120–121; Woodson, *The Rural Negro* (Washington, D.C.: Association for the Study of Negro Life and History, 1930), p. 14; Dent, "Hospital Services," pp. 326–332.

27. Dent, "Flint-Goodridge Hospital and Negro Health in New Orleans," Annual Report, 31 December 1935.

28. Ibid.

29. *Saturday Evening Post*, September 1939.

30. L. C. Spencer to Dent, 15 May 1936, copy in GEB Papers, Box 89, Folder 790.

31. Dent, Annual Report, 31 December 1935; Dent, "Flint-Goodridge Hospital Annual Report," 31 December 1942; 31 December 1943; Wanda C. Heistad, "The Development of Nurse-Midwifery Education in the United States," in *Historical Studies in Nursing*, ed. M. Louise Fitzpatrick (New York: Teachers College Press, 1978), pp. 86–103; Carnegie, *The Path We Tread*, p. 37.

32. Dent, "Flint-Goodridge Hospital Annual Report," 31 December 1937; 31 December 1940.

33. Ibid., 31 December 1940.

34. Ibid., 31 December 1975.

35. Ibid.

36. Dent, "The First Five Years," Annual Report of the Superintendent of the Flint-Goodridge Hospital, 31 December 1936; Interview Memorandum: Dent, Jackson Davis, and Mary Elizabeth Tennant, ? February 1943, GEB Papers Box 548, Folder 5864; Dent, Annual Report, 31 December 1943.

37. Dent, "The Role of a Negro Hospital in the Control of Tuberculosis in a Large Southern City," reprinted from *Transactions of the Thirty-seventh Annual Meeting of the National Tuberculosis Association* (1941); copy in GEB Papers, Box 90, Folder 802. Dent, "Flint-Goodridge Hospital Annual Report," 31 December 1935; 1936; 1937; 1938; 1939; 1940; 1941. *Saturday Evening Post*, September 1939.

38. Dent, "Flint-Goodridge Hospital Annual Report," 31 December 1936; 31 December 1938; 31 December 1940; 31 December 1943.

39. Dent to Julius Rosenwald Fund, 23 March 1940, GEB Papers, Box 90, Folder 801.

40. Dent, "The First Five Years," 31 December 1936.

41. See T. Jean Louise Mazero, "Professionalizing of Nursing in America: A Century of Struggle" (Ph.D. dissertation, University of Pittsburgh, 1972), p. 445.

42. Dent, "The First Five Years," 31 December 1936.

43. Louis T. Wright, "Address to the Graduating Class of Nurses of Harlem Hospital," *National News Bulletin* 12 (February 1939). For a graphic illustration of the "worth of a black nurse," see Black Women Oral History Project: Interview with Eunice Laurie, 10 October 1977. Copy of transcript in the Schlesinger Library, Radcliffe College.

44. Interoffice Memorandum. Re: Flint-Goodridge Hospital of Dillard University in New Orleans, La., 23 June 1936; Favrot to Arnett, 26 May 1936, GEB Papers Box 89, Folder 790.

45. Mary Beard, Interoffice Memorandum. Re: Flint-Goodridge Hospital; Dent to Favrot, 22 May 1936, GEB Papers, Box 89, Folder 790.

46. "Flint-Goodridge Hospital Annual Report," 31 December 1940; 31 December 1943; Dent, "A Request for Funds Payable over Three Years: For the Reopening of a Three-Year Nursing School and for Giving Special Instruction Including Public Health Short Courses to Graduate Nurses" (1936?). GEB Collection, Box 89, Folder 790.

47. Notes in Diary of Mary Elizabeth Tennant, 5, 6 August 1942, GEB Collection, Box 548, Folder 5864.

48. Ibid.

49. Tennant Diary, 13 August 1942, GEB Papers, Box 548, Folder 5864; Edwin R. Embree, *Investment in People: The Story of the Julius Rosenwald Fund* (New York: Harper and Brothers, 1949), pp. 110–111.

50. Robert Lambert to Jackson Davis, 22 March 1943; Memorandum of Dent's interview with Jackson Davis and M. E. Tennant, ? February 1943; William Brierley to Dent, 8 April 1943; Robert D. Calkins, Interoffice Memorandum, 4 March 1948, GEB Papers, Box 548, Folder 5864.

51. Dent to Calkins, 28 February 1949, GEB Papers, Box 548, Folder 5864.

52. Copy of "Program for Miss Rita Miller," 14 April to 12 May 1943, GEB Papers, Box 548, Folder 5865.

53. Rita E. Miller, "Negro Schools of Nursing in the South," November 1943, GEB Papers, Box 548, Folder 5864. Miller presented some of her findings at the National Conference of Hospital Administrators, Norfolk, Va., 19, 20 November 1943. Copy of the report found in the Dixie Hospital and Nurse Training School Collection, Hampton Institute Archive, Hampton, Va.

54. Memorandum of Dent interview with Davis, Tennant, ? February 1943; Dent to Tennant, 29 January 1944; Tennant Diary, 23 January 1944; Miller, "Report on the Progress Made by the Dillard University Division of Nursing, September, 1944 to September, 1945"; Miller, "Report on the Development of the Dillard University Division of Nursing, September 15, 1942 to November 22, 1943," GEB Papers, Box 548, Folder 5864.

55. Miller, "Report on the Development . . . September 15, 1942 to November 22, 1943," GEB Papers, Box 548, Folder 5864.

56. Miller, "Report of Division of Nursing, 1947; 1948"; Dent to Calkins, 14 February 1948, GEB Papers, Box 548, Folder 5864.

57. John Procope, "Flint-Goodridge Annual Report," 31 December 1943; Riddle

and Nelson, "The Negro Nurse Looks toward Tomorrow," pp. 627–629; Herbert R. Northrup, "The ANA and the Negro Nurse," *American Journal of Nursing* 50 (April 1950):207–208; Mabel K. Staupers, "Story of the National Association of Colored Graduate Nurses," *American Journal of Nursing* 51 (April 1951): 221–222.

5. Racism, Status, and the Professionalization of Black Nursing

1. Janet Wilson James, "Isabel Hampton and the Professionalization of Nursing in the 1890s," in *The Therapeutic Revolution: Essays in the Social History of American Medicine*, ed. Morris J. Vogel and Charles E. Rosenberg (Philadelphia: University of Pennsylvania Press, 1979), pp. 228–233; Richard Harrison Shryock, "Nursing Emerges as a Profession: The American Experience," *Clio Medica* 3 (1968): 136–137. The standard work on this early era is M. Adelaide Nutting and Lavinia L. Dock, *The History of Nursing: From the Earliest Times to the Present Day with Special Reference to the Work of the Past Thirty Years*, 4 vols. (New York: Putnam and Sons, 1907–1912); Celia Davies, "Professionalizing Strategies as Time- and Culture-Bound: American and British Nursing circa 1893," in *Nursing History: New Perspectives, New Possibilities*, ed. Ellen Condliffe Lagemann (New York: Teachers College, Columbia University, 1983), pp. 47–63. The literature on professionalization is voluminous. One of the most useful examinations is Magali Sarfatti Larson, *The Rise of Professionalism: A Sociological Analysis* (Berkeley: University of California Press, 1977), pp. x–xviii, 155–156; Also see Penina Migdal Glazer and Miriam Slater, *Unequal Colleagues: The Entrance of Women into the Professions, 1880–1940* (New Brunswick, N.J.: Rutgers University Press, 1987), pp. 1–23.

2. Mary N. Roberts, *American Nursing: History and Interpretation* (New York: Macmillan Co., 1961), pp. 20–30; Robert V. Piemonte, "History of the National League of Nursing Education, 1912–1932: Great Awakening in Nursing Education" (Ed.D. dissertation, Teachers College, Columbia University, 1976), pp. 15–19.

3. Roberts, *American Nursing*, pp. 20–30; two black alumnae associations belonged to the Associated Alumnae. The Lincoln Alumnae Association, organized in 1903, was accepted for membership in the New York State Nurses' Association, thus enabling Lincoln's graduate nurses to become members of the American Nurses' Association. The Freedmen's Hospital School of Nursing Alumni Association, organized in 1897, was incorporated in Washington, D.C., on May 7, 1906, as the Freedmen's Alumnae Association of Trained Nurses. *The Fifty Year Graduates of Freedmen's Hospital School of Nursing Tell Their Story* (Washington, D.C.: Freedmen's Hospital Nurses Alumni Clubs, 1986), p. 7.

4. Shryock, "Nursing Emerges as a Profession," p. 137; Marty L. Shannon, "Nurses in American History: Our First Four Licensure Laws," *American Journal of Nursing* 17 (August 1975):1327–1328; Nancy Tomes, "The Silent Battle: Nurse Registration in New York State, 1903–1920," in Lagemann, *Nursing History*, pp. 107–132.

5. M. Louise Fitzpatrick, *The National Organization for Public Health Nursing, 1912–1952: Development of a Practice Field* (New York: National League for Nursing, 1975), pp. 20–34; Mary Elizabeth Carnegie, *The Path We Tread: Blacks in Nursing, 1854–1984* (Philadelphia: J. B. Lippincott Co., 1986), pp. 101–102; Barbara Melosh, *"The Physician's Hand": Work Culture and Conflict in American Nursing* (Philadelphia: Temple University Press, 1982), pp. 122–123; Karen Buhler-Wilkerson, "False Dawn: The Rise and Decline of Public Health Nursing in America, 1900–1930," in Lagemann, *Nursing History*, pp. 89–106.

6. "Nursing Portrait: Ludie Andrews," NACGN *National News Bulletin* 14 (May 1941); Mabel Keaton Staupers, *No Time for Prejudice: The Story of the Integration of Negroes in Nursing in the United States* (New York: Macmillan Co., 1961), pp. 12, 19–20; Carnegie, *The Path We Tread*, pp. 156–157; Verdelle B. Bellamy, editor, *History of Grady Memorial Hospital School of Nursing, 1917–1964* (Atlanta, Ga.: Chi Eta Phi Sorority, c. 1985).

7. Adda Eldredge, "The Need for a Sound Professional Preparation for Colored Nurses," in *Proceedings of the Annual Congress on Medical Education, Medical Licensure, and Hospitals* (Chicago: American Medical Association, 1930), pp. 168–171.

8. Ethel Johns, "A Study of the Present Status of the Negro Woman in Nursing, 1925," unpublished report consisting of a forty-three-page typescript narrative with sixteen exhibits, usually one page in length. Each exhibit consists of descriptions of a specific institution training and employing black women nurses. Exhibit I concerns the Virginia State Board of Health, Richmond, Va. Rockefeller Foundation Archives, Box 122, Folder 1507, Rockefeller Archive Center, North Tarrytown, N.Y. For a summary of the report, see Darlene Clark Hine, "The Ethel Johns Report: Black Women in the Nursing Profession, 1925," *Journal of Negro History* 67 (Fall 1982):212–228. Also see Donelda Hamlin, "Report on Informal Study of the Educational Facilities for Colored Nurses and Their Use in Hospital, Visiting, and Public Health Nursing," the Hospital Library and Service Bureau. A copy can be found in the Rockefeller Archive Center.

9. Johns, "Negro Woman in Nursing," Exhibit N—Board of Health for Jefferson County and the city of Birmingham, Ala.; Hine, "The Ethel Johns Report," pp. 219–220.

10. Johns, "Negro Woman in Nursing," Exhibit O—the Public Health Nursing Council, Nashville, Tenn.

11. Staupers, "Story of the National Association of Colored Graduate Nurses," *American Journal of Nursing* 51 (April 1951):221–222; Elizabeth Jones, "The Negro Woman in the Nursing Profession, *Messenger* 5 (July 1923):64–65; Adah B. Thoms, *Pathfinders: A History of the Progress of Colored Graduate Nurses* (New York: McKay, 1929), pp. 201–205; Joyce Ann Elmore, "Black Nurses: Their Service and Their Struggle," *American Journal of Nursing* 76 (March 1976): 435–437.

12. Staupers, *No Time for Prejudice*, pp. 16, 19–20; Carnegie, *The Path We Tread*, p. 93; Thoms, *Pathfinders*, pp. 201–205, 237; "Articles of Incorporation and By-laws of the NACGN," 10 January 1920; NACGN, *Four Decades of Service* (New York: NACGN, 1948). Copy of this pamphlet and the articles of incorporation found in the NACGN Collection, Schomburg Library, New York City; "Nursing Portraits: Adah Belle Thoms," *National News Bulletin* 8 (June 1936). For biographies of Martha Minerva Franklin and Adah Belle Samuels Thoms, see entries by Althea T. Davis in *American Nursing: A Biographical Dictionary*, ed. Vern L. Bullough et al. (New York: Garland Publishing, 1988) pp. 120–123, 313–316.

13. Staupers, *No Time for Prejudice*, pp. 19–20.

14. Thoms's quote taken from her 1921 annual address to the National Association of Colored Graduate Nurses, which met in Washington, D.C. Reprinted in Darlene Clark Hine, ed., *Black Women in the Nursing Profession: A Documentary History* (New York: Garland Publishing, 1985), pp. 119–122; NACGN, *Four Decades of Service*; Thoms, *Pathfinders*, pp. 214–217; "Articles of Incorporation and By-laws of the NACGN."

15. "Nursing Portraits: Carrie E. Bullock," *National News Bulletin* 8 (June 1936).

16. Ibid.; Staupers, *No Time for Prejudice*, pp. 24–25.

17. "National Association of Colored Graduate Nurses Meet at Tuskegee Institute," *Southern Letter* 43 (August 1927):1.

18. Johns, "Negro Woman in Nursing," p. 6.

19. Ibid., pp. 1–2.

20. Johns, "Negro Woman in Nursing," Exhibit A—Lincoln Home and Hospital and School of Nursing, and Harlem Hospital and Nurse Training School.

21. Johns, "Negro Woman in Nursing," p. 25.

22. Ibid., Exhibit A.

23. Ibid.

24. Ibid., p. 30, Exhibit B—Municipal Board of Health, Municipal Tuberculosis Service, Chicago.

25. Ibid.

26. Jane E. Mottus, *New York Nightingales: The Emergence of the Nursing Profession at Bellevue and New York Hospital* (Ann Arbor: UMI Research Press, 1981), p. 150. By 1930, 471 black nurses out of a total of 4,986 worked in public health. Departments of health employed 248, boards of education, 20, while 203 were employed by local nursing associations and voluntary agencies. In the South only 184 black public-health nurses were reported to be employed. See Stanley Rayfield, Marjory Stimson, and Louise Tattershall, "A Study of Negro Public Health Nursing," *Public Health Nurse* 22 (October 1930):525–537.

27. Johns, "Negro Woman in Nursing," p. 27.

28. Ibid., pp. 25, 29, 30; Susan M. Reverby, *Ordered to Care: The Dilemma of American Nursing, 1850–1945* (Cambridge: Cambridge University Press, 1987), pp. 178–179.

29. Johns, "Negro Woman in Nursing," Exhibit K—Grady Hospital, Atlanta, Ga.; for more information on the history of Grady, see Bellamy, *History of Grady Memorial Hospital School of Nursing, 1917–1964*, pages are unnumbered.

30. Johns, "Negro Woman in Nursing," Exhibit N—the Tennessee Coal and Iron Company Employees Hospital, Fairfield, Ala.

31. Ibid., p. 30.

32. Ibid., p. 33.

33. John Hope Franklin, *From Slavery to Freedom*, 4th ed. (New York: Knopf, 1974), pp. 333–340.

34. Similarly, other black Americans also looked to the war as a means of proving their loyalty and service to their country with hopes that at its conclusion they would be accorded first-class citizenship. W. E. B. Du Bois, *The Autobiography of W. E. B. Du Bois* (New York: International Publishers, 1968), pp. 267–269; Elmore, "Black Nurses: Their Service and Their Struggle."

35. Julia O. Flikke, *Nurses in Action: The Story of the Army Nurse Corps* (Philadelphia: Lippincott, 1943), pp. 76–77; Bonnie Bullough and Vern L. Bullough, *The Emergence of Modern Nursing* (New York: Macmillan, 1964), pp. 168–171.

36. Mottus, *New York Nightingales*, pp. 157–158.

37. Flikke, *Nurses in Action*, pp. 76–77; Bullough and Bullough, *The Emergence of Modern Nursing*, pp. 168–171.

38. Thoms, *Pathfinders*, p. 156; Jane Delano to Isaac H. Wutter, 3 July 1918, Records of the American Red Cross, Record Group 200, National Archives, Washington, D.C.; Frances Elliott Davis, a 1912 graduate of the Freedmen's Hospital school of nursing, was the first black nurse actually to be enrolled in the American Red Cross. She served for a few months in cantonment work in Chattanooga, Tennessee. Anna B. Coles described her career briefly:

When the armistice was signed in November, 1918, she went to Detroit to take charge of the Dunbar Hospital where she organized the first training school for colored nurses in the state of Michigan and graduated the first class who took the board and were admitted to practice. She later engaged in public health work and served on the staff of the Detroit Nurses Association for 18 months, later joining the Detroit Department of Health. She was again the first colored nurse to serve in all of the departments.

"The Howard University School of Nursing in Historical Perspective," *Journal of the National Medical Association* 61 (March 1969):108; also see Susan B. DelBene and Vern L. Bullough, "Frances Elliott Davis, 1882–1965," in Bullough, *American Nursing: A Biographical Dictionary,* pp. 76–77.

39. Ibid.

40. Mabel Keaton Staupers, Memorandum on Present Status of the Negro Nurse in the Army Nursing Corps as of March 1941. Mabel K. Staupers Papers, Box 96–1, Folder 23, Moorland-Spingarn Research Center, Howard University, Washington, D.C.; transcript of a Public Health Nursing Conference luncheon held at the Rockefeller Foundation Headquarters, 16 December 1918, p. 4. Rockefeller Foundation Papers, Box 121, Folder 1494; Roy Wilkins, "Nurses Go to War," *Crisis* 50 (February 1943):42–44; Darlene Clark Hine, "The Call That Never Came: Black Women Nurses and World War I—An Historical Note," *Indiana Military History Journal* 8, (January 1983):23–27.

41. Robert R. Moton to Emmett J. Scott, Special Assistant, War Department, 20 May 1918, Records of the American Red Cross, R.G. 200.

42. "Certificate of Incorporation of the Circle for Negro War Relief, Inc.," 27 October 1917. Copy found in the Arthur B. Spingarn Papers, Box 74, Library of Congress, Manuscript Division, Washington, D.C. In correspondence the organization was also referred to as the Blue Circle for Negro War Relief. Spingarn to James Weldon Johnson, 16 November 1917; Francis M. Hugo to Spingarn, 9, 23 October 1917, Spingarn Papers, Box 74.

43. Circle Certificate of Incorporation; Minutes of the Meetings of the Directors of the Circle, 29 October 1917; Belle Davis, Secretary of the Circle, to George E. Haynes, 14 January 1921, Spingarn Papers, Box 74; copy of resolution changing the name to the Circle for Negro Relief, Inc., signed by Harrison Rhodes, president, and by the new secretary, Etnah Boutté, 19 May 1919, Spingarn Papers, Box 74; memorandum concerning request from the Circle for Negro Relief Incorporated to the Red Cross for aid in the development of black public-health nursing, 11 June 1920. For a brief historical sketch of the Circle, see "Memorandum of Understanding between the American Red Cross and the Circle for Negro War Relief, December 29, 1917," signed by E. Bigelow Hapgood, then president of the Circle, and H. D. Gibson, general manager of the American Red Cross, Papers of the American Red Cross, R.G. 200.

44. Boutté to Spingarn, 20 January, 4 February, 9 March, 5, 8 October 1920; Belle Davis to Spingarn, 20 August 1920, Spingarn Papers, Box 74; "Negro Nurse Training" includes summary of the meeting between Edwin Embree and Belle Davis, 21 April 1922, Rockefeller Foundation Papers, Box 38.

45. Summary of the several conferences concerning cooperation between the Circle for Negro Relief and the American Red Cross, 3 April 1920. Also see Conference attended by Clara Noyes, Elizabeth Fox, Jane Van de Vrede, and a (?) Holmes of the Public Health Service, Etnah Boutté and Adah Thoms in New York, 18 February 1920. Verbatim transcript of the conference found in Records of the American Red Cross, R.G. 200.

46. Spingarn to Elizabeth Fox, 14 July 1920; Fox to Boutté, 3 April 1920, Records of the American Red Cross, R.G. 200; Minutes of the Meetings of the Board of Directors of the Circle for Negro Relief, 25 February 1921, 31 March 1921, Spingarn Papers, Box 74.

47. Red Cross internal memorandum, 11 June 1920, Records of the American Red Cross, R.G. 200.

48. Ibid.

49. Ibid.

50. Thoms, *Pathfinders*, pp. 191–196.

6. The Politics of Agency and the Revitalization of the NACGN

1. Mabel Keaton Staupers, *No Time for Prejudice: The Story of the Integration of Negroes in Nursing in the United States* (New York: Macmillan Co., 1961), p. 28.

2. Midian O. Bousfield, "Bricks without Straw," guest editorial in *Opportunity Magazine* (November 1937); Staupers, *No Time for Prejudice*, p. 45.

3. Staupers, *No Time for Prejudice*, p. 28.

4. Harvard Sitkoff, *A New Deal for Blacks* (New York: Oxford University Press, 1978), pp. 32, 298–334.

5. Staupers, *No Time for Prejudice*, p. 30.

6. Ibid., p. 31.

7. Philip A. Kalisch and Beatrice J. Kalisch, *The Advance of American Nursing* (Boston: Little, Brown and Co. 1978), pp. 327–364.

8. Alma Haupt, "Statement Relative to Work of the Joint Relations Committee of the American Nurses' Association in Cooperation with the National Association of Colored Graduate Nurses," 26 January 1934, American Nurses' Association Board of Directors, ANA Papers, Box 41, Exhibit X, Mugar Library, Boston University, Boston, Mass. I would like to thank Susan Reverby for bringing this document to my attention.

9. M. Louise Fitzpatrick, *The National Organization for Public Health Nursing, 1912–1952: Development of a Practice Field* (New York: National League for Nursing, 1975), pp. 117–118.

10. Barbara Melosh, *"The Physician's Hand": Work Culture and Conflict in American Nursing* (Philadelphia: Temple University Press, 1982), pp. 114, 156; Karen Buhler-Wilkerson, "False Dawn: The Rise and Decline of Public Health Nursing, 1900–1930" (Ph.D. dissertation, University of Pennsylvania, 1984), pp. 195–252.

11. Stanley Rayfield, Marjory Stimson, and Louise Tattershall, "A Study of Negro Public Health Nursing," *Public Health Nurse* 22 (October 1930):527.

12. Fitzpatrick, *The National Organization for Public Health Nursing*, pp. 151, 152.

13. Susan Armeny, "Organized Nurses, Women Philanthropists, and the Intellectual Bases for Cooperation among Women, 1898–1920," in *Nursing History: New Perspectives, New Possibilities*, ed. Ellen Condliffe Lagemann (New York: Teachers College, Columbia University, 1983), pp. 26, 28; Melosh, *"The Physician's Hand,"* p. 122.

14. Haupt, "Statement Relative to Work of the Joint Relations Committee."

15. Ibid.

16. Ibid.

17. Melosh, *"The Physician's Hand,"* pp. 114, 123, 124.

18. Haupt, "Statement Relative to Work of the Joint Relations Committee."

19. Ibid.

20. Susan Reverby, "'Something besides Waiting': The Politics of Private Duty Nursing Reform in the Depression," in *Nursing History: New Perspectives, New Possibilities*, ed. Ellen Condliffe Lagemann (New York: Teachers College, Columbia University, 1983), p. 137.

21. Ibid., pp. 134–137. Also see Susan M. Reverby, *Ordered to Care: The Dilemma of American Nursing, 1850–1945* (Cambridge: Cambridge University Press, 1987), pp. 187–188.

22. Armeny, "Organized Nurses, Women Philanthropists," p. 28; David Loth, *A Long Way Forward: The Biography of Congresswoman Frances P. Bolton* (New York: Longmans, Green and Co. 1957), pp. 2, 3, 189, 191.

23. Quote in Loth, *A Long Way Forward*, p. 225; Mabel K. Staupers to Frances Payne Bolton, 3 January 1946, Frances Payne Bolton Papers, Box 3, Folder 3, Western Reserve Historical Society, Cleveland, Ohio; Staupers to M. O. Bousfield, Associate for Negro Health of the Julius Rosenwald Fund, 27 August 1936, General Education Board (GEB) Papers, Box 549, Folder 5876, Rockefeller Foundation Archive Center, Pocantico Hills, North Tarrytown, N.Y.

24. Bousfield to Estelle Massey Riddle, 4 June 1936; Bousfield to Staupers, 29 June 1936; Staupers to Bousfield, 27 June 1936; W. W. Brierley to Staupers, 30 January 1937; Mary Beard to Jackson Davis, 5 January 1937; GEB Papers, Box 549, Folder 5867.

25. Staupers, *No Time for Prejudice*, pp. 31–36.

26. Ibid., p. 32.

27. Edna Yost, *American Women of Nursing* (New York: J. B. Lippincott Co., 1947), pp. 96–118; Biographical Sketch of Estelle Massey Riddle, Akron, Ohio, in National Association for the Advancement of Colored People (NAACP) Papers, Box C-278, Administration Files, Manuscript Division, Library of Congress, Washington, D.C.

28. Biographical Data, Mabel Keaton Staupers Papers, Box 96–1, Moorland-Spingarn Research Center, Howard University, Washington, D.C.; W. Montague Cobb, "Mabel Keaton Staupers, R.N., 1890–," *Journal of the National Medical Association* 9 (March 1969):198–199; Anna B. Coles, "The Howard University School of Nursing in Historical Perspective," *Journal of the National Medical Association* 9 (March 1969):105–118; Helen S. Miller and Ernest D. Mason, ed., *Contemporary Minority Leaders in Nursing: Afro-American, Hispanic, Native American Perspectives* (Kansas City, Mo.: American Nurses' Association, 1983), pp. 122–125.

29. Oral interview with Lillian H. Harvey, conducted and transcribed by Patricia Sloan, deputy dean and professor of nursing at Hampton University, 8 January 1976. Copy at the M. Elizabeth Carnegie Nursing Archive, Hampton University, Hampton, Va. I am grateful to Professor Sloan for sharing her collection of oral interviews with black nurses.

30. Staupers, *No Time for Prejudice*, pp. 32–33; Mary Elizabeth Carnegie, *The Path We Tread: Blacks in Nursing, 1854–1984* (Philadelphia: J. B. Lippincott Co., 1986), p. 96.

31. *National News Bulletin*, October–November 1937, copies in NACGN Papers, Schomburg Library, New York City Public Library; Staupers to Favrot, 20 January 1937, GEB Papers, Box 549, Folder 5876; Report of NACGN Accounts, 31 July 1943, copy found in Bolton Papers, Box 3, Folder 3, Western Reserve Historical Society.

32. Reverby, *Ordered to Care*, pp. 136–139, 196–198, 216, 232.

33. Staupers, *No Time for Prejudice*, p. 33; conference reported on in *National News Bulletin* 7 (December 1935).

34. Estelle Massey Riddle, "Does Your Community Know You?" *National News Bulletin*, October 1936, repeated in January 1941.

35. Staupers to Bousfield, 27 August 1936; Staupers to Bousfield, 1 February 1937, GEB Papers, Box 549, Folder 5876.

36. Staupers to Favrot, 19 October 1937, GEB Papers, Box 549, Folder 5876; Staupers, *No Time for Prejudice*, pp. 40–45, for other critical developments of the year. For example, she notes that the NOPHN accredited the public-health-nursing program at the Medical College of Virginia. The most disturbing problem that continued to dog black nursing leaders was the persistence of educational discrimination and segregation on the graduate level. She wrote, "In certain universities that did admit Negro nurses, these nurses were being discouraged by student advisors from taking courses in administration and teaching. They were told that jobs in these categories were seldom available to Negro nurses," p. 43.

37. *National News Bulletin*, December 1936; ibid., December 1941; Staupers to Bousfield, 29 June 1936; 27 August 1936; 1 February 1937, GEB Papers, Box 549, Folder 5876.

38. Riddle, "Does Your Community Know You?"

39. Staupers to Favrot, 20 January 1937, GEB Papers, Box 549, Folder 5876.

40. Ruth S. Fitzgerald, "Problems with the Bulletin," *National News Bulletin*, October–November 1937. Also see the following issues of the *National News Bulletin* for a running commentary on its problems and changes: December 1935, November 1938, August 1942. See whole issue, *Opportunity: Journal of Negro Life* 15 (November 1937).

41. *National News Bulletin*, October–November 1937. Also see Susan M. Hartman, "Women's Organizations during World War II: The Interaction of Class, Race, and Feminism," in *Woman's Being, Woman's Place: Female Identity and Vocation in American History*, ed. Mary Kelley (Boston: G. K. Hall, 1979), pp. 314–318.

42. *National News Bulletin*, October–November 1937; Staupers, *No Time for Prejudice*, p. 53; NACGN, "The National Health Act of 1939," A Special News Bulletin, June 1939, Claude Barnett Papers, Box 305, Folder 2, Chicago Historical Society, Chicago, Ill.

43. Interview with Adele Logan Alexander, niece of Ruth Logan Roberts, 1 October 1986, Washington, D.C.; Ruth Logan Roberts, "To the Board of the National Association of Colored Graduate Nurses," 1941, Staupers Papers, Box 96-2, Folder 5; "Minutes of the Advisory Council of the National Association of Colored Graduate Nurses, Inc.," Held in the Committee Room of the American Nurses' Association, 3 November 1939. Claude Barnett Papers, Box 305, Folder 2; Staupers to Favrot, 19 October 1937; Staupers to Mary Beard, 22 April 1937, GEB Papers, Box 549, Folder 5876.

44. Roberts, "To the Board of the National Association of Colored Graduate Nurses," 1941.

45. Staupers to Bolton, 11 January 1944, Bolton Papers, Box 3, Folder 3.

46. Diary of Mary Beard, 9 October 1937, GEB Papers, Box 549, Folder 5876.

47. Ibid., 23 March 1938, GEB Papers, Box 549, Folder 5876.

48. Mary A. Hickey to Riddle, 28 March 1938, GEB Papers, Box 549, Folder 5876; Minutes of the National Advisory Council, 3 November 1939, Barnett Papers, Box 305, Folder 2.

49. Riddle to Walter White, 13 April 1939, NAACP Papers, Box C-278, Administrative Files.

50. Ibid.

51. Ibid.

52. Lylis Burgess to Riddle, 13 April 1939. Copy in NAACP Papers, Box C-278, Administrative Files.

53. Riddle to White, 13 April 1939, ibid.

54. White to Riddle, 17 April 1939, ibid.

55. Ruth Logan Roberts to Julia C. Stimson, 15 April 1939. Copy in ibid.

56. Reverby, *Ordered to Care*, pp. 193–195.

7. Black Women in White

1. Interview with Lillian Harvey, 8 January 1976, conducted by Patricia Sloan. Original transcript is at the M. Elizabeth Carnegie Nursing History Archive, Hampton University School of Nursing, Hampton, Va. For a critique of the idealized images and unrealistic expectations of nurses, see Janet Muff, "Of Images and Ideals: A Look at Socialization and Sexism in Nursing," in *Images of Nurses: Perspectives from History, Art, and Literature*, ed. Anne Hudson Jones (Philadelphia: University of Pennsylvania Press, 1988), pp. 197–200.

2. Interview with Eunice Rivers [Laurie], 10 October 1977, Schlesinger Library Black Women's Oral History Project, Radcliffe College, Cambridge. Mass.

3. Interview with Lillian Harvey, 8 June 1976, conducted by Sloan. Copy of the transcript is at the Carnegie Nursing History Archive, Hampton University. Harvey retired as dean of the School of Nursing at Tuskegee in 1973; "Lillian H. Harvey," in *Contemporary Minority Leaders in Nursing: Afro-American, Hispanic, Native American Perspectives*, ed. Helen S. Miller and Ernest D. Mason (Kansas City, Mo.: American Nurses' Association, 1983), pp. 53–57.

4. Jean Maddern Pitrone, *Trailblazer: Negro Nurse in the American Red Cross* (New York: Harcourt, Brace and World, 1969), pp. 26, 44; Anna B. Coles, "The Howard University School of Nursing in Historical Perspective," *Journal of the National Medical Association* 61 (March 1969): 105–118; Susan B. DelBene and Vern L. Bullough, "Francis Elliott Davis, 1882–1965," in *American Nursing: A Bibliographical Dictionary*, ed. Vern L. Bullough et al. (New York: Garland Publishing, 1988), pp. 76–77.

5. Pitrone, *Trailblazer*, pp. 69, 77, 80–81.

6. DelBene and Bullough, "Francis Elliot Davis," p. 77.

7. Salaria Kee O'Reilly, "While Passing Through" (1938). This forty-five-page typescript autobiography was apparently written by O'Reilly as copy for a pamphlet published by the Negro Committee to Aid Spain with the Medical Bureau and North American Committee to Aid Spanish Democracy. The committee's pamphlet is called *A Negro Nurse in Republican Spain* (New York: Negro Committee to Aid Spain, 1938). (The Bay Area Post, Veterans of the Abraham Lincoln Brigade, reissued the pamphlet on February 6, 1977). There are several differences between the typed and published documents. Many of the personal data concerning her childhood, education, and family relationships were not included in the published document. In this discussion of O'Reilly's nursing career, I draw upon both documents. I owe special thanks to Barbara Melosh at the National Museum of American History, Smithsonian Institution, for sending copies of these and other items to me.

8. O'Reilly, "While Passing Through," p. 6.

9. Ibid., p. 7.

10. Ibid., p. 8.

11. Ibid., pp. 8–9.

12. *A Negro Nurse in Republican Spain*, p. 6.

13. O'Reilly, "While Passing Through," pp. 13–14.

14. *A Negro Nurse in Republican Spain*, p. 7.

15. Tom Burns, "Abraham Lincoln Brigade Vets Hold a Reunion," *Washington Post*, 5 October 1983.

16. Blake Green, "The Angels of the Last 'Pure War,'" *San Francisco Chronicle*, 10 February 1977.

17. O'Reilly, "While Passing Through," p. 13; "Abraham Lincoln Brigade," 5 October 1983.

18. O'Reilly, "While Passing Through," pp. 9, 23.

19. *A Negro Nurse in Republican Spain*, p. 14.

20. Philip A. Kalisch and Beatrice J. Kalisch, *The Advance of American Nursing* (Boston: Little, Brown and Co., 1978), p. 561.

21. Interview with Lillian Harvey, 8 January 1976, conducted by Sloan.

22. Ibid.

23. Ibid.

24. Interview with Henrietta Smith Chisholm, 17 July 1976, conducted by Sloan.

25. Ibid.

26. Interview with Elizabeth Sharpe, 17 July 1976, conducted by Sloan.

27. Mary Elizabeth Carnegie, *The Path We Tread: Blacks in Nursing, 1854–1984* (Philadelphia: J. B. Lippincott Co., 1986), p. 154; *Mercy Hospital and School for Nurses Annual Report, 1923–1924* (Philadelphia), pp. 24–25. Copy of this annual report and the *Bi-annual Report, 1924–1926* found in the Moorland-Spingarn Library, Howard University,.

28. Interview with Elizabeth Sharpe, 17 July 1976, conducted by Sloan.

29. L. Bibb, "Problems of Student Adjustment to Nursing School Life," *National News Bulletin*, October-November 1937.

30. Kalisch and Kalisch, *The Advance of American Nursing*, p. 565; Janie E. Price to Walter White, 27 November 1930, NAACP Papers, Box C-275, Administrative Files, Manuscript Division, Library of Congress. Price, a black graduate nurse at Lincoln Hospital, wrote of the white director of nurses, Elizabeth Miller, "She does not talk to us as another graduate nurse but as a slave. I wrote her a letter. She refused to answer." NAACP Attorney William C. Andrews to Armitage Whitman, Chairman of the Committee of Management for the Lincoln Hospital, 2 August 1930, about other complaints, NAACP Papers, Box C-275.

31. Marion Rottman to Alyce Eugenia Greene, 24 September 1934, ibid. The writer continued, "I should advise you to make inquiries concerning such a course at St. Philip's Hospital, Richmond, Virginia."

32. Roy Wilkins to S. S. Goldwater, 25 October 1934, ibid.

33. Walter White to S. S. Goldwater, 2 November 1934; "Memorandum" of conversation at the Municipal Building in New York City between Goldwater and White, 1 November 1934, ibid. For a statement of Goldwater's personal conviction that "Negro nurses do not function as efficiently as a large number of the other group," see Staupers, *No Time for Prejudice*, p. 77.

34. NAACP Press Release, "Urge Congressional Backing in Hiring Negro Nurses in D.C.," 11 August 1939, NAACP Papers, Administrative Files, Box C-384.

35. NAACP press release, "House District Committee Chairman Says Negro Nurses Will Get Jobs in D.C.," 19 August 1939, ibid.

36. George E. DeMar, "Negro Women Are American Workers, Too," *Opportunity* 21, no. 2 (April 1943):41–43, 77; Susan M. Hartman, "Women's Organizations

during World War II: The Interaction of Class, Race, and Feminism," in *Woman's Being, Woman's Place: Female Identity and Vocation in American History*, ed. Mary Kelley (Boston: G. K. Hall, 1979); Karen Tucker Anderson, "Last Hired, First Fired: Black Women Workers during World War II," *Journal of American History* 69 (June 1982):96–97; D'Ann Campbell, *Women at War with America: Private Lives in a Patriotic Era* (Cambridge: Harvard University Press, 1984), pp. 128–129. Also see Lois Rita Helmbold, "Making Choices, Making Do: Black and White Working-Class Women's Lives during the Great Depression" (Ph.D. dissertation, Stanford University, 1982).

37. DeMar, "Negro Women Are American Workers, Too," pp. 41–43, 77. The experiences of black nurses are best viewed as a microcosm of the overall oppression and exclusion of black women from substantial participation in American economic life during the 1930s and 1940s. In the latter decade, 20.9 percent of the 1,656,000 black women workers were employed in agriculture, while 57.0 percent worked in domestic service. By 1944 the respective percentages had dropped to 10.9 percent and 43.7 percent. The percentage working in industrial jobs increased from 5.8 to 17.6 percent. The percentage in the professional rank remained virtually unchanged, 4.1 percent in 1940 and 4.2 percent in 1944. Of course, by 1944 the total number of black women workers had exploded to 2,345,000. Seymour L. Wolfbein, "Postwar Trends in Negro Employment," *Monthly Labor Review* 65 (December 1947):664; Campbell, *Women at War with America*, p. 240; Ruth Milkman, *Gender at Work: The Dynamics of Job Segregation by Sex during World War II* (Urbana: University of Illinois Press, 1987), p. 55.

38. I. Malinde Havey, National Director, Public Health Nursing and Home Hygiene, to Gladys Lowe, 13 May 1933, Records of the American Red Cross, Record Group 200, Box No. 1, Folder 003, National Archives, Washington, D.C.

39. John R. Barreau to the NAACP, 27 March 1939; Ruth Logan Roberts to Barreau, 12 April 1939, NAACP Papers, Box C-384, Administrative Files.

40. Effie J. Taylor to Towns, 27 March 1941, Frances Payne Bolton Papers, Box 3, Folder 3, Western Reserve Historical Society, Cleveland, Ohio.

41. Cornelia A. Erf to Harriet M. Towns, 15 March 1941, ibid.

42. Mabel K. Staupers, *No Time for Prejudice: The Story of the Integration of Negroes in Nursing in the United States* (New York: Macmillan Co., 1961), pp. 59, 60, 61.

43. Mabel K. Staupers to T. Arnold Hill, 11 June 1941, National Youth Administration, Record Group 119, Division of Negro Affairs, Box 2, National Archives, Washington, D.C.

44. Hill to Anson Phelps Stokes, 9 June 1941, Record Group 119, Box 3, National Youth Administration.

45. Roberts to Frances Payne Bolton, 18 April 1941, Bolton Papers, Box 3, Folder 3.

46. Bolton to Roberts, 1, 22 April 1941, ibid.

47. Roberts to Bolton, 30 April 1941, ibid.

48. Staupers, *No Time for Prejudice*, p. 59.

49. Bolton to Roberts, 5 May 1941, Bolton Papers, Box 3, Folder 3.

50. Roberts to Bolton, 30 April 1941, ibid.

51. Carnegie, *The Path We Tread*, p. 145.

52. Staupers, *No Time for Prejudice*, p. 61.

53. Estelle Massey Riddle Osborne, "Status and Contribution of the Negro Nurse," *Journal of Negro Education* 18 (Summer 1949):364–369. The 7,065 black nurses in America in 1970, according to Riddle, were concentrated primarily in

fifteen states. New York led with 1,709; Georgia followed with 569; Alabama, Missouri, North Carolina, and Virginia each had more than 400; while Washington, D.C., Florida, Pennsylvania, South Carolina, Tennessee, Texas, and Illinois numbered between 200 and 300 black nurses. Six states, California, Louisiana, Maryland, Michigan, Mississippi, and New Jersey, each had only slightly more than 100 black nurses.

54. Ibid.; Mabel K. Staupers, "Story of the National Association of Colored Graduate Nurses," *American Journal of Nursing* 51 (April 1951):221–223; Campbell, *Women at War*, p. 51; Kalisch and Kalisch, *The Advance of American Nursing*, p. 445.

55. Staupers, *No Time for Prejudice*, p. 109.

56. David Loth, *A Long Way Forward: The Biography of Congresswoman Frances P. Bolton* (New York: Longmans, Green and Co., 1957), p. 216.

57. Carnegie, *The Path We Tread*, p. 46.

58. Kalisch and Kalisch, *The Advance of American Nursing*, p. 564.

59. *Pittsburgh Courier*, 14 August 1943; NACGN "Newsletter," 19 August 1943, vol. 1, no. 13. Copy found in Bolton Papers, Box 3, Folder 3: Bolton Bill (Public Law 74–78th Congress). Signed by President Franklin Delano Roosevelt on 15 June 1943.

60. Kalisch and Kalisch, *The Advance of American Nursing*, p. 563.

61. Osborne, "Status and Contribution of the Negro Nurse," p. 364.

62. Gerald A. Spencer, *Medical Symphony: A Study of the Contributions of the Negro to Medical Progress in New York* (New York: Arlain Printing Co., 1947), p. 101.

63. Edwin R. Embree, *Investment in People: The Story of the Julius Rosenwald Fund* (New York: Harper and Brothers, 1949), p. 118.

64. Interview with Henrietta Smith Chisholm, 17 July 1976, conducted by Sloan.

65. Spencer, *Medical Symphony*, p. 107.

66. Interview with Eunice Rivers Laurie, 10 October 1977, Schlesinger Library Black Women's Oral History Project.

67. Ibid.

68. Ibid. James H. Jones, *Bad Blood: The Tuskegee Syphilis Experiment* (New York: Free Press, 1981), p. 160.

69. Jones, *Bad Blood*, pp. 164–167.

70. Interview with Henrietta Smith Chisholm, 17 July 1976, conducted by Sloan.

71. Estelle Massey Riddle and Josephine Nelson, "The Negro Nurse Looks toward Tomorrow," *American Journal of Nursing* 45 (August 1945):627–630.

72. Interview with Henrietta Smith Chisholm, 17 July 1976, conducted by Sloan.

73. Ibid.

74. Interview with Mary L. Steele Reives, 17 July 1976, conducted by Sloan.

75. Quoted from *Nurses' Settlement News*, 1906, in Carnegie, *The Path We Tread*, p. 149.

76. Interview with Mary L. Steele Reives, 17 July 1976, conducted by Sloan.

77. Ibid.

78. Ibid.

8. "We Shall Not Be Left Out"

1. Richard M. Dalifume, "The 'Forgotten Years' of the Negro Revolution," *Journal of American History* 55 (June 1968):90–106; Darlene Clark Hine, *Black*

Victory: The Rise and Fall of the White Primary in Texas (New York: Kraus-Thomson Organization, 1979), pp. 233–242.

2. George E. DeMar, "Negro Women Are American Workers, Too," *Opportunity* 21, no. 2 (April 1943):41–43, 77; Susan M. Hartman, "Women's Organizations during World War II: The Interaction of Class, Race, and Feminism," in *Woman's Being, Woman's Place: Female Identity and Vocation in American History*, ed. Mary Kelly (Boston: G. K. Hall, 1979), pp. 313–328; William H. Chafe, *The American Woman: Her Changing Social, Economic, and Political Roles, 1920–1978* (New York: Oxford University Press, 1972), p. 142; Karen Tucker Anderson, "Last Hired, First Fired: Black Women Workers during World War II," *Journal of American History* 69 (June 1982):96–97.

3. Herbert Garfinkel, *When Negroes March: The March on Washington Movement in the Organizational Politics for FEPC* (New York: Atheneum, 1969).

4. Bonnie Bullough and Vern L. Bullough, *The Emergence of Modern Nursing* (New York: Macmillan, 1964), p. 187; Philip A. Kalisch and Beatrice J. Kalisch, *The Advance of American Nursing* (Boston: Little, Brown and Co. 1978), p. 449. Ruth Logan Roberts to Frances Payne Bolton, 25 September 1940, Frances Payne Bolton Papers, Box 3, Folder 3; Western Reserve Historical Society, Cleveland, Ohio; National Nursing Council for War Services, Incorporated, By-laws, Article I, Membership: four representatives each from the American Nurses' Association, the National League of Nursing Education, and the National Organization for Public Health Nursing; one each from the NACGN and the Association of Collegiate Schools of Nursing; One each from the National Committee on the American Red Cross Nursing Service and the Subcommittee on Nursing of the Office of Defense Health and Welfare Services. Record Group 171, Box 23, Folder-National Nursing Council, National Archives, Suitland, Md.

5. Memorandum from Colonel R. Cross: Subject, H.R. 2651, 79th Congress, 17 July 1945. Record Group 165, War Department; Memorandum: Subject, Bill to provide for drafting nurses through the selective service system, 12 January 1945. Record Group 165, War Department, File 2912, National Archives, Suitland, Md.

6. Roberts to Bolton, 25 September 1940; Frances Foulkes Gaines to Bolton, 27 February 1940; Bolton to Mabel Keaton Staupers, 9 December 1940, Bolton Papers; Staupers to Claude Barnett, 1 October 1940, Claude Barnett Papers, Box 305, Folder 2, Chicago Historical Society; Kalisch and Kalisch, *The Advance of American Nursing*, pp. 560–561.

7. Estelle Massey Riddle Osborne, "Status and Contribution of the Negro Nurse," *Journal of Negro Education* 18 (Summer 1949):364–369.

8. William H. Hastie, Memorandum to Undersecretary of War Robert P. Patterson, 10 January 1941, Record Group 112, Surgeon General's Office; Memorandum for Colonel Cross, 12 January 1945, Record Group 165, War Department, National Archives.

9. Mabel Keaton Staupers, *No Time for Prejudice: The Story of the Integration of Negroes in Nursing in the United States* (New York: Macmillan Co., 1961), p. 100; Staupers to Barnett, 27 January 1941, Barnett Papers, Box 305, Folder 2.

10. Magee to Ellison D. Smith, 9 January 1943; Memorandum for Col. James E. Wharton of the War Department, Re: Plan for Use of Colored Personnel in the Medical Department, 5 May 1941; Memorandum to William H. Hastie from Brigadier General William E. Shedd, 7 January 1941; Magee to the Secretary of War, 15 June 1941, Records of the Office of the Surgeon General of the United States Army, Record Group 112.

11. Robert P. Patterson to Charles C. Morrison, editor of the *Christian Century*, May 1942, Records of the Surgeon General's Office, R.G. 112.

12. Walter White, *A Man Called White: An Autobiography* (New York: Viking Press,1948).

13. James Magee to Undersecretary of War Patterson, 15 January 1941; Magee to Mary Beard, 8 April 1941, Records of the Surgeon General's Office, R.G. 112.

14. Staupers to Beard, 27 January 1941. Mabel K. Staupers Papers, Box 96–1, Folder 23, Moorland-Spingarn Research Center, Howard University, Washington, D.C. See Charles Herbert Garvin, "The Negro in the Special Services of the United States Army: Medical Corps, Dental Corps, and Nurses' Corps," *Journal of Negro Education* 12 (Summer 1943):335–344; Ulysses Lee, *The Employment of Negro Troops: U.S. Army in WW II* (Washington, D.C.: GPO, 1966), p. 84.

15. Franklin Delano Roosevelt to Walter White, 25 October 1940, Franklin Delano Roosevelt Papers, Official Files 93, Container 3, Folder "Colored Matters," Franklin Delano Roosevelt Archive, Hyde Park, N.Y.

16. National Medical Association Liaison Committee to Franklin Delano Roosevelt, 1 October 1940, Claude Barnett Papers, Box 304, Folder 1.

17. Mary McLeod Bethune to Eleanor Roosevelt, 5 October 1940, F. D. Roosevelt Papers, Official Files 93, Container 3.

18. Staupers to FDR, 26 October 1940; FDR to Staupers, 7 November 1940, F. D. Roosevelt Papers, Official Files 93, Container 3.

19. Robert P. Patterson to Chiefs of All Supply Arms and Services, Memorandum: Procedures in cases involving discrimination by War Department contractors and subcontractors, 24 September 1941, Records of the Surgeon General, R.G. 112.

20. Staupers to Beard, 4 January 1941, Staupers Papers, Box 96–1, Folder 3.

21. Staupers to Barnett, 27 January 1941, Barnett Papers, Box 305, Folder 2.

22. Staupers to Beard, 4 April 1941; Magee to Beard, 8 April 1941, Record Group 112, Surgeon General's Office, National Archives; *Philadelphia Tribune*, 7 February 1942. An editorial declared, "It has become apparent to onlookers in Washington, that at least some of the difficulties which have been experienced by Negro professionals in the medical branches of the armed forces have their origin in the office of one man. He is Major General James C. Magee, Surgeon General of the United States Army."

23. R. Cross, Memorandum for the Executive, 17 July 1945; Howard E. Kessinger in the Undersecretary of War's Office to Staupers, 16 September 1944, Records of the War Department and Special Staff G–1, R.G. 165, File 2912, National Archives.

24. Staupers, *No Time for Prejudice*, p. 101.

25. Staupers to Hastie, 21 March 1941, Staupers Papers, Box 96–1, Folder 23; also see Staupers to Barnett, 1 October 1940, Barnett Papers, Box 305, Folder 2.

26. Staupers to Marian Seymour, 27 January 1941; Staupers to Sylvia Daily Hines, 28 January 1941, Staupers Papers, Box 96–1, Folder 23.

27. "Army Nurses Humiliated before German Prisoners," *St. Louis Argus*, 26 January 1945.

28. Virginia Dunbar to Staupers, 26 June 1939; 7 June 1941, Staupers Papers, Box 96–1, Folder 23.

29. Lester Granger to J. L. Fieser, 8 September 1942, National Urban League Manuscript Collection, Box 4, Library of Congress, Washington, D.C.; James E.

Wharton, Memorandum to Surgeon General: Attention Col. Lull, 18 January 1941, Records of the Surgeon General's Office, R.G. 112. Wharton wrote, "Hastie does not consider the American Red Cross as an entirely reliable agency for use in procurement of Negro nurses and hinted that if they were procured only through the American Red Cross, there might be some discrimination against them by that organization."

30. Staupers to Seymour, 27 January 1941, Staupers Papers, Box 96–1, Folder 23.

31. Staupers to Beard, 1 April 1941, ibid.

32. Staupers to Dunbar, 28 April 1941, ibid.

33. Dunbar to Staupers, 7 June 1941; Staupers to Della Raney, 23 June 1941, ibid.

34. Barnett to Staupers, 21 October 1942, Barnett Papers, Box 305, Folder 2.

35. Magee to Bolton, 14 February 1942; Rufus C. Holman to Magee, 5 March 1942; Magee to Holman, 10 March 1942; Records of the Surgeon General's Office of the United States Army, R.G. 112.

36. Phyllis Baileau, Marian Young, Melbourne M. Barrow to the Secretary of War, 31 December 1942, Records of the Surgeon General's Office of the United States Army, R.G. 112.

37. John A. Rogers to Adjutant General, 8 September 1942, Re: Policy regarding separation of army nurses from services. Records of the Surgeon General's Office, R.G. 112.

38. Kalisch and Kalisch, *The Advance of American Nursing*, p. 453.

39. Ibid., p. 457; Bonnie Bullough, "The Lasting Impact of World War II on Nursing," *American Journal of Nursing* 76 (January 1976):119–120.

40. Staupers, *No Time for Prejudice*, p. 103.

41. Wade H. Haislip to William H. Hastie, 6 March 1941.

42. S. G. Marshall, Memorandum, 1 December 1941, quoted in Lee, *The Employment of Negro Troops*, pp. 140–141.

43. Ibid., p. 171.

44. Lt. Commander Sue S. Dauser, quoted in Julia O. Flikke, *Nurses in Action: The Story of the Army Nurse Corps* (Philadelphia: Lippincott, 1943), pp. 217–219.

45. R. W. Wood to Staupers, 5 August 1943, Staupers Papers, Box 96–1, Folder 25.

46. Staupers to Beard, 1 April 1941, Staupers Papers, ibid., Folder 23.

47. D. Dow to Malvina C. Thompson, 31 October 1944. Copy of the letter sent to Eleanor Roosevelt by Staupers with heading, "Written by a Colored Army Nurse." Eleanor Roosevelt to Norman T. Kirk, 14 November 1944, Eleanor Roosevelt Papers, Container 1687, Folder 100, General Correspondence, FDR Library, Hyde Park, N.Y.; see also "Army Nurses Humiliated before German Prisoners," *St. Louis Argus*, 26 January 1945.

48. Roosevelt to Henry L. Stimson, 20 November 1943, Eleanor Roosevelt Papers, Box 890, Folder 70.

49. Stimson to E. Roosevelt, 21 December 1943, Box 890, Folder 70; Beard to E. Roosevelt, 30 November 1943; Thompson to Elmira B. Wickenden, 12 January 1944; Wickenden to E. Roosevelt, 4 January 1944, E. Roosevelt Papers, Box 1181, Folder 90.

50. Thompson (Secretary to E. Roosevelt) to Staupers, 31 October 1944, E. Roosevelt Papers, Box 2619, Folder 170; Anna Arnold Hedgeman to E. Roosevelt, 26 October 1944, ibid., Box 1759, Folder 100.

51. Staupers to E. Roosevelt, 3 November 1944; Staupers to Bolton, 30 Novem-

ber 1944, Staupers Papers, Box 96–1, Folder 23; Eventually the army instituted a plan of rotation for duty in the prisoner-of-war camps. De Haven Hinkson to Staupers, 1 January 1945, ibid., Folder 15; *St. Louis Argus*, 26 January 1945.

52. E. Roosevelt to Kirk, 12 December 1944, 14 November 1944; Thompson to Kirk, 17 January 1945, 20 February 1945, E. Roosevelt Papers, Box 1787, Folder 100.1; Kalisch and Kalisch, *Advance of American Nursing*, p. 567.

53. *The People's Voice*, 13 January 1945; Chicago *Defender*, 27 January 1945; *Boston Guardian*, 20 January 1945.

54. Kalisch and Kalisch, *Advance of American Nursing*, p. 567.

55. *Boston Guardian*, 20 January 1945.

56. Mary M. Roberts, *American Nursing: History and Interpretation* (New York: Macmillan Co., 1961), pp. 376–377; Major General S. G. Henry, Memorandum for the Chief of Staff, Re: The Need of the Army for More Nurses, 29 December 1944; S. G. Marshall, Chief of Staff, to Stimson, Secretary of War, 29 December 1944; Records of the Department of War, R.G. 165.

57. Cleveland *Call and Post*, 20 January 1945; *Amsterdam-Star News*, 27 January 1945; Chicago *Defender*, 13 January 1945; Kalisch and Kalisch, *Advance of American Nursing*, p. 568.

58. Thelma M. Dale to President Franklin Delano Roosevelt, 23 January 1945, F. D. Roosevelt Papers, Official Files 4675–7, Folder "Nurses." Copies of all the telegrams found in Record of the War Department, R.G. 165. See Files 291.2.

59. Staupers to Bolton, 26 January 1945; Staupers Papers, Box 96–1, Folder 16; Staupers to E. Roosevelt, February Papers; *Boston Guardian*, 20 January 1945; New York *Age*, 3 February 1945.

60. Staupers to Bolton, 11 January 1944, Frances Payne Bolton Papers, Box 3, Folder 3, Western Reserve Historical Society, Cleveland, Ohio; Bullough, "The Lasting Impact of World War II on Nursing," p. 119.

61. NACGN, *Four Decades of Service* (1948); Roberts to Barnett, 25 September 1940, Barnett Papers, Box 305, Folder 2; Roberts, "Report Submitted to the Board of NACGN," 1941, Staupers Papers, Box 96–2, Folder 35.

62. *National News Bulletin* 3 (January 1949); Staupers, "Story of the NACGN," *American Journal of Nursing* 51 (April 1951):221–222; NACGN, *Four Decades of Service* (1948); Editorial, "Negro Nurses in the ANA," *American Journal of Nursing* 48 (October 1948):750.

63. *National News Bulletin* 2 (September 1948). Herbert R. Northrup, "The ANA and the Negro Nurse," *American Journal of Nursing* 50 (April 1950): 207–208; Mary E. Carnegie and Estelle M. (Riddle) Osborne, "Integration in Professional Nursing," *Crisis* 69 (January 1962):5–9.

64. W. Montague Cobb, "The Negro Nurse and the Nation's Health," *Journal of Negro Education* 20 (1951):216–230.

65. Staupers, "The Story of the NACGN," pp. 221–222; Alma Vessels John to Carrie E. Bullock, 8 March 1951, Staupers Papers, Box 96–1, Folder 16; Carnegie and Osborne, "Integration in Professional Nursing," p. 8.

66. Esther Lucille Brown, *Nursing for the Future: A Report Prepared for the National Nursing Council* (New York: Russell Sage Foundation, 1948), quoted in Estelle Massey Riddle Osborne, "Status and Contribution of the Negro Nurse," *Journal of Negro Education* 18 (Summer 1949):364–369.

67. Roberts, *American Nursing*, p. 473; T. Jean Louise Mazero, "Professionalizing of Nursing in America: A Century of Struggle" (Ph.D. dissertation, University of Pittsburgh, 1972), pp. 459–469.

68. NACGN, "Press Release on the Dissolution of the NACGN" (January 1951),

in the NACGN Collection; Staupers, "Story of the NACGN," NACGN Collection, pp. 221–222; Staupers, *No Time for Prejudice*, p. 17.

69. Ralph J. Bunche, "Greetings to the Delegates and Guests Attending the Testimonial Dinner of the NACGN," Staupers Papers, Box 96–2, Folder 35.

70. Walter White, quoted in Carnegie and Osborne, "Integration in Professional Nursing."

71. Copy of speech delivered by Judge William H. Hastie, 26 January 1951. Testimonial Dinner of the NACGN. Staupers Papers, Box 96–2, Folder 35.

72. Alma C. Haupt to Staupers, 1 February 1951, ibid., Box 96–1, Folder 15.

73. Antoinette Martina Ricks Demby to Staupers, ibid., Folder 11.

74. Mary Ella Adams to Staupers, 26 July 1951, ibid., Folder 8.

75. Channing H. Tobias to Staupers, 31 May 1951, ibid., Folder 24.

Conclusion

1. For a complete discussion of black nurses who have achieved outstanding recognition since the dissolution of the NACGN, see Mary Elizabeth Carnegie, *The Path We Tread: Blacks in Nursing, 1854–1984* (Philadelphia: J. B. Lippincott, 1986), pp. 108, 109–160.

2. Ibid., p. 33.

3. Ibid., p. 62.

4. Ibid., pp. 103–105. Carnegie notes that membership in the organization is open to all registered nurses, licensed practical nurses, licensed vocational nurses, and student nurses.

5. Ibid., p. 105; Gloria R. Smith, "From Invisibility to Blackness: The Story of the National Black Nurses' Association," *Nursing Outlook* 23 (April 1975):225–229. Smith notes that the members of the NBNA felt that "the greater emphasis of their organization [was] on health care delivery rather than on establishing and maintaining professional standards," p. 229.

Bibliography

Manuscript Collections

Amistad Research Center, Tulane University, New Orleans, Louisiana.
    Mabel Keaton Staupers Papers
Chicago Historical Society, Chicago, Illinois
    Claude Barnett Papers
Fisk University, Nashville, Tennessee
    Julius Rosenwald Fund Papers
Franklin Delano Roosevelt Library, Hyde Park, New York
    Eleanor Roosevelt Papers
    Franklin Delano Roosevelt Papers
Hampton University, Hampton, Virginia
    Dixie Hospital Manuscript Collections
    M. Elizabeth Carnegie Nursing History Archives Collection
Library of Congress, Washington, D.C.
    National Association for the Advancement of Colored People Papers
    National Urban League Papers
    Arthur B. Spingarn Papers
    Mary Church Terrell Papers
    Booker T. Washington Papers
Moorland-Spingarn Research Center, Howard University, Washington, D.C.
    Mabel Keaton Staupers Papers
National Archives, Washington, D.C.
    Records of the American Red Cross
    Records of the Bureau of Refugees, Freedmen and Abandoned Lands
National Archives, Suitland, Maryland
    Records of the Office of the Surgeon General of the United States
    Records of the Department of War
    Records of the War Department and Special Staff

Rockefeller Foundation Archive and Research Center, Pocantico Hills, New York
    General Education Board Papers
    Laura Spelman Rockefeller Memorial Fund Papers
    Rockefeller Foundation Papers
Schomburg Center for Research in Black Culture, New York, New York
    National Association of Colored Graduate Nurses Manuscript Collection
University of Chicago, Chicago, Illinois
    Julius Rosenwald Papers
Waring Historical Library, Medical College of Charleston, South Carolina
    McClennan-Banks Memorial Hospital Manuscript Collection
Western Reserve Historical Society, Cleveland, Ohio
    Frances Payne Bolton Papers
    Jane Edna Hunter Papers

Government Documents

United States Census of Population: 1950. Washington, D.C.: Government Printing Office.
"Professional Nursing Schools in the United States, 1850–1950." In *Historical Statistics of the United States: Colonial Times to 1970*, Bicentennial Edition. Washington, D.C.: Government Printing Office, 1975.

Reports and Pamphlets

Flint-Goodridge Hospital. Annual Reports, 1916, 1935–1943, 1975.
Frederick Douglass Memorial Hospital and Nurse Training School. Annual Reports, 1905–1906.
Freedmen's Hospital. Annual Report, 1900.
Hampton Training School for Nurses and Dixie Hospital. Annual Reports, 1895–1896, 1896–1897, 1901–1902, 1903–1904.
The Hospital Herald: A Journal Devoted to Hospital Work, Nurse Training, and Domestic and Public Hygiene, December 1898, January 1899, July 1899, November 1899. McClennan-Banks Memorial Hospital, Charleston, S.C.
Mercy Hospital and School for Nurses. Annual Reports, 1923–1926.
Negro Hospitals: A Compilation of Available Statistics. Chicago: Julius Rosenwald Fund, 1931.
Provident Hospital and Training School. Annual Report, 1913.
Tuskegee Normal and Industrial Institute. *Annual Catalogues*, 1894–1895, 1896–1897, 1902–1903, 1906–1907.
Hamlin, Donalda. "Report on Informal Study of the Educational Facilities for Colored Nurses and Their Use in Hospital, Visiting, and Public Health Nursing." Chicago: Hospital Library and Service Bureau, 1924–1925. Copy found in the Rockefeller Archive Center.
Johns, Ethel. "A Study of the Present Status of the Negro Woman in Nursing." New York: Rockefeller Foundation, 1925.
Miller, Rita E. "Negro Schools of Nursing in the South." New York: General Education Board, 1943.
O'Reilly, Salaria Kee. "While Passing Through." New York: Negro Committee to Aid Spain, 1938.
Williams, W. T. B. "Hospital and Training School for Nurses." New York: Rockefeller Foundation, 1905.

Interviews and Oral Histories

Alexander, Adele Logan. Interview, 1 October 1986, Washington, D.C.

Chisholm, Henrietta Smith. Interview with Patricia Sloan, 17 July 1976, Hampton, Va. Transcript located in the M. Elizabeth Carnegie Nursing History Archive, Hampton University School of Nursing, Hampton. Va.

Dent, Albert W. Interview, 15 October 1980, New Orleans, La.

Harvey, Lillian H. Interview with Patricia Sloan, 8 January 1976, Hampton. Va. Transcript located in the M. Elizabeth Carnegie Nursing History Archive, Hampton University School of Nursing, Hampton, Va,

Kemp, Lillian. Interview with Patricia Sloan, 14 June 1976, Hampton, Va. Transcript located in the M. Elizabeth Carnegie Nursing History Archive, Hampton University School of Nursing, Hampton, Va.

Laurie, Eunice Rivers. Oral history, 10 October 1977, Cambridge. Transcript located in the Schlesinger Library Black Women's Oral History Project, Radcliffe College, Cambridge.

Osborne, Estelle Massey Riddle. Interview with Patricia Sloan, 21 June 1976, Hampton, Va. Transcript located in the M. Elizabeth Carnegie Nursing History Archive, Hampton University School of Nursing, Hampton, Va.

Reives, Mary L. Steele. Interview with Patricia Sloan, 17 July 1976, Hampton, Va. Transcript located in the M. Elizabeth Carnegie Nursing Archive, Hampton University School of Nursing, Hampton, Va.

Sharpe, Elizabeth. Interview with Patricia Sloan, 17 July 1976, Hampton, Va. Transcript located in the M. Elizabeth Carnegie Nursing History Archive, Hampton University School of Nursing, Hampton, Va.

Staupers, Mabel K. Interview, October 18, 1980, Washington, D.C.

Newspapers and Periodicals

Amsterdam-Star News
Boston Guardian
Chicago *Defender*
Cleveland *Call and Post*
Kansas Citian
New York Age
People's Voice
Philadelphia Tribune
Pittsburgh Courier
Richmond Planet
Saint Louis Argus
San Francisco Chronicle
Saturday Evening Post
Times Picayune, New Orleans, La.
Washington Post

Journals

American Journal of Nursing, 1900–1950.
Crisis, NAACP, New York, 1920–1965.
Dillard Bulletin, Dillard University, New Orleans, La., 1937–1950.
Hospital Herald, organ of the Hospital and Nurse Training School, Charleston, S.C., 1896–98.
Journal of the National Medical Association, 1910–1986.

Journal of Negro Education, Howard University, Washington, D.C., 1935–1950.
National News Bulletin, organ of the National Association of Colored Graduate Nurses, New York, 1934–1948.
Opportunity, organ of the National Urban League, New York, 1930–1938.
Southern Letter, Tuskegee Institute, Tuskegee, Ala., 1917–1923.
Southern Workman, Hampton Institute, Hampton, Va., 1891–1925.

Books

Abrams, Ruth J., ed. *"Send Us a Lady Physician": Women Doctors in America, 1835–1930.* New York: W. W. Norton, 1985.
Anderson, James D. *The Education of Blacks in the South, 1860–1935.* Chapel Hill: University of North Carolina Press, 1988.
Beardsley, Edward H. *A History of Neglect: Health Care for Blacks and Mill Workers in the Twentieth-Century South.* Knoxville: University of Tennessee Press, 1987.
Bellamy, Verdelle B., ed. *History of Grady Memorial Hospital School of Nursing, 1917–1964.* Atlanta, Ga.: Chi Eta Phi Sorority, circa 1985).
Berkin, Carol, and Norton, Mary Beth. *Women of America: A History.* Boston: Houghton Mifflin Co., 1979.
Blassingame, John W. *Black New Orleans, 1860–1880.* Chicago: University of Chicago Press, 1973.
Boyd, William Kenneth. *The Story of Durham: City of the New South.* Durham: Duke University Press, 1925.
Brandt, Allan M. *No Magic Bullet: A Social History of Venereal Disease in the United States since 1880.* New York: Oxford University Press, 1985.
Bridgeman, Margaret. *Collegiate Education for Nursing.* New York: Russell Sage Foundation, 1953.
Brown, Birdie E. *Face It with a Smile.* New York: Vantage Press, 1976.
Brown, Esther Lucille. *Nursing for the Future: A Report Prepared for the National Nursing Council.* New York: Russell Sage Foundation, 1948.
Buckler, Helen. *Daniel Hale Williams, Negro Surgeon.* New York: Putnam, 1968.
Bullough, Bonnie, and Bullough, Vern L. *The Emergence of Modern Nursing.* New York: Macmillan, 1964.
Bullough, Vern L., et al., eds. *American Nursing: A Biographical Dictionary.* New York: Garland Publishing, 1988.
Campbell, D'Ann. *Women at War with America: Private Lives in a Patriotic Era.* Cambridge: Harvard University Press, 1984.
Carnegie, Mary Elizabeth. *The Path We Tread: Blacks in Nursing, 1854–1984.* Philadelphia: J. B. Lippincott Co., 1986.
Chafe, William H. *The American Woman: Her Changing Social, Economic, and Political Roles, 1920–1978.* New York: Oxford University Press, 1972.
Cobb, W. Montague. *Medical Care and the Plight of the Negro.* New York: NAACP, 1947.
Dannett, S. G. L. *Profiles of Negro Womanhood.* Vol. 2, *Twentieth Century.* New York: Negro Heritage Library, Educational Heritage, 1966.
Davis, Elizabeth Lindsay. *Lifting As They Climb.* Washington, D.C.: NACW, circa, 1933.
Du Bois, W. E. B. *The Autobiography of W. E. B. Du Bois.* New York: International Publishers, 1968.
Duffy, John. *The Healers: A History of American Medicine.* Urbana: University of Illinois Press, 1976.

Embree, Edwin R. *Investment in People: The Story of the Julius Rosenwald Fund*. New York: Harper and Brothers, 1949.

The Fifty Year Graduates of Freedmen's Hospital School of Nursing Tell Their Story. Washington, D.C.: Freedmen's Hospital Nurses Alumni Clubs, 1986.

Fitzpatrick, M. Louise. *The National Organization for Public Health Nursing, 1912–1952: Development of a Practice Field*. New York: National League for Nursing, 1975.

Flikke, Julia O. *Nurses in Action: The Story of the Army Nurse Corps*. Philadelphia: Lippincott, 1943.

Fosdick, Raymond B. *Adventure in Giving: The Story of the General Education Board*. New York: Harper and Row, 1962.

Fox, Daniel M. *Health Policies, Health Politics: The British and American Experience, 1911–1965*. Princeton: Princeton University Press, 1986.

Franklin, John Hope. *From Slavery to Freedom*. 4th ed. New York: Knopf, 1974.

————, and August Meier, eds. *Black Leaders in the Twentieth Century*. Urbana: University of Illinois Press, 1982.

Franklin, Vincent P. *The Education of Black Philadelphia*. Philadelphia: University of Pennsylvania Press, 1979.

Fredrickson, George M. *The Black Image in the White Mind: The Debate on Afro-American Character and Destiny, 1817–1914*. New York: Harper Torch Books, 1971.

Gamble, Vanessa. *Black Community Hospitals: A Historical Perspective*. New York: Garland Publishing, 1987.

Garfinkel, Herbert. *When Negroes March: The March on Washington Movement in the Organizational Politics for FEPC*. New York: Atheneum, 1969.

Glazer, Penina Migdal, and Slater, Miriam. *Unequal Colleagues: The Entrance of Women into the Professions, 1890–1940*. New Brunswick, N.J.: Rutgers University Press, 1987.

Glenton, Mary V. *The Story of a Hospital*. Hartford, Conn.: Church Missions Publishing Co., 1923.

Hair, William Ivy. *Carnival of Fury: Robert Charles and the New Orleans Race Riot of 1900*. Baton Rouge: Louisiana State University Press, 1976.

Hine, Darlene Clark. *Black Women in the Nursing Profession: A Documentary History*. New York: Garland Publishing, 1985.

————. *The State of Afro-American History: Past, Present, and Future*. Baton Rouge: Louisiana State University Press, 1986.

Holt, Thomas; Smith-Parker, Cassandra; Terborg-Penn, Rosalyn. *A Special Mission: The Story of Freedmen's Hospital, 1862–1962*. Washington, D.C.: Howard University Press, 1975.

Johnson, Charles S. *Into the Main-stream: A Survey of Best Practices in Race Relations in the South*. Chapel Hill: University of North Carolina Press, 1947.

————. *The Negro in American Civilization: A Study of Negro Life and Race Relations in the Light of Social Research*. New York: Henry Holt and Co., 1936.

Jones, Anne Hudson, ed. *Images of Nurses: Perspectives from History, Art, and Literature*. Philadelphia: University of Pennsylvania Press, 1988.

Jones, James H. *Bad Blood: The Tuskegee Syphilis Experiment*. New York: Free Press, 1981.

Jones, Woodrow, Jr., and Rice, Mitchell F., eds. *Health Care Issues in Black America: Policies, Problems, and Prospects*. Westport, Conn.: Greenwood Press, 1987.

Kalisch, Philip A., and Kalisch, Beatrice J. *The Advance of American Nursing*. Boston: Little, Brown and Co., 1978.

Kelley, Mary, ed. *Woman's Being, Woman's Place: Female Identity and Vocation in American History*. Boston: G. K. Hall, 1979.

Kenney, John A. *The Negro in Medicine*. Tuskegee, Ala.: Tuskegee Institute, 1912.

Lagemann, Ellen Condliffe, ed. *Nursing History: New Perspectives, New Possibilities*. New York: Teachers College, Columbia University, 1983.

Larson, Magali Sarfatti. *The Rise of Professionalism: A Sociological Analysis*. Berkeley: University of California Press, 1977.

Leavitt, Judith Walzer, ed. *Women and Health in America*. Madison: University of Wisconsin Press, 1984.

Lee, Ulysses. *The Employment of Negro Troops: U.S. Army in WW II*. Washington, D.C.: Government Printing Office, 1966.

Lerner, Gerda, ed. *Black Women in White America: A Documentary History*, New York: Random House, 1973.

Logan, Rayford W., and Winston, Michael R. *Dictionary of American Negro Biography*. New York: W. W. Norton and Co., 1982.

Loth, David. *A Long Way Forward: The Biography of Congresswoman Frances P. Bolton*. New York: Longmans, Green and Co., 1957.

Maynard, Aubre de L. *Surgeons to the Poor: The Harlem Hospital Story*. New York: Appleton-Century-Crofts, 1978.

Melosh, Barbara. *"The Physician's Hand": Work Culture and Conflict in American Nursing*. Philadelphia: Temple University Press, 1982.

Miller, Helen S. *The History of Chi Eta Phi Sorority, Inc., 1932–1967*. Washington, D.C.: Association for the Study of Afro-American Life and History, 1968.

————. *Mary Eliza Mahoney, 1845–1926: America's First Black Professional Nurse*. Atlanta: Wright Publishing Co., 1986.

————, and Mason, Ernest D., eds. *Contemporary Minority Leaders in Nursing: Afro-American, Hispanic, Native American Perspectives*. Kansas City, Mo.: American Nurses' Association, 1983.

Moore, Judith. *A Zeal for Responsibility: The Struggle for Professional Nursing in Victorian England, 1868–1883*. Athens: University of Georgia Press, 1988.

Morais, Herbert M. *The History of the Negro in Medicine*. Washington, D.C.: Association for the Study of Afro-American Life and History, 1967.

Mossell, Mrs. Nathan F. *The Work of the Afro-American Woman*. Freeport, N.Y.: Books for Libraries Press, 1971. Reprint.

Mottus, Jane E. *New York Nightingales: The Emergence of the Nursing Profession at Bellevue and New York Hospital*. Ann Arbor: UMI Research Press, 1981.

Mullan, Fitzhugh. *White Coats, Clenched Fists: The Political Education of an American Physician*. New York: Macmillan, 1976.

Neverdon-Morton, Cynthia. *Afro-American Women of the South and the Advancement of the Race, 1895–1925*. Knoxville: University of Tennessee Press, 1989.

Newman, Dorothy K., et al. *Protest, Politics, and Prosperity: Black Americans and White Institutions, 1940–1975*. New York: Pantheon Books, 1978.

Nutting, M. Adelaide, and Dock, Lavinia L. *The History of Nursing: From the Earliest Times to the Present Day with Special Reference to the Work of the Past Thirty Years*. 4 vols. New York: Putnam and Sons, 1907–1912.

Osofsky, Gilbert. *Harlem: The Making of a Ghetto, 1890–1930*. New York: Harper and Row, 1966.

Perry, John Edward. *Forty Cords of Wood: Memoirs of a Medical Doctor*. Jefferson City, Mo.: Lincoln University Press, 1947.

Pitrone, Jean Maddern. *Trailblazer: Negro Nurse in the American Red Cross*. New York: Harcourt, Brace and World, 1969.

Read, Florence Matilda. *The Story of Spelman College*. Princeton, N.J.: Princeton University Press, 1961.

Reverby, Susan M. *Ordered to Care: The Dilemma of American Nursing, 1850–1945*. Cambridge: Cambridge University Press, 1987.

Richardson, Clement, ed. *The National Cyclopedia of the Colored Race*. Vol. 1. Montgomery: National Publishing Co., 1919.

Roberts, Mary M. *American Nursing: History and Interpretation*. New York: Macmillan Co., 1961.

Rosenberg, Charles E. *The Care of Strangers: The Rise of America's Hospital System*. New York: Basic Books, 1987.

Rosner, David. *A Once Charitable Enterprise: Hospitals and Health Care in Brooklyn and New York, 1885–1915*. Princeton, N.J.: Princeton University Press, 1982.

Savitt, Todd L. *Medicine and Slavery: The Disease and Health Care of Blacks in Antebellum Virginia*. Urbana: University of Illinois Press, 1978.

Shryock, Richard H. *The History of Nursing: An Interpretation of the Social and Medical Factors Involved*. Philadelphia: Saunders, 1959.

Sitkoff, Harvard. *A New Deal for Blacks*. New York: Oxford University Press, 1978.

Smith, J. Lynn, and Hitt, Homer L. *People of Louisiana*. Baton Rouge: State University Press, 1952.

Spear, Allan H. *Black Chicago: The Making of a Negro Ghetto, 1890–1920*. Chicago: University of Chicago Press, 1967.

Spencer, Gerald A. *Medical Symphony: A Study of the Contributions of the Negro to Medical Progress in New York*. New York: Arlain Printing Co., 1947.

Starr, Paul. *The Social Transformation of American Medicine*. New York: Basic Books, 1982.

Staupers, Mabel Keaton. *No Time for Prejudice: The Story of the Integration of Negroes in Nursing in the United States*. New York: Macmillan Co., 1961.

Sterling, Dorothy. *We Are Your Sisters: Black Women in the Nineteenth Century*. New York: W. W. Norton, 1984.

Stewart, Isabel M. *The Education of Nurses*. New York: Macmillan, 1943.

Street, Margaret M. *Watchfires on the Mountain: The Life and Writings of Ethel Johns*. Toronto: University of Toronto Press, 1973.

Taylor, Susie King. *Reminiscences of My Life in Camp with the 33rd United States Colored Troops Late 1st South Carolina Volunteers*. Boston: privately printed, 1902.

Thoms, Adah B. *Pathfinders: A History of the Progress of Colored Graduate Nurses*. New York: McKay Co., 1929.

Vicinus, Martha. *Independent Women: Work and Community for Single Women, 1850–1920*. Chicago: University of Chicago Press, 1985.

Vogel, Morris J. *The Invention of the Modern Hospital: Boston, 1870–1930*. Chicago: University of Chicago Press, 1980.

White, Walter. *A Man Called White: An Autobiography*. New York: Viking Press, 1948.

Woodson, Carter G. *The Negro Professional Man and the Community*. Washing-

ton, D.C.: Association for the Study of Negro Life and History, 1969 Reprint.
————. *The Rural Negro.* Washington, D.C.: Association for the Study of Negro Life and History, 1930.
Worcester, Alfred. *Small Hospitals: Establishment and Maintenance.* New York: John Wiley and Sons, 1909.
Work, Monroe N. *Negro Year Book and Annual Encyclopedia of the Negro.* Tuskegee, Ala.: Tuskegee Normal and Industrial Institute, 1921.
Yost, Edna. *American Women of Nursing.* New York: J. B. Lippincott Co., 1947.

Articles

Anderson, Karen Tucker. "Last Hired, First Fired: Black Women Workers during World War II." *Journal of American History* 69 (June 1982):82–97.
Armeny, Susan. "Organized Nurses, Women Philanthropists, and the Intellectual Bases for Cooperation among Women, 1898–1920." In *Nursing History: New Perspectives, New Possibilities,* edited by Ellen Condliffe Lagemann, pp. 13–45. New York: Columbia University Press, 1983.
Bacon, Alice. "The Hampton Training School for Nurses." In *Fourth Annual Report of the Training School for Nurses and Dixie Hospital.* Hampton, Va., 1895–1896.
Banks, Anna De Costa. "The Work of a Small Hospital and Training School in the South." In *Eighth Annual Report of the Hampton Training School for Nurses and Dixie Hospital,* pp. 23–28. Hampton, Va., 1898–1899.
Beardsley, E. H. "Making Separate, Equal: Black Physicians and the Problems of Medical Segregation in the Pre–World War II South." *Bulletin of the History of Medicine* 57 (Fall 1983):382–396.
Bennett, Emily W. "The Work of a Rosenwald Nurse." *Public Health Nurse* 23 (March 1931):119–120.
Bernard, Jacqueline De. S. "Sojourner Truth, 1797?–1883." In *Dictionary of American Negro Biography,* edited by Rayford W. Logan and Michael R. Winston, pp. 605–606. New York: W. W. Norton, 1982.
Bullough, Bonnie. "The Lasting Impact of World War II on Nursing." *American Journal of Nursing* 76 (January 1976):119–120.
Carnegie, Mary Elizabeth. "Are Negro Schools of Nursing Needed Today?" *Nursing Outlook* 12 (1964):52–56.
————. "Nurse Training Becomes Nursing Education at Florida A. & M. College." *Journal of Negro Education* 17 (September 1948):200–204.
————. "The Path We Tread." *International Nursing Review* 9 (September/October 1962):25–33.
————, and Osborne, Estelle M. (Riddle). "Integration in Professional Nursing." *Crisis* 69 (January 1962):5–9.
Cobb, W. Montague. "The Negro Nurse and the Nation's Health." *Journal of Negro Education* 20 (1951):216–230.
————. "Mabel Keaton Staupers, R.N., 1890–." *Journal of the National Medical Association* 69 (March 1969):198–199.
————. "Nathan Francis Mossell, M.D., 1856–1946." *Journal of the National Medical Association* 46 (March 1954):118–129.
————. "Saint Agnes Hospital, Raleigh, North Carolina, 1896–1961." *Journal of the National Medical Association* 53 (September 1961):439–442.
————. "Henry McKee Minton, 1870–1946." *Journal of the National Medical Association* 47 (July 1955):285–286.
Coles, Anna B. "Mary Mahoney, 1845–1926." In *Dictionary of American Negro*

Biography, edited by Rayford Logan and Michael R. Winston, pp. 420–421. New York: W. W. Norton, 1982.

———. "The Howard University School of Nursing in Historical Perspective." *Journal of the National Medical Association* 61 (March 1969):105–118.

Cooper, Edward S. "The Mercy-Douglass Hospital." *Journal of the National Medical Association* 53 (January 1961):3.

Dalifume, Richard M. "The 'Forgotten Years' of the Negro Revolution." *Journal of American History* 55 (June 1968):90–106.

Daniel, Pete. "Black Power in the 1920s: The Case of Tuskegee Veterans Hospital." *Journal of Southern History* 36 (1970):368–388.

Davies, Celia. "Professionalizing Strategies as Time- and Culture-Bound: American and British Nursing circa 1893." In *Nursing History: New Perspectives, New Possibilities*, edited by Ellen Condliffe Lagemann, pp. 47–63. New York: Columbia University, 1983.

Davis, Althea T. "Adah Belle Samuels Thoms, 1870–1943." In *American Nursing: A Biographical Dictionary*, edited by Vern L. Bullough et al., pp. 313–316. New York: Garland Publishing, 1988.

———. "Martha Minerva Franklin, 1870–1968." In *American Nursing: A Biographical Dictionary*, edited by Vern L. Bullough et al., pp. 122–123. New York: Garland Publishing, 1988.

———. "Mary Eliza Mahoney, 1845–1926." In *American Nursing: A Biographical Dictionary*, edited by Vern L. Bullough et al., pp. 226–228. New York: Gerland Publishing, 1988.

Davis, Fred; Olesen, Virginia L.; and Whittaker, Elni Waik. "Problems and Issues in Collegiate Nursing Education." In *The Nursing Profession: Five Sociological Essays*, edited by Fred Davis, pp. 138–175. New York: John Wiley and Sons, 1966.

DelBene, Susan B., and Bullough, Vern L. "Frances Elliot Davis, 1882–1965." In *American Nursing: A Biographical Dictionary*, edited by Vern L. Bullough et al., pp. 76–77. New York: Garland Publishing, 1988.

DeMar, George E. "Negro Women Are American Workers, Too." *Opportunity* 21, no. 2 (April 1943):41–43.

Deming, Dorothy. "The Negro Nurse in Public Health." *Opportunity: Journal of Negro Life* 15 (November 1937):333–335.

Dent, Albert W. "Hospital Services and Facilities Available to Negroes in the United States." *Journal of Negro Education* 18, no. 3 (1949):326–332.

———. "The Role of a Negro Hospital in the Control of Tuberculosis in a Large Southern City." In *Transactions of the Thirty-seventh Annual Meeting of the National Tuberculosis Association*, 1941.

Dibble, Eugene H., Jr.; Rabb, Louis A.; and Ballard, Ruth B. "John A. Andrew Memorial Hospital." *Journal of the National Medical Association* 53 (March 1961):103–105.

Eldredge, Adda. "The Need for a Sound Professional Preparation for Colored Nurses." *Proceedings of the Annual Congress on Medical Education, Medical Licensure, and Hospitals* 94 (1930):168–171.

Eleazer, R. B. "Flint-Goodridge Hospital." *Crisis* 40 (July 1933):151–153.

Elmore, Joyce Ann. "Black Nurses: Their Service and Their Struggle." *American Journal of Nursing* 76 (March 1976):435–437.

Folsom, Cora M. "The Dixie Hospital: In the Beginning." *Southern Workman* 55 (March 1926):121–126.

Gage, Nina D., and Haupt, Alma C. "Some Observations on Negro Nursing in the South." *Public Health Nursing* 24 (December 1932):674–680.

Garvin, Charles Herbert. "The Negro in the Special Services of the United States Army: Medical Corps, Dental Corps, and Nurses' Corps." *Journal of Negro Education* 12 (Summer 1943):335–344.

Giffin, William. "The Mercy Hospital Controversy among Cleveland's Afro-American Civic Leaders, 1927." *Journal of Negro History* 61 (1976): 327–350.

Goldstein, Moise H., and MacLean, B. C. "A Hospital That Serves as a Center of Negro Medical Education." *Modern Hospital* 39 (November 1932):1–8.

Green, H. M. "A Plea for the Small Hospital for Negroes." *Trained Nurse and Hospital Review*, August 1926, p. 172.

Haller, John, S., Jr. "Race, Mortality, and Life Insurance: Negro Vital Statistics in the Late Nineteenth Century." *Journal of the History of Medicine* 25 (1970):247–261.

Hartman, Susan M. "Women's Organizations during World War II: The Interaction of Class, Race, and Feminism." In *Woman's Being, Woman's Place: Female Identity and Vocation in American History*, edited by Mary Kelley. Boston: G. K. Hall, 1979.

Harvey, Basil C. H. "Provision for Training Colored Medical Students." *Journal of the American Medical Association* 94 (May 1930):1415.

Heistad, Wanda C. "The Development of Nurse-Midwifery Education in the United States." In *Historical Studies in Nursing*, edited by Louise Fitzpatrick, pp. 86–103. New York: Teachers College Press, 1978.

Hine, Darlene Clark. "From Hospital to College: Black Nurse Leaders and the Rise of Collegiate Nursing Schools." *Journal of Negro Education* 51 (Summer 1982):223–237.

———. "Lifting the Veil, Shattering the Silence: Black Women's History in Slavery and Freedom." In *The State of Afro-American History: Past, Present, and Future*, pp. 223–249. Baton Rouge: Louisiana State University Press, 1982.

———. "The Call That Never Came: Black Women Nurses and World War I—An Historical Note." *Indiana Military History Journal* 8, no. 1 (January 1983):23–27.

———. "The Ethel Johns Report: Black Women in the Nursing Profession, 1925." *Journal of Negro History* 67 (Fall 1982):212–228.

———. "Mabel K. Staupers and the Integration of Black Nurses into the Armed Forces." In *Black Leaders of the Twentieth Century*, pp. 241–257. Urbana: University of Illinois Press, 1982.

———. "Co-laborers in the Work of the Lord: Nineteenth-Century Black Women Physicians." In *"Send Us a Lady Physician": Women Doctors in America, 1835–1930*, edited by Ruth Abrams, pp. 107–120. New York: W. W. Norton, 1985.

"Investigation of Negro Hospitals." *Journal of the American Medical Association* 80 (April 1923).

James, Janet Wilson. "Isabel Hampton and the Professionalization of Nursing in the 1890s." In *The Therapeutic Revolution: Essays in the Social History of American Medicine*, edited by Morris J. Vogel and Charles E. Rosenberg, pp. 201–244. Philadelphia: University of Pennsylvania Press, 1979.

Jones, Elizabeth. "The Negro Woman in the Nursing Profession." *Messenger* 5 (July 1923):64–65.

Kalisch, Philip A., and Kalisch, Beatrice J. "Untrained but Undaunted: The Women Nurses of the Blue and the Gray." *Nursing Forum* 15, no. 1 (1976).

Karl, Barry D., and Katz, Stanley N. "The American Private Philanthropic Foundation and the Public Sphere, 1890–1930." *Minerva* 19, no. 2 (Summer 1981):236–270.

Kenney, John A. "Some Facts concerning Negro Nurse Training Schools and Their Graduates." *Journal of the National Medical Association* 11 (April–June 1919):53–68.

———. "The Negro Hospital Renaissance." *Journal of the National Medical Association* 23 (July–September 1930):109.

Kerber, Linda K. "Separate Spheres, Female Worlds, Woman's Place: The Rhetoric of Women's History." *Journal of American History* 75 (June 1988):9–39.

Knight, Captain H. W. "Flint-Goodrich [*sic*] Hospital." *Journal of the National Medical Association* 22 (July-September 1930):130–131.

Kousser, J. Morgan. "Separate but *Not* Equal: The Supreme Court's First Decision on Racial Discrimination in Schools." *Journal of Southern History* 46 (February 1980):17–44.

Lerner, Gerda. "Early Community Work of Black Club Women." *Journal of Negro History* 59 (1974):158–167.

Logan, Rayford W. "Adah B. Samuels Thoms, 1863?–1943." In *Dictionary of American Negro Biography*, edited by Rayford W. Logan and Michael R. Winston, p. 589. New York: W. W. Norton, 1982.

Malveaux, Julianne, and Englander, Susan. "Race and Class in Nursing Occupations." *Sage* 3 (Spring 1986):41–45.

Matthews, Henry B. "Provident Hospital—Then and Now." *Journal of the National Medical Association* 53 (May 1961):209.

Melosh, Barbara. "Every Woman Is a Nurse: Work and Gender in the Emergence of Nursing." In *"Send Us a Lady Physician": Women Doctors in America, 1835–1930*, edited by Ruth Abrams, pp. 121–127. New York: W. W. Norton, 1985.

Minton, Russell F. "The History of Mercy-Douglass Hospital." *Journal of the National Medical Association* 43 (1951):153–159.

Muff, Janet. "Of Images and Ideals: A Look at Socialization and Sexism in Nursing." In *Images of Nurses: Perspectives from History, Art, and Literature*, edited by Anne Hudson Jones, pp. 197–220. Philadelphia: University of Pennsylvania Press, 1988.

Murray, Peter Marshall. "Hospital Provision for the Negro Race." *Journal of the American Medical Association* 94 (May 1930):1414.

"National Association of Colored Graduate Nurses Meet at Tuskegee Institute." *Southern Letter* 43 (August 1927).

"Negro Nurses in the ANA." Editorial. *American Journal of Nursing* 48 (October):750.

"No Negro Nurses Wanted." *Crisis* 52 (February 1945):40.

Northrup, Herbert R. "The ANA and the Negro Nurse." *American Journal of Nursing* 50 (April 1950):207–208.

Norton, Mary Beth. "The Paradox of 'Women's Sphere.'" In *Women of America: A History*, edited by Carol Berkins and Mary Beth Norton, pp. 139–149. Boston: Houghton Mifflin Co., 1979.

Osborne, Estelle Massey Riddle. "Status and Contribution of the Negro Nurse." *Journal of Negro Education* 18 (Summer 1949):364–369.

Peters, William H. "Negro Health and Race Relations." *Cincinnati Journal of Medicine*, May 1925, pp. 149–152.

Pitter, Evelyn. "The Colored Nurse in Public Health." *American Journal of Nursing* 26 (September 1926):719–720.

Rann, Emery L. "The Good Samaritan Hospital of Charlotte, North Carolina." *Journal of the National Medical Association* 56 (May 1916):223–225.

Rayfield, Stanley; Stimson, Marjory; and Tattershall, Louise. "A Study of Negro Public Health Nursing." *Public Health Nurse* 22 (October 1930):525–537.

Reverby, Susan. "From Aide to Organizer: The Oral History of Lillian Roberts." In *Women of America: A History*, edited by Carol Ruth Berkin and Mary Beth Norton, pp. 289–317. Boston: Houghton Mifflin Co., 1979.

———. "'Something besides Waiting': The Politics of Private Duty Nursing Reform in the Depression." In *Nursing History: New Perspectives, New Possibilities*, edited by Ellen Condliffe Lagemann, pp. 133–156. New York: Columbia University Press, 1983.

———. "The Search for the Hospital Yardstick: Nursing and the Rationalization of Hospital Work." In *Health Care in America: Essays in Social History*, edited by David Rosner and Susan Reverby, pp. 206–225. Philadelphia: Temple University Press, 1979.

Riddle, Estelle Massey. "The Training and Placement of Negro Nurses." *Journal of Negro Education* 4 (1935):42–48.

———. "Negro Nurses: The Supply and Demand." *Opportunity* 15 (November 1937):327–329.

———. "Sources of Supply of Negro Health Personnel, Section C: Nurses." *Journal of Negro Education* 6 (1937):483–492.

———, and Nelson, Josephine. "The Negro Nurse Looks toward Tomorrow." *American Journal of Nursing* 45 (August 1945):627–630.

Roberts, Abbie. "Nursing Education and Opportunities for the Colored Nurse." In *Proceedings of the National Conference of Social Work*, pp. 183–185. Chicago: University of Chicago Press, 1928.

Rodgers, Samuel U. "Kansas City General Hospital No. 2: A Historical Perspective." *Journal of the National Medical Association* 54 (September 1962): 527–528.

Rosenberg, Charles E. "Inward Vision and Outward Glance: The Shaping of the American Hospital, 1880–1914." *Bulletin of the History of Medicine* 53 (1979):346–391.

Rothman, Sheila. "Women's Special Sphere." In *Women and the Politics of Culture: Studies in the Sexual Economy*, edited by Michele Wender Zak and Patricia P. Moots. New York: Longman, 1983.

Rudwick, Elliott, M. "A Brief History of Mercy-Douglass Hospital in Philadelphia." *Journal of Negro Education* 20 (January 1951):50–66.

Shannon, Marty L. "Nurses in American History: Our First Four Licensure Laws." *American Journal of Nursing* 17 (August 1975):1327–1328.

Shryock, Richard H. Nursing Emerges as a Profession: The American Experience." *Clio Medica* 3 (1968):131–147.

Sloan, Patricia E. "Geneva Estelle Massey Riddle Osborne, 1901–1981," In *American Nursing: A Biographical Dictionary*, edited by Vern L. Bullough et al., pp. 250–252. New York: Garland Publishing, 1988.

Smith, Gloria R. "From Invisibility to Blackness: The Story of the National Black Nurses' Association." *Nursing Outlook* 23 (April 1975):225–229.

Staupers, Mabel K. "Story of the National Association of Colored Graduate Nurses." *American Journal of Nursing* 51 (April 1951):221–223.

———. "The Negro Nurse in America." *Opportunity: Journal of Negro Life* 15 (November 1937):339–341, 349.

Stein, Alice P. "Harriet (Araminta) Ross Tubman, 1820–1913." In *American*

Nursing: A Biographical Dictionary, edited by Vern L. Bullough et al., pp. 321–322. New York: Garland Publishing, 1988.

Stewart, Isabel M. "Next Step in the Education of Nurses." *National News Bulletin* 13 (December 1939).

Taylor, Eola Lyons. "The Training of Negro Nurses in the South." *Opportunity: Journal of Negro Life* 15 (November 1937):330–331.

Terry, C. E. "The Negro: His Relation to Public Health in the South." *American Journal of Public Health* 9 (April 1913):300–310.

Thompson, W. Arthur, and Greenidge, Robert. "The Negro in Medicine in Detroit." *Journal of the National Medical Association* 55 (November 1963): 475–479.

Thoms, Adah. "Annual Address of the National Association of Colored Graduate Nurses, 1921." In *Black Women in the Nursing Profession: A Documentary History*, edited by Darlene Clark Hine, pp. 119–122. New York: Garland Publishing, 1985.

———. "President's Address, National Association of Colored Graduate Nurses." *Journal of the National Medical Association* 12 (October–December 1920): 73–74.

Tomes, Nancy. "'Little World of Our Own': The Pennsylvania Hospital Training School for Nurses, 1895–1907." *Journal of the History of Medicine and Allied Sciences* 33 (October 1978):507–530.

———. "The Silent Battle: Nurse Registration in New York State, 1903–1920." In *Nursing History: New Perspectives, New Possibilities*, edited by Ellen Condliffe Lagemann, pp. 107–132. New York: Columbia University Press, 1983.

Venable, H. Phillip. "The History of Homer G. Phillips Hospital." *Journal of the National Medical Association* 53 (November 1961):541–551.

Walsh, William H. "Report of the Committee on Hospitalization of Colored People—1930." *Transactions of the American Hospital Association* 32 (1930): 53–61.

Washington, Booker T. "Training Colored Nurses at Tuskegee." *American Journal of Nursing* 10 (December 1910):167–171.

Wilkins, Roy. "Nurses Go to War." *Crisis* 50 (February 1943):42–44.

Williams, Daniel Hale. "Afro-Americans as Surgeons and Nurses." *AME Church Review* 10 (January 1894):425–431.

———. "The Need of Hospitals and Training Schools for the Colored People of the South." *AME Church Review* 17 (July 1900):9–18.

Williams, Lorraine A. "Harriet Tubman, c. 1821–1913." In *Dictionary of American Negro Biography*, edited by Rayford W. Logan and Michael R. Winston, pp. 606–607. New York: W. W. Norton Co., 1982.

Wolfbein, Seymour L. "Postwar Trends in Negro Employment." *Monthly Labor Review* 65 (December 1947):664.

Wood, Ann Douglas. "The War within a War: Women Nurses in the Union Army." *Civil War History* 18 (1979):197–222.

Theses, Dissertations, and Unpublished Writings

Bennett, Alisan M. "A History of the Harlem Hospital School of Nursing: Its Emergence and Development in a Changing Urban Community, 1923–1973." Ed.D. dissertation, Teachers College, Columbia University, 1984.

Buhler-Wilkerson, Karen. "False Dawn: The Rise and Decline of Public Health

Nursing in America, 1900–1930." Ph.D. dissertation, University of Pennsylvania, 1984.

Elmore, Joyce Ann. "A History of Freedmen's Hospital Training School for Nurses in Washington, D.C., 1894–1909." M.A. thesis, Catholic University, 1965.

Gamble, Vanessa Lee. "The Provident Hospital Project: An Experiment in Black Medical Education." University of Pennsylvania Seminar Paper, September 1980.

Helmbold, Lois Rita. "Making Choices, Making Do: Black and White Working-Class Women's Lives during the Great Depression." Ph.D. dissertation, Stanford University, 1982.

Mazero, T. Jean Louise. "Professionalizing of Nursing in America: A Century of Struggle." Ph.D. dissertation, University of Pittsburgh, 1972.

Mitchell, Delora. "Provident Hospital: A Black Institution Survives." Master's thesis, Northeastern Illinois University, 1962.

Piemonte, Robert V. "History of the National League of Nursing Education, 1912–1932: Great Awakening in Nursing Education." Ed.D. dissertation, Teachers College, 1976.

Reverby, Susan M. "The Nursing Disorder: A Critical History of the Hospital-Nursing Relationship, 1860–1945." Ph.D. dissertation, Boston University, 1982.

Sloan, Patricia E. "Black Hospitals and Nurse Training Schools: Spelman, Provident, Hampton, and Tuskegee." Ed.D. dissertation, Teachers College, Columbia University, 1978.

Smith, Susan Lynn. "The Black Women's Club Movement: Self-improvement and Sisterhood, 1890–1915." Master's thesis, University of Wisconsin, 1986.

Index

Abraham Lincoln Battalion, blacks in, 139
Accreditation laws, state: and longer nursing school terms, 54
Administrators, xviii, 89; in nursing institutions, 64, 80; public-health, 189
Administrators, hospital, 98, 189; of black hospitals, 20–21, 22, 26, 42
Admissions standards: advocated by white nurse leaders, 89; of black nursing schools, 49–51, 95
Age-requirements: for armed-forces nurses, 173; for nursing students, 49, 219 n.4
Agnew, Rear Adm. W. J. C., 179, 181
Alumnae associations and ANA membership requirements, 91
American Academy of Nursing: black nurse members of, 191
American College of Surgeons: approval of black hospitals, 10, 31
American Hospital Association: 1930 report on black hospitals, 213 n.15
American Medical Association (AMA), 4, 184; on black hospitals, 31, 66, 213 n.15
American Medical Bureau to Aid Spanish Democracy, 140
American Nurses' Association (ANA), 90, 115, 192–93; black exclusion from, 94, 109, 114, 115–16, 129–31, 190; integration of black nurses in, xix, 111–16, 183, 190–91; invitation to Riddle to attend New Orleans meeting, 130–31; membership requirements, 91, 92, 225 n.3; and the NACGN, 110, 115, 125, 129, 184; and nurses for military service, 102–103, 181
American Nurses' Association House of Delegates: acceptance of black members, 183
American Red Cross: and Circle for Negro Relief affiliation attempt, 105–106; Davis as first black nurse in, 134, 136; discrimination during World War I era, 102–104
American Red Cross Nursing Service: as recruitment center, 167, 171, 178, 237–38 n.29
Anderson, Karen Tucker, 146

Andrews, Ludie Clay, xx-xxii, 92–93; Mary Mahoney Award, 126
Antilynching legislation, NACGN support for, 128
Anti-poll tax legislation, NACGN support for, 128
Antisegregation campaigns of black nurses, 190
Armed Forces Nurse Corps, 140, 174; discriminatory policies of, 102, 188; marital status of members, 173; use of black nurses in World War II, 167, 170, 181. See also Army Nurse Corps; Navy Nurse Corps
Armour, Philip D., 28, 30
Armour and Company, 31
Army Nurse Corps: officers' relative rank, 174; Red Cross as official auxiliary of, 102–104; use of black nurses in World War II, 84, 167, 172, 179, 181
"Art and Value of X-Ray as Anesthesia, The" (NACGN session paper), 98
Associate nurses: membership in NACGN, 95
Associate nursing degree programs, 191, 222 n.9
Association for the Study of Negro Life and History, 30
Association of Collegiate Schools of Nursing (ACSN), 63
Atlanta Baptist Female Seminary, 8–9. See also Spelman College
Autonomy, professional: enjoyed by public-health nurses, 189

Baccalaureate degrees: at Dillard University, 69, 81; at Florida A&M, 65
Bacon, Alice Mabel, 16–17
Bacon, Francis, 17
Banks, Anna De Costa, 16, 22, il. 23
Barbour, Warren W., 151
Barnett, Claude: publicity for black nurses, 126–77, 172–73
Barreau, John R., 147